14

CURRENT CLINICAL TOPICS IN INFECTIOUS DISEASES

14

CURRENT CLINICAL TOPICS IN INFECTIOUS DISEASES

Edited by

JACK S. REMINGTON, MD

Professor of Medicine
Division of Infectious Diseases and Geographic Medicine
Stanford University School of Medicine

Marcus A. Krupp Research Chair and
Chairman, Department of Immunology
and Infectious Diseases, Research Institute
Palo Alto Medical Foundation

MORTON N. SWARTZ, MD

Professor of Medicine
Harvard Medical School

Chief, James Jackson Firm
Medical Services
Massachusetts General Hospital
Infectious Disease Unit
Massachusetts General Hospital

Blackwell
Science

Blackwell Science
  Editorial offices
238 Main Street, Cambridge, Massachusetts
  02142, USA
Osney Mead, Oxford OX2 0EL, England
25 John Street, London, WC1N 2BL, England
23 Ainslie Place, Edinburgh EH3 6AJ, Scotland
54 University Street, Carlton, Victoria 3053,
  Australia
Arnette SA, 1 rue de Lille, 75007 Paris, France
Blackwell Wissenschaft-Verlag GmbH,
  Kurfürstendamm 57, 10707 Berlin, Germany
Blackwell MZV, Feldgasse 13, A-1238 Vienna,
  Austria

Distributors:
North America
  Blackwell Science, Inc.
  238 Main Street
  Cambridge, Massachusetts 02142
  (Telephone orders: 800-215-1000 or
    617-876-7000)

Australia
  Blackwell Science Pty Ltd.
  54 University Street
  Carlton, Victoria 3053
  (Telephone orders: 03-347-5552 or
    03-347-0300)

Outside North America and Australia
  Blackwell Science, Ltd.
  c/o Marston Book Services Ltd.
  PO Box 87
  Oxford OX2 0DT
  England
  (Telephone orders: 44-1865-791155)

Typeset by Huron Valley Graphics, Inc.
Printed and bound by Braun-Brumfield, Inc.

Library of Congress Cataloging-in-
  Publication Data
The LIbrary of Congress has catalogued this serial
publication as follows:
Current clinical topics in infectious diseases.
1-
  New York. McGraw-Hill Book Co.,
  © 1980–1988
  Boston, Blackwell Scientific Publications,
  © 1989–
    v. ill. 25 cm.
    Annual
    Key title: Current clinical topics in
    infectious diseases, ISSN 0195-3842.
    1. Communicative diseases—
    Periodicals.
    DNLM: 1. Communicable Diseases—
    Periodicals. W 1 CU786T
  RC111.C87   616.9'05
    80-643590
  ISBN 0-86542-359-8

To our fellows

Contents

Preface   ix

Contributors   xi

Foot Infections in Diabetes: Evaluation and Management   1
Adolf W. Karchmer and Gary W. Gibbons

**Splenic Abcess: Pathogenesis, Clinical Features, Diagnosis,
and Treatment**   23
J. Davis Allan

Azithromycin and Clarithromycin   52
Ellen Eisenberg and Michael Barza

**Biologic and Geographic Factors in Prevention and Treatment
of Malaria**   80
Godfred L. Masinde and Donald J. Krogstad

**Automated Antimicrobial Susceptibility Testing: What the Infectious
Diseases Subspecialist Needs to Know**   103
Mary Jane Ferraro

Hepatitis C Virus and Chronic Liver Disease   120
Stanley M. Lemon and Edwin A. Brown

**Nodular Lymphangitis: Clinical Features, Differential Diagnosis
and Management**   142
Howard M. Heller and Morton N. Swartz

Human Herpesvirus 6   159
William S. Robinson

**Methicillin-Resistant *Staphylococcus aureus:* The Persistent
Resistant Nosocomial Pathogen**   170
Michael A. Martin

How Vaccines Are Developed   192
R. Gordon Douglas Jr.

Bacillary Angiomatosis and *Rochalimaea* species   205
David A. Relman

**Prevention of Human Immunodeficiency Virus Infection among
Hospital Personnel**   220
Julie Louise Gerberding

Cytokine Therapy of Infectious Diseases   228
Miles H. Beaman

Intelligent Dosing of Antimicrobials   252
Charles H. Nightingale, Richard Quintiliani and David P. Nicolau

Ethical Issues in Infectious Diseases   266
Jerome H. Kim and David T. Durack

Preface

As literature in the field of infectious diseases has increased in complexity and volume, a need has become evident for timely, concise summaries and critical commentaries on subjects pertinent to the student and practitioner of medicine, the specialist in infectious diseases, and those in allied fields. It is our intention that this series provide the reader with a true update of information in very specific areas of infectious diseases which require reevaluation.

Each author was requested to confine his/her chapter to a relatively narrow subject, to deal only with contemporary questions and problems, to gather and synthesize the information on recent advances which is often spread diffusely among numerous journals, to offer critical evaluation of this information, to place the information into perspective by defining its present status, and to point out deficiencies in the information and thereby indicate directions for further study. All of this was to be done within the most rigid deadlines to ensure that the chapters be written and published in less than a year. We are extremely grateful to the contributing authors, each of whom is a recognized authority in the particular field, for consenting to undertake such an admittingly difficult task.

Current Clinical Topics in Infectious Diseases: 14 is the fourteenth volume of a series which is published annually. Each text in the series consists of updates of a variety of subjects covering the wide scope of clinical infectious disease problems, including bacteriology, mycology, virology, parasitology, and epidemiology.

JACK S. REMINGTON
MORTON N. SWARTZ

Contributors

J. Davis Allan, MD
Assistant Professor of Medicine, Harvard Medical School; Staff Physician, Infectious Disease Section, New England Deaconess Hospital, Boston, Massachusetts

Michael Barza, MD
Professor of Medicine, Tufts University School of Medicine; Associate Chief, Division of Geographic Medicine and Infectious Diseases, New England Medical Center, Boston Massachusetts

Miles H. Beaman, MD
Senior Lecturer in Medicine, University of Western Australia, Nedlands; Fremantle Hospital, Fremantle, Australia

Edwin A. Brown, MD
Clinical Instructor, Department of Medicine, Division of Infectious Diseases, University of North Carolina at Chapel Hill, Chapel Hill, North Carolina

R. Gordon Douglas Jr., MD
Clinical Professor of Medicine, Cornell University Medical College; Attending Physician, The New York Hospital; President, Merck Vaccine Division, Merck and Company, New York, New York

David T. Durack, MD, DPhil
Professor of Medicine and Microbiology; Chief, Division of Infectious Diseases and International Health, Duke University Medical Center, Durham, North Carolina

Ellen Eisenberg, MD
Staff Physician, Quincy and Milton Hospitals; Private Practice in Infectious Diseases, Quincy, Massachusetts

Mary Jane Ferraro, PhD
Associate Professor of Pathology and Medicine, Harvard Medical School; Director of Clinical Microbiology, Massachusetts General Hospital, Boston, Massachusetts

Julie Louise Gerberding, MD, MPH
Assistant Professor of Medicine (Infectious Diseases) and Epidemiology and Biostatistics, University of California at San Francisco; Director, Center for Hospital Epidemiology and Infection Prevention, San Francisco General Hospital, San Francisco, California

Gary W. Gibbons, MD
Associate Clinical Professor of Surgery, Harvard Medical School; Clinical Chief, Division of Vascular Surgery, New England Deaconess Hospital, Boston, Massachusetts

Howard M. Heller, MD
Instructor in Medicine, Harvard Medical School; Assistant Physician, Massachusetts General Hospital, Boston, Massachusetts

Adolf W. Karchmer, MD
Associate Professor of Medicine, Harvard Medical School; Chief, Division of Infectious Diseases, New England Deaconess Hospital, Boston, Massachusetts

Jerome H. Kim, MD
Senior Scientist, Department of Retroviral Research, Walter Reed Army Institute of Research, Rockville, Maryland

Donald J. Krogstad, MD
Henderson Professor and Chair, Department of Tropical Medicine, Tulane School of Public Health and Tropical Medicine; Professor of Medicine, Tulane School of Medicine, New Orleans, Louisiana

Stanley M. Lemon, MD
Professor of Medicine and Microbiology and Immunology, Associate Chairman for Research, Department of Medicine; Attending Physician, University of North Carolina Hospital, Chapel Hill, North Carolina

Michael A. Martin, MD
Assistant Professor of Medicine and Epidemiology, Oregon Health Sciences University School of Medicine, and Hospitals and Clinics, Portland, Oregon

Godfred L. Masinde, MSC
Department of Tropical Medicine, Tulane School of Public Health and Tropical Medicine, New Orleans, Louisiana

David P. Nicolau, PharmD
Assistant Clinical Professor, School of Pharmacy, University of Connecticut; Coordinator for Research, Department of Medicine, Division of Infectious Diseases and Allergy, and Department of Pharmacy Services, Hartford Hospital, Hartford, Connecticut

Charles H. Nightingale, PhD
Research Professor, University of Connecticut School of Pharmacy; Vice President for Research, Hartford Hospital, Hartford, Connecticut

Richard Quintiliani, MD
Professor of Medicine, University of Connecticut School of Medicine; Director, Division of Infectious Diseases and Allergy Immunology, Hartford Hospital, Hartford, Connecticut

David A. Relman, MD
Assistant Professor of Medicine (Infectious Diseases and Geographic Medicine) and of Microbiology and Immunology, Stanford University School of Medicine; Staff Physician, Department of Veterans Affairs Medical Center, Palo Alto, California

William S. Robinson, MD
Professor of Medicine, Division of Infectious Diseases and Geographic Medicine, Stanford University School of Medicine, Stanford, California

Morton N. Swartz, MD
Professor of Medicine, Harvard Medical School; Chief, James Jackson Firm Medical Services, Massachusetts General Hospital, Infectious Disease Unit, Massachusetts General Hospital, Boston, Massachusetts

Other Volumes in the Series

CURRENT CLINICAL TOPICS IN INFECTIOUS DISEASES 1

The role of CT Scanning in Diagnosis of Infections of the Central Nervous System
Staphylococcus aureus Bacteremia
Cytomegalovirus Infection in Transplant and Cancer Patients
Diagnosis and Management of Meningitis Due to Gram-Negative Bacilli in Adults
Infection Prevention during Granulocytopenia
Infant Botulism
The Role of Surgery in Infective Endocarditis
Treatment of Bacterial Infections of the Eye
Giardiasis: The Rediscovery of an Ancient Pathogen
Legionnaires' Disease
Antibiotic-Associated Diarrhea
Antibiotic-Resistant Pneumococci
The Cancer Patient with Fever and Pulmonary Infiltrates: Etiology and Diagnostic Approach
Q Fever: An Update

CURRENT CLINICAL TOPICS IN INFECTIOUS DISEASES 2

Acute Epiglottitis, Laryngitis, and Croup
Urinary Tract Infections in the Female: A Perspective
Treatment of Cryptococcal, Candidal, and Coccidiodal Meningitis
Bacteriology, Clinical Spectrum of Disease, and Therapeutic Aspects in Coryneform Bacterial Infection
Rocky Mountain Spotted Fever: A Clinical Dilemna
The Doctor's Dilemna: Have I Chosen the Right Drug? An Adequate Dose Regimen? Can Laboratory
    Tests Help in my Decision?
Shock in Gram-Negative Bacteremia: Predisposing Factors, Pathophysiology, and Treatment
The Management of Patients with Mycotic Aneurysm
A Review of the "New" Bacterial Strains Causing Diarrhea
Endocarditis Complicating Parenteral Drug Abuse
The Cephalosporins and Cephamycins: A Perspective
The Diagnosis and Treatment of Gangrenous and Crepitant Cellulitis
Management of Acute and Chronic Otitis Media

CURRENT CLINICAL TOPICS IN INFECTIOUS DISEASES 3

Sexually Transmitted Enteric Disease
Nucleotide Derivatives and Interferons as Antiviral Agents

Prophylaxis and Treatment of Malaria
Guillain-Barré Syndrome
Newer Antifungal Agents and their Use, Including an Update on Amphotericin B and Flucytosine
Role of Ultrasound and Computed Tomography in the Diagnosis and Treatment of Intraabdominal
   Abscess
Treatment of Infections Due to Atypical Mycobacteria
Combination of Single Drug Therapy for Gram-Negative Sepsis
Deep Infections Following Total Hip Replacement
Treatment of the Child with Bacterial Meningitis
Diagnosis and Management of Meningitis Associated with Cerebrospinal Fluid Leaks
Prophylactic Antibiotics for Bowel Surgery
Infections Associated with Intravascular Lines
Diagnosis and Treatment of Cutaneous Leishmaniasis
Candida Endophthalmitis

CURRENT CLINICAL TOPICS IN INFECTIOUS DISEASES 4

Diagnosis and Management of Septic Arthritis
Kawasaki's Disease
A Critical Review of the Role of Oral Antibiotics in the Management of Hematogenous Osteomyelitis
When Can the Infected Hospital Employee Return to Work?
Endocardiography and Infectious Endocarditis
Orbital Infections
The Use of White Blood Cells Scanning Techniques in Infectious Disease
Antimicrobial Prophylaxis in the Immunosuppressed Cancer Patient
The Diagnosis of Fever Occurring in a Postpartum Patient
Management at Delivery of Mother and Infant When Herpes Simplex, Varicella-Zoster, Hepatitis, or
   Tuberculosis Have Occurred during Pregnancy
"Nonspecific Vaginitis," Vulvovaginal Candidiasis, and Trichomoniasis: Clinical Features, Diagnosis and
   Management
Radionuclide Imaging in the Management of Skeletal Infections
Comparison of Methods for Clinical Quantitation of Antibiotics
What is the Clinical Significance of Tolerance to B-lactam Antibiotics?
A Critical Comparison of the Newer Aminoglycosidic Aminocyclitol
The Third Generation Cephalosporins

CURRENT CLINICAL TOPICS IN INFECTIOUS DISEASES 5

Prostatitis Syndromes
Staphylococcus epidermidis: The Organism, Its Diseases, and Treatment
Management of Nocardia Infections
Current Issues in Toxic Shock Syndrome
Isolation and Management of Contagious, Highly Lethal Diseases
Nutrition and Infection
Infections Associated with Hemodialysis and Chronic Peritoneal Dialysis
New Perspectives on the Epstein-Barr Virus in the Pathogeneis of Lymphoproliferative Disorders
Staphyloccal Teichoic Acid Antibodies
Current Status of Granulocyte Transfusion Therapy
Infections Associated With Intrauterine Devices
Hospital Epidemiology: An Emerging Discipline
The Viridians Streptococci in Perspective
Current Status of Prophylaxis for *Haemophilus influenzae* Infections
Acute Rheumatic Fever: Current Concepts and Controversies

CURRENT CLINICAL TOPICS IN INFECTIOUS DISEASES 6

The Acquired Immunodeficiency Syndrome
Health Advice and Immunizations for Travelers

Travelers' Diarrhea: Recent Developments
Bacterial Adherence and Anticolonization Vaccines
Clinically Significant Phagocytic Cell Defects
Metronidazole in the Treatment of Anaerobic Bacterial Infections
Bacteremia in Febrile Children Managed Out of Hospital
Non-A, Non-B Hepatitis
Viral Gastroenteritis
Infections in Chronic Peritoneal Dialysis Patients
Infection in Recipients of Bone Marrow Transplants
Infections Involving Fascial Compartments and Tendon Sheaths of the Hand
Toxoplasmosis of the Central Nervous System

CURRENT CLINICAL TOPICS IN INFECTIOUS DISEASES 7

Hyperinfection Syndrome with Strongyloidiasis
Nonepidemic (Endemic) Meningococcal Disease: Pathogenic Factors and Clinical Features
Infections Complicating Cystic Fibrosis
Current Problems in Diagnosis and Treatment of Amebic Infections
Disseminated *Mycobacterium Avium-Intracellulare* Disease and Therapy
Rapid Tests for the Diagnosis of Bacterial Meningitis
Cost-Effective Clinical Microbiology and Newer Tests of Importance to the Practicioner
Newer Developments in Diagnosis and Treatment of Pneumocystis Infections
The Controversy about Pertussis Vaccine
Nosocomial Legionellosis: Current Epidemiological Issues
Approach to the Patient with Suspected Histoplasmosis
Diagnosis and Treatment of Cysticercosis
CT of Infections of the Spine

CURRENT CLINICAL TOPICS IN INFECTIOUS DISEASES 8

Diagnosis and Management of Infection in the Pleural Space
Management of Animal and Human Bites and Resulting Human Infections
Penicillin-Binding Proteins and Beta-Lactamases: Their Effects on the Use of Cephalosporins and Other
    New Beta-Lactams
Approach to the Patient with Chronic Osteomyelitis
Hepatitis D (Delta) Virus
Cryptosporidiosis and Immune Enteropathy: A Review
What the Infectious Disease Subspecialist Should Know about Dermatophytes
The Management of the Carrier of Methicillin-Resistant *Staphylococcus aureus*
Respiratory Tract Infections Due to *Branhamella catarrhalis* and *Neisseria* Species
Current Antimicrobial Management of Tuberculosis
Oropharyngeal Space Infections
Management of Patients with Intraabdominal Infection Due to Colonic Perforation

CURRENT CLINICAL TOPICS IN INFECTIOUS DISEASES 9

Antimicrobial Prophylaxis for Infection in Neutropenic Patients
Infections in Cardiac Pacemakers
Management of the Ambulatory Patient with a Sore Throat
An Approach to Urinary Tract Infections in Ambulatory Women
Chronic Fatique Syndrome: A Manifestation of Epstein-Barr Virus Infection?
Evaluation and Management of an Asymptomatic Patient with a Positive VDRL Reaction
Clinical Indications for Virologic Diagnosis
Choices of New Penicillins and Cephalosporins in the DRG Era
Infections of Mechanical Cerebrospinal Fluid Shunts
Delayed Hypersensitivity Skin Testing: Uses and Pitfalls
Management of Infection in Total Knee Replacement
Epidemiology and Prevention of Nosocomial Pneumonia

CURRENT CLINICAL TOPICS IN INFECTIOUS DISEASES 10

Genital Herpes and the Pregnant Woman
Home Management of Antibiotic Therapy
Serum Bactericidal Test: Past, Present and Future Use in the Management of Patients with Infections
Lyme Borreliosis
The Role of MR Imaging in the Diagnosis of Infections of the Central Nervous System
Imipenem and Aztreonam: Current Role in Antimicrobial Therapy
Progressive Multifocal Leukoencephalopathy
Campylobacter pylori: Its Role in Gastritis and Peptic Ulcer Disease
Nucleic Acid Probes in Infectious Diseases
Norfloxacin, Ciprofloxacin, and Ofloxacin: Current Clinical Roles
Liposomes in Infectious Disease: Present and Future
Antibiotic Prophylaxis: Non-abdominal Surgery
Prevention of *Haemophilus influenzae* type b Disease: Vaccines and Passive Prophylaxis

CURRENT CLINICAL TOPICS IN INFECTIOUS DISEASES 11

The Chlamydial Pneumonias
Human Immunodeficiency Virus (HIV)-Associated Pneumocystosis
Fever of Unknown Origin-Reexamined and Redefined
Echinococcal Disease
The Epidemiology of AIDS: A Decade of Experience
Antibiotic Resistance Among Enterococci: Current Problems and Management Strategies
Intraocular Infections: Current Therapeutic Approach
Bronchiectasis: A Current View
Infection of Burn Wounds: Evaluation and Management
Colonic Diverticulitis: Microbiologic, Diagnostic, and Therapeutic Considerations
Echocardiography in the Management of Patients with Suspected or Proven Endocarditis
The Clinical Spectrum of Human Parvovirus B19 Infections

CURRENT CLINICAL TOPICS IN INFECTIOUS DISEASES 12

Viral Aseptic Meningitis in the United States: Clinical Features, Viral Etiologies, and Differential
   Diagnosis
Aeromonas Species: Role as Human Pathogens
Neurologic Complications of Bacterial meningitis in Children
Purulent Pericarditis
Diagnosis and Management of Infections of Implantable Devices Used for Prolonged Venous Access
Pancreatic Abcess and Infected Pseudocyst: Diagnosis and Treatment
Approach to the Febrile Traveler Returning from Southeast Asia and Oceania
Management of Septic Shock: New Approaches
The Increasing Prevalence of Resistance to Antituberculosis Cheotherapeutic Agents: Implications for
   Global Tuberculosis Control
Use of Immune Globulins in the Prevention and Treatment of Infections
Mycobacterium avium Complex in AIDS
Hepatitis B Immunization: Vaccine Types, Efficacy, and Indications for Immunization
Therapy of Cytomegalovirus Infections with Ganciclovir: A Critical Appraisal
Evaluation of Cryptic Fever in a Traveler to Africa

CURRENT CLINICAL TOPICS IN INFECTIOUS DISEASES 13

The Pathogenesis, Prevention, and Management of Urinary Tract Infection in Patients with Spinal Cord
   Injury
Epidemiologic Considerations in the Evaluation of Undifferentiated Fever in a Traveler Returning from
   Latin America or the Caribbean
Fever in a Recent Visitor to the Middle East
Fluconazole and Intraconazole: Current Status and Prospects for Antifungal Therapy
Genital Warts: Diagnosis, Treatment, and Counseling for the Patient

Varicella in a Susceptible Pregnant Woman
Evaluation and Treatment of Patients with Prior Reactions to B-Lactam Antibiotics
Periodontal Disease: Gingivitis, Juvenile Periodontis, Adult Periodontis
Diagnosis and Management of Perianal and Perirectal Infection in the Granulocytopenic Patient
Hemolytic Uremic Syndrome: Clinical Picture and Bacterial Connection
Clinical Features and Treatment of Infection Due to Myobacterium Fortuitum/Chelonae Complex
Fish and Shellfish Poisoning
Management of Infectious Complications Following Liver Transplantation
The Management of Cryptococcal Disease in Patients with AIDS
Magnetic Resonance Imaging Update on Brain Abscess and Central Nervous System Aspergillosis
Prophylaxis and Treatment of Infection in the Bone Marrow Transplant Recipient
Toxoplasmosis in the Non-AIDS Immunocompromised Host

14

CURRENT CLINICAL TOPICS IN INFECTIOUS DISEASES

Foot infections in diabetes: evaluation and management

ADOLF W. KARCHMER
GARY W. GIBBONS

INTRODUCTION

Amputation of the lower extremity, a major morbidity associated with diabetes mellitus, is often precipitated by infection acting alone or in combination with severe vascular insufficiency. More than 50,000 lower extremity amputations are performed annually among diabetic patients in the United States. Hospital discharge data indicate that 45% of all lower extremity amputations are performed on the 5% of the United States population with diabetes and that the risk of amputation among persons with diabetes is increased 15 times as compared with that in nondiabetic individuals (1). Moreover, amputations in diabetic patients increased by 50% from 1980 to 1987, age-adjusted rates increased from 6 to 8 per 1,000 persons with diabetes (2). In a study of 92 unselected diabetic patients (mean age, 59.6 yr; mean duration of diabetes, 13.9 yr), 15 had been hospitalized a total of 1,480 days because of pedal ulcerations or amputation. The prevalence of hammer toe deformity, reduced cutaneous pressure sensation, and vascular insufficiency was significantly increased in these patients as contrasted to those without a history of ulceration or amputation (3). Furthermore, Reiber and colleagues (4) found that reduced transcutaneous oxygen tension (<20 mm Hg below knee and dorsal foot), a history of peripheral vascular disease, the absence of lower leg vibratory sensation, and the lack of education regarding diabetic foot care were independent variables associated with an increased risk for amputation. Although presented as risk factors for lower extremity amputations, these factors predispose patients to nonhealing ulcers, which then serve as a portal of entry for local soft-tissue infection. In turn, pedal infection is at least an additional risk for amputation; it may aggravate a nonhealing ulcer by further tissue necrosis, precipitate local gangrene, or, if extensive and causing severe systemic toxicity, necessitate an emergency guillotine amputation as a life-saving procedure. Prompt effective treatment of pedal infections, or even better prevention of these infections, can significantly reduce the morbidity and cost associated with diabetes mellitus. With reduced morbidity as our goal, we review the evaluation of pedal infections, as well as their medical and surgical therapy.

1

PATHOGENESIS

Although ulceration of the foot is not the only factor in the pathogenesis of pedal infections in diabetic patients, it is often a seminal event. As a consequence of a distal sensory neuropathy, the relatively or often markedly insensate foot is at high risk of ulceration due to repetitive mild trauma or an acute physical injury (3–5). Foot deformities that arise from motor neuropathy–induced muscle imbalance across small joints create points of increased weight bearing that further enhance the likelihood of ulceration (3). The importance of these bony prominences in the pathogenesis of ulceration and secondary infection is demonstrated by the salutary effect of their resection on healing and the prevention of recurrent ulcers (6). Finally, autonomic neuropathy may contribute to pedal infections by causing abnormalities in skin hydration and associated skin fissures.

Occlusive atherosclerotic peripheral vascular disease, which in diabetic patients involves not only the proximal arteries but also the infrapopliteal vessels and the tibial and peroneal arteries, contributes to the occurrence of ulceration and to delayed wound healing (3–5). Although inadequate delivery of antimicrobial agents to infected tissues in the foot is frequently cited as a further mechanism by which vascular disease abets pedal infection, the evidence for this relationship is scanty (7). It seems unlikely that delivery of therapeutic concentrations of antimicrobial agents is impaired when blood supply is sufficient to support tissue viability.

Hyperglycemia has been associated with impairment of polymorphonuclear leukocyte chemotaxis, phagocytosis, and bactericidal activity *in vitro* and in animal models (8–10). Diabetic patients with untreated pedal infections are typically hyperglycemic; thus these defects may contribute to the severity of infection on presentation. However, a role for hyperglycemia and polymorphonuclear leukocyte dysfunction in the initiation of these infections has not been demonstrated. Furthermore, that these defects are reversible with the restoration of euglycemia, raises questions regarding their clinical significance when insulin and anti-infective therapy reverse the hyperglycemia associated with untreated pedal infections.

Finally, intercurrent events may contribute to the genesis of foot infection. Skin fissuring in the web space due to tinea pedis may result in limb-threatening infection. Similarly, injuries associated with unskilled foot care (e.g., trimming of toenails and calluses), as well as accidental injuries, including burns, puncture wounds, and blunt trauma, may precipitate limb-threatening infection (11).

CLINICAL PRESENTATIONS

Foot infections in the diabetic population have varied presentations; they are affected by portal of entry, local extension with or without abscess formation, the invading organisms, the integrity of the vascular supply to the foot, and the occurrence of metastatic infections in remote sites. Many features of the infected foot reflect the isolated or combined manifestations of neuropathy and vascular insufficiency. Although an appreciation of these features is essential to optimal management, attention to them is beyond the scope of this article.

Although the classification of foot infections proposed by Wagner (12) is perhaps the best known, for practical considerations we divide these infections into 2 groups: (1) nonlimb-threatening infections, which typically can be treated without hospitalization; and (2) limb-threatening infections, which warrant immediate hospitalization (13). A similar classification and approach to therapy has been suggested by Tan and File (14). Patients with nonlimb-threatening infections have superficial infection, lack systemic toxicity, and have minimal cellulitis (<2 cm extension from the portal of entry). If an ulceration is present, it does not penetrate fully through skin. In addition, these patients do not have bone or joint involvement, nor is there significant ischemia. In contrast, patients with limb-threatening infection have more extensive cellulitis (>2 cm extension from the portal of entry) and lymphangitis, and often have ulcers that penetrate through skin into subcutaneous tissue. Infection of contiguous bones or joints occurs frequently in this group, and significant ischemia with or without gangrene may be present. Although hyperglycemia is virtually universal among patients in both groups, fever is not. In fact, only 35% of patients with limb-threatening infection have significant fever (>100°F) on hospitalization (15). Fever is seen in patients with extensive soft-tissue involvement, deep plantar space abscess, bacteremia, or hematogenously seeded remote sites of infection.

The classification of these infections into limb-threatening and nonlimb-threatening also accommodates the anatomic presentations that Bose (16) used to categorize foot infections. Cellulitis of the dorsum of the foot, often with accompanying lymphangitis, commonly takes origin from the nail margin. Although generally superficial and limited to the distal foot, it can be extensive and complicated by involvement of fascial planes (fasciitis). Web space infections and infection complicating deep penetrating plantar ulcers over the second through fourth metatarsal heads or the prominent aspect of the collapsed arch of the rocker bottom foot may extend proximally along the intermediate plantar muscular compartment. In this circumstance, the foot is typically swollen, the longitudinal arch is lost, and systemic toxicity, including fever and chills, is noted. Compromise of the digital arteries may result in toe gangrene. Similar infection, albeit usually more limited, may develop in the medial and lateral muscular compartments of the foot due to penetrating ulcers. Neuropathic foot ulcers, known as *mal perforans* (Figure 1.1), occur over bony prominences, especially metatarsal heads despite relatively intact vascular supply. When not extending proximally along the plantar spaces, infections of these ulcers may be indolent but nevertheless remain limb-threatening. Even though these ulcers may extend to tendon sheath, bone, or even into the joint space, and be surrounded by a rim of cellulitis, fever is commonly absent or minimal.

A foul, so called fetid, smell characterizes some of the more extensive foot infections and usually indicates the participation of anaerobic bacteria. Gas formation in deep tissues (away from the immediate ulcer) may be detected as crepitus on clinical examination or radiologically. This gas is usually the consequence of a mixed infection caused by facultative gram-negative bacilli and anaerobes. Gas formation in this setting rarely reflects infection caused by *Clostridium* spp.

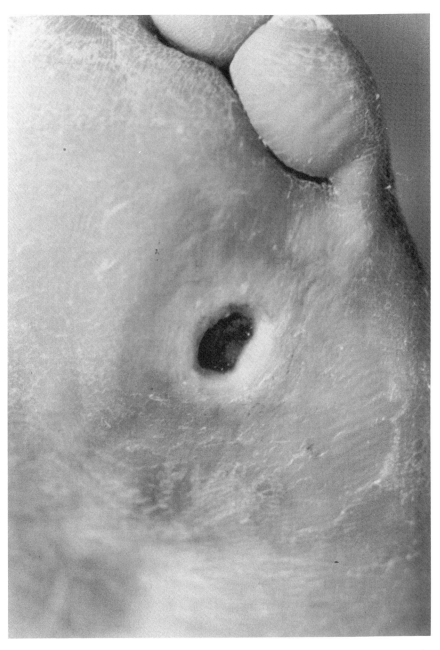

Figure 1.1 Uninfected neuropathic ulcer, *mal perforans*, occurring over the fourth metatarsal head.

MICROBIOLOGY

It is difficult to establish the precise microbial cause of foot infections in patients with diabetes. The portal of entry for infection and a seemingly appropriate site for culture is often an ulcer that is potentially contaminated by extensive contact with the environment. Alternatively, abscesses that can be aspirated are infrequent, and obtaining specimens from deep sites of infection by aspiration or biopsy through uncontaminated tissue is impractical as well as potentially hazardous. Sapico and colleagues (17), in a study of patients with severe lower extremity infection, compared the microbiologic yields procured from aerobic and anaerobic culture of specimens obtained by swab from the ulcer base, by curettage of the previously cleansed ulcer base, by aspiration of infected tissue (with or without injecting sterile saline), and by excising a piece of necrotic infected deep tissue that was not in direct communication with the ulcer. Concordance of isolates from specimens obtained by various modalities with those from deep tissue was best for specimens obtained by aspiration and curettage and was approximately 50%; more extensive discrepancies occurred among anaerobic bacteria. Of note, in 20% of patients, potential pathogens recovered from curettage and deep-tissue specimens were not recovered from aspirates. In a similar study, Wheat and associates (18) found poor concordance between organisms isolated from specimens recovered through ulcers compared with those from specimens obtained by routes that were not in direct communication with the ulcer. For purposes of patient care, there remains some debate regarding the need for precisely defining the organisms causing foot infections. With better general knowledge of the cause of pedal infections in diabetic patients and the availability of relatively nontoxic broad-spectrum antimicrobial agents, effective therapy of these infections can be provided without precisely defining the etiological agents.

In patients with nonlimb-threatening infection, *Staphylococcus aureus* is the major pathogen; these organisms are isolated from 50% of the infections and are recovered in pure culture from 35% (13,19). Aerobic streptococci were recovered from slightly more than one third of patients, often in a polymicrobial infection. Facultative gram-negative bacilli and anaerobic organisms are infrequent isolates. In half these patients, the infections are monomicrobial.

In contrast, limb-threatening infection is generally polymicrobial, with a broad array of bacterial species implicated (Table 1.1). Both gram-positive cocci and gram-negative bacilli are commonly isolated from a single infection, and in 40% of patients, both anaerobic and aerobic bacteria are isolated (11,13,15,17,18). *S. aureus* and streptococci, especially group B streptococci, and facultative gram-negative bacilli are prominent pathogens in this setting. Anaerobic gram-positive cocci and *Bacteroides* species, including those of the *B. fragilis* group, are also frequently implicated. In general, *Clostridium* species are recovered infrequently. Of note, the spectrum of isolates that are recovered may be altered by prior antimicrobial therapy, and nosocomially acquired pedal infections are often caused by more antibiotic-resistant bacteria (15). Wheat and colleagues (18) noted that *Pseudomonas aeruginosa* and *Acinetobacter* spp. were recovered more frequently from cultures obtained from ulcers than from cultures of material that did not communicate with the ulcer; the increased frequency with which these

Table 1.1 Microbiology of limb-threatening pedal infections in patients with diabetes*

Organisms	Percent of patients (ref) (Number patients)					
	Gibbons et al (13) (42)	Wheat et al (18) (54)	Hughes et al (22) (50)	Bamberger et al (55) (51)	Scher et al (11) (65)	Grayson et al (15) (96)
Aerobic						
S. aureus	22	20	25	22	23	54
S. epidermidis	12	17	14	19	18	12
Enterococcus spp.	16	15	17			28
Streptococcus spp.	13	23	20	41	54	55
Corynebacterium spp.	7	11		8		
E. coli	7	5	3	1	19	6
Klebsiella spp.	4	6	7	4	10	5
Proteus mirabilis	11	9	11	5	36	9
Enterobacter spp.	3	4	7	7		9
Other Enterobactereaceae	2	15	5	7	50	17
P. aeruginosa	3	4	0	5	15	8
Acinetobacter spp.	1	0	0	0		7
Anaerobic						
Gram-positive cocci	21	30	40	14	52	12
Bacteroides fragilis		2	5	4		
Bacteroides melaninogenicus		3	11			
Other Bacteroides spp.	6	12	2	5	55	30
Clostridium spp.	2	3	1	3	23	
Other anaerobes			13	2	20	14
Number isolates/infection	2.76	3.31	3.62	2.88	5.76	2.77

*Specimens obtained by various routes, including deep ulcer swabs, curettage of the ulcer base, aspiration or tissue biopsy, except Wheat et al, who excluded specimens obtained through the ulcer cavity.

organisms were recovered from ulcers probably reflects their role as a contaminant and not as an invasive pathogen (18).

The role of relatively avirulent bacteria often isolated from limb-threatening infections is uncertain. *Staphylococcus epidermidis* is recovered from 15% to 35% of these infections. Because these organisms, which are dominant elements of skin flora, are often recovered from specimens obtained through the ulcer, their role as pathogens has been questioned. Nevertheless, Wheat and associates (18), examining specimens obtained by aspiration or biopsy with minimal contamination with ulcer content, noted that *S. epidermidis* and *S. aureus* were recovered with similar frequency. Enterococci, viridans streptococci, and *Corynebacterium* spp., organisms usually considered to be skin contaminants and not primary pathogens in skin and soft-tissue infection, are also isolated frequently from these infections. Although often disregarded, it is notable that these avirulent organisms may be recovered from uncontaminated specimens and occasionally are the only organisms recovered from these infections (18,19). These observations suggest that on occasion these organisms, either alone or by acting synergistically in mixed infections, have a significant etiologic role.

Except for the general differences in the microbiology of limb-threatening and nonlimb-threatening infections, the clinical features of pedal infections do not provide meaningful clues to their etiology (13,18,19). Fetid, foul smelling infections suggest that anaerobic bacteria have a role, and gas in deep tissues suggests infection caused by a mixture of gram-negative bacilli and gram-positive cocci, including anaerobes (20). Similarly, necrotizing infection has been associated with recovery of *Bacteroides* spp. The organisms associated with these unique clinical features frequently cause infection without these clinical findings. Thus, even these clinical clues are not sufficient to predict the microbiology of an infection.

We and others have developed a practical approach to the microbiologic assessment of these infections (15,18). After cleansing the skin and debriding any overlying eschar, and before initiating antibiotic therapy, specimens for culture are obtained by swab (or curettage if there is tissue necrosis) from the base of the ulcer. Bullae or fluctuant collections are aspirated for culture as well. Specimens are collected and handled to allow processing as routine wound cultures and as primary anaerobic cultures. In patients who are febrile or have a history of fever with this infection, blood cultures are also obtained. During the initial days of hospitalization, deep tissue or purulent necrotic material, including exposed bone, is cultured. Although concurrent antimicrobial therapy may limit isolation of susceptible organisms from these follow-up cultures, resistant organisms, potentially missed on the initial cultures, can be recovered at this time. We do not routinely aspirate or biopsy unexposed bone when osteomyelitis is suspected because of radiologic findings. Careful follow-up of these suspect bones will often resolve the question of osteomyelitis without the potential hazard of an invasive procedure. This approach to microbiologic evaluation, combined with an approach to antimicrobial therapy that will be outlined, provides a satisfactory basis for management of these polymicrobial infections while avoiding the debate over the adequacy of given specimens or the role of particular organisms.

ANTIMICROBIAL TREATMENT

Antimicrobial therapy for foot infections in patients with diabetes is initiated empirically and subsequently revised as necessary based on clinical response and microbiologic data. Selection of effective empiric therapy requires knowledge of the microorganisms that usually cause these infections, as well as the alterations in etiologic agents that might be induced in selected circumstances. The potential toxicity of antimicrobial agents must also be considered. Accordingly, the availability of broad-spectrum non-nephrotoxic antimicrobials renders the aminoglycosides relatively unnecessary and certainly less desirable for standard treatment in this population because of the increased frequency of underlying renal disease.

With regard to the selection of empiric therapy, it is reasonable to consider patients with nonlimb-threatening infection as a group. The treatment of these patients, many of whom can be safely treated at home, is directed primarily at staphylococci and streptococci. In a randomized comparative study of patients with these infections who had not received antimicrobial therapy within the preceding 2 weeks and who were not febrile, Lipsky and associates (19) demonstrated that oral administration of clindamycin or cephalexin for 2 weeks resulted in a satisfactory clinical outcome in 96% and 86% of the patients treated, respectively. In 14 of these patients, the initial culture yielded 1 or more organisms resistant to the administered antimicrobial agent. Nevertheless, improvement and ultimate healing was noted in 13 of these 14 patients. This response not only raises questions about the pathogenetic role of these resistant organisms but also suggests that local wound care is important in treatment. The observed outcomes also suggest that other antimicrobial agents targeted at gram-positive cocci (e.g., oral semi-synthetic penicillinase-resistant penicillins [dicloxacillin, cloxacillin] and erythromycin) might also be effective. In addition, although wounds had not healed in 33 of 52 patients in this trial at the conclusion of 2 weeks of antibiotic therapy, ulcers healed in 19 (58%) of these 33 and 75% of all patients without surgical intervention. Furthermore, antimicrobial therapy in addition to the initial 2-week regimen was rarely required. When treating patients with superficial ulcers but with cellulitis that warrants hospitalization and parenteral antibiotics, we have found cefazolin to be effective.

For initial empiric antimicrobial treatment of polymicrobial limb-threatening infection, parenterally administered broad-spectrum antibiotics are used. The microbiology of these infections suggests that initial therapy should be effective against S. aureus; streptococci (especially group B streptococci); Enterobacteriacae, including E. coli, Proteus mirabilis, and Klebsiella spp.; anaerobic gram-positive cocci; and Bacteroides spp., including the B. fragilis group. Multi-drug regimens that included clindamycin and an aminoglycoside were previously utilized to treat these patients. These regimens, however, have been replaced by broad-spectrum beta-lactam antibiotics effective against a large proportion of the bacteria isolated from these infections. Although not all of the potentially effective antimicrobials have been evaluated for treatment of this entity, a variety of regimens could be anticipated to provide effective antimicrobial therapy. Fierer and colleagues (21), in a small study, demonstrated efficacy of cefoxitin in the treatment of these infections. Subsequently, Hughes and associates (22), in a randomized double-blind trial, achieved satisfactory responses in 82% of patients treated with ceftizoxime and in 68% of cefoxitin recipients (mean daily dose of each agent, 8.1 gm). Peterson and colleagues (23), using prolonged treatment with oral ciprofloxacin (1,500 or 2,000 mg daily) noted an initial response in 43 (91%) of 47 patients and a 60% satisfactory response after long-term follow-up. Other investigators have shown ciprofloxacin to be effective in the treatment of limb-threatening infections (24). Nevertheless, the potential role of Bacteroides spp. in these infections, the increasing resistance to ciprofloxacin among S. aureus from these infections, and failures of therapy associated with the emergence of resistance to ciprofloxacin raise concerns regarding the use of ciprofloxacin alone in the treatment of these infections (23,25). Grayson and associates (15), in a randomized, double-blind comparison of ampicillin-sulbactam and imipenem-cilastatin treatment of limb-threatening infection, found improvement in 94% and 98% of patients, respectively, after 5 days of therapy; at the conclusion of parenteral therapy, clinical cures were noted in 81% of patients treated with ampicillin-sulbactam (mean ± SD, 13 ± 6.5 days) and 85% of imipenem-cilastatin recipients (14.8 ± 8.6 days).

Unless a failure of prior antimicrobial therapy or nosocomial acquisition of infection suggest the presence of unusually antibiotic-resistant pathogens, we advocate selecting initial empiric therapy for limb-threatening infection from these regimens: ampicillin-sulbactam; ticarcillin-clavulanate; a third-generation cephalosporin plus clindamycin; or a fluoroquinolone plus clindamycin. Undoubtedly, other comparable regimens can be designed. Although the recommended regimens are not effective against every pathogen potentially encountered in these infections, each regimen should provide excellent antimicrobial activity against the major pathogens: S. aureus, aerobic strepto-cocci, the commonly encountered Enterobacteriaceae, anaerobic gram-positive cocci, and Bacteroides spp., including the B. fragilis group. Contingent on the clinical response to the initial treatment, the microbiologic data from deep ulcer cultures obtained prior to therapy or the cultures of debrided tissue or purulent drainage obtained during the initial days of therapy can be used to revise the empiric regimen. For example, if a satisfactory clinical response is coupled with isolation of pathogens that do not require broad-spectrum therapy, it is reasonable to complete treatment with more specifically targeted antibiotics. Alternatively, if a satisfactory clinical response is achieved despite recovering bacteria that are resistant to the empiric regimen, it is not necessary to expand the therapy.

Satisfactory outcomes have been noted with various regimens despite the recovery of bacteria in pretherapy cultures that are resistant to the administered regimen (15,19). This satisfactory response may indicate that the resistant organisms are not functioning as pathogens, that the pathogenicity of the resistant organism is contingent on the synergistic effect of coinfecting bacteria eradicated by the initial therapy, or that wound care (surgery, sterile dressings) and host defenses have a major role in eradicating infection. In contrast, when bacteria that are resistant to the current treatment are isolated and the response of pedal infection is not fully satisfactory, it is necessary to expand therapy to encompass these bacteria. Although a definite pathogenetic role cannot be assigned to the resistant organisms, pending detection and correction of other factors impacting adversely on the clinical response (e.g., inadequate drainage and debridement, ischemia, poorly controlled carbohydrate metabolism), this expansion of therapy is warranted. Although this approach—using cultures obtained from material deep in ulcers—may on occasion result in unnecessarily broad therapy, it is practical and obviates the need for invasive sampling in the absence of clinically apparent abscesses (18).

The need to treat relatively less virulent organisms such as enterococci, viridans streptococci, coagulase-negative staphylococci, and corynebacteria should be viewed in the context of this discussion. As noted earlier, these organisms are not likely pathogens. Nevertheless, they are occasionally recovered as the sole isolate from unexposed deep sites of pedal infection, a circumstance that strongly suggests a role as a pathogen, or as the residual bacteria in an infection that has not responded adequately. In these settings, these less virulent bacteria should be treated. Although it seems reasonable to withhold treatment for selected bacteria whose pathogenic role is questionable, the preeminent role of S. *aureus* in pedal infections makes it unwise to ignore this organism.

The appropriate duration of antibiotic treatment (parenteral and oral) for soft-tissue infections in the feet of patients with diabetes has not been established. For infections limited to soft tissues, parenteral therapy has been administered on average for 10 to 14 days (15,22). Oral antibiotics have often been continued for prolonged periods in patients with unhealed ulcers. Peterson and colleagues (23) concluded that more favorable outcomes were achieved by continuing antibiotic therapy until ulcers heal. In addition, antibiotics have been used in the treatment of uninfected *mal perforans*. However, studies have not demonstrated a benefit from prolongation of antibiotic therapy beyond that required to eliminate infection or from the treatment of uninfected ulcers (26). Lipsky and associates (19), in treating nonlimb-threatening infections, noted that patients with ulcers that persisted after infections had responded satisfactorily to a 2-week course of oral antibiotics generally healed without additional antibiotic treatment. After eradicating infection, the healing of ulcers is primarily the consequence of wound care, adequate blood supply and oxygen delivery, avoiding local trauma from weight bearing, satisfactory nutrition, and control of carbohydrate metabolism (6,27).

Bacteremia in patients with foot infections, although not common, is usually due to S. *aureus* or *Bacteroides* spp. (28). Diabetic patients with S. *aureus* bacteremia despite a primary focus of infection are at particular risk for infective endocarditis or other metastatic infections and require careful evaluation (29). Hematogenously seeded S. *aureus* infections require more prolonged courses of parenteral antimicrobial therapy than uncomplicated soft-tissue foot infections.

In patients who appear severely ill (e.g., have life-threatening infection, including those with ketoacidosis or extensive necrotizing or gas-forming infection), more inclusive empiric antibiotic coverage is indicated (18). As a consequence of severe metabolic derangement or overwhelming sepsis, these patients are at risk of dying, thus warranting initial empiric antimicrobial therapy designed to encompass virtually all of the pathogens encountered in this infection. We suggest using one of these or a comparable regimen in this setting: imipenem-cilastatin; ampicillin-clindamycin (or ampicillin-sulbactam) and gentamicin; or vancomycin, aztreonam, and metronidazole.

SURGICAL MANAGEMENT

Surgical management begins with inspection of the infected foot to identify a wound that serves as a portal of entry for infection and to determine the extent and severity of infection. Because neuropathy is common and severe in these patients, inspection, including probing the depths of ulcers and debriding necrotic tissue, can be done at the bedside with little or no anesthesia. Good light and a sterile wound dressing kit containing forceps, scissors, and a probe are required. It is imperative to unroof all encrusted areas and to inspect the wound using the probe to determine the extent of deep-tissue destruction and possible involvement of bone, joint, or tendon. Advise the patient and family of the importance of inspecting and debriding an eschar or necrotic tissue.

Furthermore, describe the findings to the patient and family so that they will not misconstrue the debridement as having caused the ulcer.

Regardless of the extent of infection, it is essential to rest the foot. The healing of ulcers on weight-bearing surfaces requires that patients be restricted from weight bearing on that surface. Because neuropathy prevents patients from accurately assessing the degree of weight bearing, partial weight bearing is not a realistic program. Contact casting and felted foam dressing, often used to protect an uninfected *mal perforans* in patients who cannot remain off the foot, are unsuitable for infected ulcers. Open ulcers are gently packed 1 to 3 times daily with sterile plain gauze moistened with normal saline or dilute isotonic antiseptic solutions (one-quarter strength betadine). Full-strength solutions, astringents, enzymatic debriding agents, whirlpools, soaks, and heat in any form should not be used because they may potentially injure tissues. Although the use of platelet-derived or recombinant tissue growth factors has been advocated to promote healing, neither the clinical efficacy nor the cost benefit of these agents has been adequately demonstrated. Patients with nonlimb-threatening infection who are treated at home (Figure 1.2) should be re-evaluated within 48 hours, and those failing to improve should be hospitalized. Patients with larger, deeper ulcers extending into subcutaneous tissues and with spreading cellulitis or lymphangitis or deep-tissue necrosis and purulence require immediate hospitalization (Figure 1.3). Surgical debridement and drainage of infection in the operating room should be carried out as expeditiously as possible. Neither systemic toxicity nor local infection will improve until adequate surgical debridement and drainage have been performed. Control of carbohydrate metabolism should be pursued vigorously, which will generally require administration of insulin in excess of

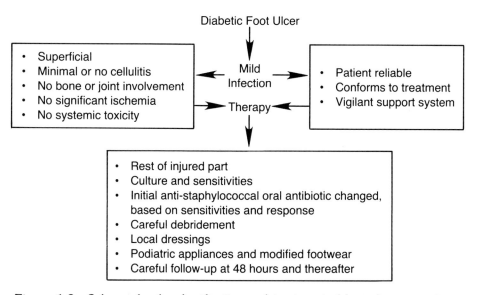

Figure 1.2 Schema for the classification and treatment of foot ulcers complicated by mild, nonlimb-threatening infection.

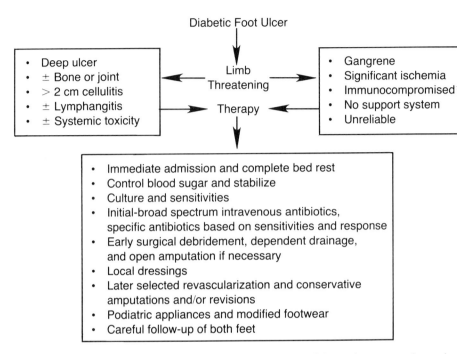

Figure 1.3 Schema for classification and treatment of foot ulcers complicated by limb-threatening infection.

previous baseline doses. Edema should be eliminated by elevating the foot with bed rest or, when it is a component of congestive heart failure, by diuretic therapy.

Patients with diabetes do not tolerate undrained purulence and infection. Deep necrotizing infection cannot be adequately debrided and drained through small stab wounds or by the placement of drains (Figure 1.4). Initial surgical treatment, although assuring adequate drainage and debridement, must be performed in a manner that maximizes the potential for later reconstruction and limb salvage. Carefully placed incisions that allow dependent drainage and sharp debridement yet that conserve as much healthy tissue as possible are required even if this means multiple visits to the operating room (30). The location of the ulcer, the extent of the infection, and the adequacy of the circulation will determine the final result in the infected foot. Occasionally, muscle flaps, skin grafts, and even free-tissue transfers are required to close these wounds (31). Although infection must be controlled initially regardless of the circulatory status, an infected neuropathic foot with adequate circulation is managed differently than the same infection in an ischemic foot.

Patients with infection that has destroyed much of the foot architecture and weight-bearing capability are managed by amputation. Patients must be prepared emotionally to accept this recommendation. In patients with life-threatening, extensive infection, emergency open guillotine amputation may be necessary. When an amputation is required because of infection, an open guillotine procedure followed by a definitive

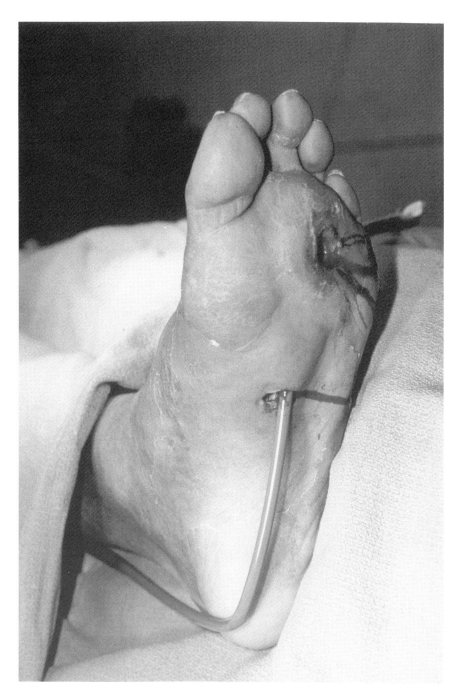

Figure 1.4 (a) Limb-threatening infection that has dissected along the intermediate plantar muscle compartment from an ulcer over the third metatarsal head. This infection has been inadequately drained by placement of a catheter.

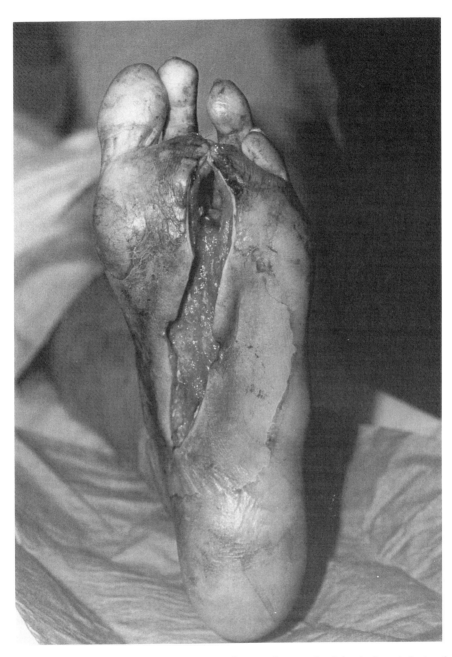

Figure 1.4 **(b)** The infection has now been adequately debrided and drained, with resection of the third ray because of osteomyelitis involving the metatarsal head and the proximal phalanx.

revision is preferred. The frequency of primary healing is higher with the 2-stage procedure than with a 1-stage definitive amputation (32).

MANAGEMENT OF ISCHEMIA

Critical ischemia is strongly associated with nonhealing ulceration and amputation in diabetic patients with foot infections (4,33). Unrecognized or inadequately treated ischemia increases the risk for major amputation (33,34). With an ischemic extremity, the initial surgical debridement and drainage is rarely definitive. Once infection has been controlled, assessment of the circulation to the foot is required to ascertain the surgical treatment that will provide patients with a usable foot. Clinical judgment remains most important in determining the severity of vascular insufficiency of the diabetic lower extremity. All noninvasive tests, including transcutaneous oxygen determinations, are complimentary to clinical judgment. No diabetic patient should undergo a foot amputation solely on the basis of unfavorable results from noninvasive testing (34). Before denying a diabetic patient a chance for foot salvage by arterial reconstruction, arteriography that visualizes the tibial, peroneal, and foot arteries is mandatory.

In diabetic patients, there is a predilection for macrovascular arterial occlusive disease to involve the tibial and peroneal vessels (35–37). Furthermore, diabetics tend to have less occlusive arterial disease in the foot than nondiabetics (35–37). Thus, tissue perfusion in the ischemic foot of patients with diabetes can be restored by appropriate vascular reconstructive surgery (38–40). Although the specifics of vascular reconstruction are beyond the scope of this discussion, autogenous vein bypass grafting to foot arteries in diabetics is successful, with patency and limb-salvage rates of 88% and 92% at 3 years, respectively (39). After control of infection with broad-spectrum antibiotics, local debridement, or open partial forefoot amputation, autogenous vein bypass grafting to pedal arteries is a safe, effective technique for restoration of blood flow (40,41). This aggressive approach to arterial reconstruction allows incorporation of aggressive drainage and debridement of infected soft tissue or bone into the strategy for surgical management of pedal infection and is the cornerstone for increased limb salvage in patients with diabetes.

OSTEOMYELITIS

Among the most challenging and unresolved problems in the management of foot infection in patients with diabetes are the diagnosis and treatment of osteomyelitis. The occurrence of a neuro-osteoarthropathy, often called diabetic osteopathy or Charcot's changes, in the feet of these patients generates confusion in the diagnosis of osteomyelitis. This phenomenon, which is thought to be the consequence of severe neuropathy, repetitive trauma, and reflex alterations in circulation to the foot, is encountered with greatest frequency in the phalanges but with the most severity in the metatarsal and tarsal bones. Osteopathy can be associated with notable radiologic changes, including fractures, bone destruction and resorption, bone sclerosis, and periosteal new bone formation, some of which can easily be mistaken for osteomyelitis (42,43). With severe disruption and dislocation of bones and articular surfaces, the foot becomes deformed, resulting in areas of excessive weight bearing with secondary ulceration and infection that can extend to bone. Alternatively, infection extending from neuropathic ulcers may be complicated by osteomyelitis in contiguous bones in the absence of osteopathy.

Pedal osteomyelitis complicates a substantial portion of limb-threatening infection in diabetics. Of 96 limb-threatening infections treated in an antibiotic trial, osteomyelitis was noted by Grayson and colleagues (15) in 58 (60%); it was confirmed histopathologically in 52 of these infections. Seldin and associates (44), in a retrospective study, confirmed pedal osteomyelitis in 12 (52%) of 23 patients with infected ulcers. In a prospective evaluation of 41 diabetic patients with foot ulcers, Newman and colleagues (45) reported pedal osteomyelitis in 28 (68%) patients; bone infection was suspected clinically in only 9 of these patients. The diagnosis of osteomyelitis in 13 patients in this study was based on isolation of bacteria from a bone biopsy in the absence of diagnostic histopathologic abnormalities, a finding that could be accounted for by soft-tissue infection adjacent to bone rather than bone infection. Even if the diagnosis of osteomyelitis is not accepted in these 13 patients, 15 foot ulcers in the 41 patients (37%), a still notable frequency, were complicated by osteomyelitis. Of note in this study, shallow ulcers (<3 mm deep) were less frequently associated with bone infection than were deep ulcers (45).

Because effective treatment of pedal osteomyelitis in diabetic patients differs from that advocated for soft-tissue infection in the foot, a precise diagnosis is important. Unfortunately, no current clinical, radiographic, or scintigraphic technique is sufficient to accurately diagnose pedal osteomyelitis, in particular to detect bone infection early and to reliably distinguish it from osteopathy (Table 1.2). Most evaluations of diagnostic tests suffer from a retrospective design, inclusion of small numbers of patients with osteopathy, or imprecisely specified definitions of osteomyelitis. Bone changes indicative of osteomyelitis on plain radiographs are not only delayed in developing but also are difficult to distinguish from osteopathy, causing radiographs to be both insufficiently sensitive and nonspecific (44–48). Triple-phase bone scans are notably more sensitive than radiographs; however, uninfected osteopathic lesions are not distinguishable from infected bone with this technique. Therefore, these scintigrams often yield false-positive results, reducing the specificity and positive predictive value of the tests (44, 46–49, 50). Although bone scans in patients with pedal osteomyelitis are occasionally negative in the setting of severe ischemia and bone necrosis, a negative bone scan argues strongly against osteomyelitis. The utility of the gallium-67 citrate scan has been limited by its poor spatial definition of lesions as well as by uptake in sites of osteopathy (50). Although it does not provide optimal spatial localization, indium-111-labeled leukocyte imaging has been found to be sensitive, specific, and to have high predictive values (45, 48–50). Computed tomography, although useful in defining soft-tissue collections in various anatomic compartments of the foot, has not enhanced our ability to diagnose osteomyelitis (43). Initial studies with magnetic resonance imaging indicate promise in detecting both localized soft-tissue infection and osteomyelitis (47,51). Yuh and associates (47), in a study of 44 pedal bones wherein

Table 1.2   The reliability of tests in the diagnosis of osteomyelitis complicating foot infections in patients with diabetes

Test, Author (Reference) (Number Studied)	PERCENTAGE				
	Sensitivity*	Specificity*	Positive predictive value*	Negative predictive value*	Accuracy*
Plain radiograph					
Park (46) (39)	62	69	80	47	64
Seldin (44) (25)	93	50	74	83	76
Yuh (47) (39)	75	60	75	60	69
Keenan (48) (88)	69	76	75	77	76
Newman (45) (37)	28	92	87	38	49
Triple-phase bone scan					
Park (46) (36)	83	75	87	69	80
Seldin (44) (30)	94	79	83	92	87
Schauwecker (49) (35)	100		49		49
Maurer (50) (13)	75	56	43	83	61
Yuh (47) (29)	94	18	65	66	65
Keenan (48) (94)	100	38	52	100	63
Indium-111 leukocyte scan					
Schauwecker (49) (35)	100	83	85	100	91
Maurer (50) (13)	75	89	75	89	85
Keenan (48) (46)	100	78	76	100	87
Newman (45) (39)	89	69	85	75	82

*Sensitivity = true positive/true positive + false negative; specificity = true negative/true negative + false positive; positive predictive value = true positive/true positive + false positive; negative predictive value = true negative/true negative + false negative; accuracy = true positive + true negative/entire population studied.

there was a clinical suspicion of infection, found magnetic resonance imaging to be sensitive (100%), specific (90%), and to have high positive (93%) and negative (100%) predictive values for osteomyelitis. Although the marrow signal from osteomyelitic bone could be distinguished from that of subacute to chronic osteopathy, marrow changes in acutely traumatized bone (e.g., fracture, recent surgery) was indistinguishable from that associated with osteomyelitis.

Lipsky and colleagues (52) advocated culture of a bone specimen obtained through a route that does not intersect the ulcer tract as the most accurate means to diagnose osteomyelitis. Specimens can be obtained surgically or by percutaneous needle biopsy. Newman and associates (45) obtained bone for culture and histologic examination by biopsy with a 15-gauge trochar placed through a 5-mm incision. In addition to the impracticality and potential risk associated with these invasive techniques, aspiration or biopsy with a needle or trochar is subject to both sampling errors and, in the absence of histopathologic findings diagnostic of osteomyelitis, the inability to distinguish bacteria isolated from infected soft tissue adjacent to bone from those isolated from osteo-myelitic bone.

The diagnosis of osteomyelitis requires judicious clinical evaluation and careful use of diagnostic tests as well as long-term observation. Detecting bone in the depths of an infected ulcer by gently probing the base of the ulcer with a blunt surgical probe, although not a sensitive test, has been associated with a high predictive positive value (53). Among 76 patients with infected limb-threatening foot ulcers, probing to bone detected 66% of proven episodes of osteomyelitis (sensitivity); furthermore, in 89% of patients with bone probed in the ulcer base, osteomyelitis was confirmed (positive predictive value). Newman and associates (45) reported that exposed bone in an ulcer (visible in 6 and probed in 3 patients) was uniformly associated with osteomyelitis. Accordingly, for purposes of patient management, it has been our practice to accept the diagnosis of osteomyelitis when bone can be probed at the base of ulcers and we have not relied on other costly diagnostic modalities for confirmation. Plain radiographs should be obtained routinely in patients with limb-threatening foot infections. If radiographic changes possibly associated with osteomyelitis are noted in probe-negative bone adjacent to a moderately deep ulcer, the bone should either be further evaluated with an In-111 leukocyte scan or magnetic resonance imaging, or the patient should be treated with antibiotics and monitored carefully using clinical observations and serial plain radiographs to confirm or refute the diagnosis. We do not routinely recommend scintigraphic studies of infected feet, nor do we routinely advise percutaneous needle or trochar biopsy of suspected but unexposed bony abnormalities.

Two recent reports of the treatment of pedal osteomyelitis in patients with diabetes have generated controversy. The classic article by Waldvogel and colleagues (54) suggested that surgical debridement was required for successful therapy of chronic osteomyelitis wherein there was devitalized bone, and that debridement, often necessitating amputation, was particularly important in the effective therapy of pedal osteomyelitis occurring in association with vascular insufficiency. Recently, Bamberger and associates (55) concluded, after studying 51 diabetic patients, that osteomyelitis, in the absence of extensive necrosis and gangrene, usually responds to prolonged antibiotic therapy (given for at least 4 weeks intravenously or for 10 weeks intravenously or orally) without surgical ablation. Notably, however, the diagnosis of osteomyelitis was substantiated histopathologically in only 8 patients (at least 6 of whom had the infected bone amputated); in remaining patients, the diagnoses were based on plain radiographs or triple-phase bone scans, tests noted previously to inadequately discriminate between infection and osteopathy. Ultimately, 15 (29%) and 9 (18%) patients underwent below-knee or toe-ray amputations, respectively. Thus, 27 (53%) patients with presumed osteomyelitis responded to prolonged or repetitive courses of antibiotics without extensive surgical debridement. Subsequently, Peterson and colleagues (23) treated 31 patients for osteomyelitis, having based the diagnosis on radiography and triple-phase bone scan. Ciprofloxacin was given orally for at least 3 months, but significant surgical debridement was not performed. Nineteen (61%) of these patients with presumed osteomyelitis were considered to have been successfully treated. The imprecise documentation of osteomyelitis makes it difficult to accept these studies as having demonstrated the efficacy of prolonged antibiotic therapy alone in the treatment of pedal osteomyelitis in diabetics.

If by osteomyelitis one refers to infected bone with areas of devitalization and necrosis, as opposed to periostitis, based on our experience we advocate a more aggressive surgical approach to its treatment. We reviewed our experience with 110 patients with pedal osteomyelitis (96% confirmed histopathologically). Of 86 patients with infection involving the phalanges or the metatarsal heads, or both, 76 were cured with a combined limited surgical procedure (i.e., resection of a toe or ray or a transmetatarsal amputation) and antibiotic therapy. Because all infected bone was resected, parenteral antibiotic therapy was administered for only an average (± SD) of 16 ± 10 days (median, 14 days). A weight-bearing foot was preserved in all patients. The remaining 10 patients with forefoot osteomyelitis underwent below-knee amputation. Of these, 2 underwent emergency guillotine amputations for life-threatening infection and 8 required a foot amputation because severe unreconstructable vascular insufficiency precluded the healing of distal wounds. An additional 5 patients with osteomyelitis involving the tarsal bones or calcaneous, and with either severe ischemia or disrupted foot architecture, also underwent foot amputation. Prolonged parenteral antibiotic therapy was attempted in 19 patients. Of 7 with forefoot or midfoot osteomyelitis, 5 ultimately underwent limited foot-salvaging surgical procedures and 2 underwent foot amputations. Of 12 patients with calcaneous osteomyelitis, 7 with palpable pedal pulses were cured with piecemeal debridement and prolonged parenteral antibiotic therapy (mean [± SD], 33 ± 11 days; median, 34 days). Four patients with hindfoot osteomyelitis did not respond to antibiotic therapy and ultimately underwent below-knee amputation; none had palpable pedal pulses. One patient died during therapy. Although this surgical approach to osteomyelitis of the forefoot may appear unduly aggressive, others have advocated this approach when it can be accomplished without loss of the functional integrity of the foot (52,56). In addition to removing infected bone, these resections eliminate points of undue weight bearing that, if not remodeled, would likely lead to recurrent ulceration and infection (6). Finally, although precise definition of the microbiology of bone infection is required if antibiotic therapy supplemented by piecemeal debridement is employed, the resection en bloc of all the infected bone allows antimicrobial therapy to be focused on residual soft-tissue infection and based on the bacteria isolated from serial deep wound cultures. As in patients with infection limited to soft tissues, the ability to aggressively debride infections complicated by pedal osteomyelitis is founded on the ability, if necessary, to restore blood flow to the foot through arterial reconstruction (38–40).

THE CHALLENGE

Loss of vision or loss of an extremity are dread complications of diabetes. The United States Department of Health and Human Services has set as an objective for the year 2,000 a 40% reduction in the frequency of lower extremity amputations among patients with diabetes. In pursuing this objective, the challenge for all health care systems and practitioners is to manage lower extremity problems of diabetics in a clinically and cost effective manner and thereby reduce the frequency of major amputations in an era of reduced health care dollars. To this end, the medical and surgical approaches to the infected foot in diabetics that have been presented in this review can be implemented by a team of providers including a vascular surgeon, podiatrist, infectious disease specialist, a diabetologist and a cardiologist, the latter assisting with the perioperative management of patients with co-existing coronary artery disease who are to undergo major surgery. Through the aggressive and effective implementation of these approaches, especially extreme distal arterial reconstruction, we have reduced the rate of amputations at all levels among our diabetic patients (57). Additionally, this has been accomplished while reducing the average length of stay among diabetics hospitalized with limb threatening ischemia and infection treated in 1990 by 33% as compared to those treated in 1984 (58). This experience suggests that high quality care can be provided in a reduced cost-of-care environment.

REFERENCES

1 **Most RS, Sinnock P.** The epidemiology of lower extremity amputations in diabetic individuals. *Diabetes Care* 1983;6:87–91.

2 **U.S. Department of Health and Human Services, Publication Service.** *Diabetes Surveillance 1980–1987: Policy and Program Research; 1990 Annual Report.* Atlanta, GA: Centers for Disease Control, 1990.

3 **Holewski JJ, Moss KM, Stess RM, Graf PM, Grunfeld C.** Prevalence of foot pathology and lower extremity complications in a diabetic outpatient clinic. *J Rehab Res Dev* 1989;26:35–44.

4 **Reiber GE, Pecoraro RE, Koepsell TD.** Risk factors for amputation in patients with diabetes mellitus: a case control study. *Ann Intern Med* 1992;117:97–105.

5 **Sims DS Jr, Cavanagh PR, Ulbrecht JS.** Risk factors in the diabetic foot: recognition and management. *Phys Ther* 1988;68:1887–1902.

6 **Tillow T, Giurini J, Habershaw G, Chrzan J, Rowbotham J.** Review of metatarsal osteotomies for the treatment of neuropathic ulcerations. *J Am Podiat Med Assoc* 1990;80:211–217.

7 **Seabrook GR, Edmiston CE, Schmitt DD, Krepel C, Bandyk DF, Towne JB.** Comparison of serum and tissue antibiotic levels in diabetes-related foot infections. *Surgery* 1991; 110:671–677.

8 **Mowat A, Baum J.** Chemotaxis of polymorphonuclear leukocytes from patients with diabetes mellitus. *N Engl J Med* 1971;284:621–627.

9 **Nolan CN, Beaty HN, Bagdade JD.** Further characterization of the impaired bactericidal function of granulocytes in patients with poorly controlled diabetes. *Diabetes* 1978;27:889–894.

10 **Drachman RH, Root RK, Wood WB Jr.** Studies on the effect of experimental non-ketotic diabetes mellitus on antibacterial defenses: demonstration of a defect in phagocytosis. *J Exp Med* 1966;124:227–240.

11 **Scher KS, Steele FJ.** The septic foot in patients with diabetes. *Surgery* 1988;104:661–666.

12 **Wagner FW Jr.** The diabetic foot and amputation of the foot. In: Mann RA, ed. *Surgery of the Foot, ed. 5.* St. Louis: CV Mosby, 1986: 421–455.

13 **Gibbons GW, Eliopoulos GM.** Infection of the diabetic foot. In: GP Kozak, Hoar CS Jr, Rowbotham RL, et al, eds. *Management of Diabetic Foot Problems.* Philadelphia: W. B. Saunders, 1984:97–102.

14 **Tan JS, File TM Jr.** Diagnosis and treatment of diabetic foot infections. *Comp Ther* 1988;14: 52–62.

15 **Grayson ML, Gibbons GW, Habershaw GM, et al.** Ampicillin/sulbactam vs. imipenem/cilastatin in the treatment of limb-threatening foot infections in diabetic patients. *Clin Infect Dis* (In Press)

16 **Bose KA.** A surgical approach for the infected diabetic foot. *Int Orthop* 1979;3:177–181.

17 **Sapico FL, Canawati HN, Witte JL, Montgomerie JZ, Wagner FW Jr, Bessman AN.** Quantitative aerobic and anaerobic bacteriology of infected diabetic feet. *J Clin Microbiol* 1980;12:413–420.

18 **Wheat LJ, Allen SD, Henry M, et al.** Diabetic foot infections: bacteriologic analysis. *Arch Intern Med* 1986;146:1935–1940.

19 **Lipsky BA, Pecoraro RE, Larson SA, Hanley ME, Ahroni JH.** Outpatient management of uncomplicated lower-extremity infections in diabetic patients. *Arch Intern Med* 1990;150: 790–797.

20 **Sapico FL, Witte JL, Canawati HN, Montgomerie JZ, Bessman AN.** The infected foot of the diabetic patient: quantitative microbiology and analysis of clinical features. *Rev Infect Dis* 1984;6:S171–S176.

21 Fierer J, Daniel D, Davis C. The fetid foot: lower-extremity infections in patients with diabetes mellitus. *Rev Infect Dis* 1979;1:210–217.

22 Hughes CE, Johnson CC, Bamberger DM, et al. Treatment and long-term follow-up of foot infections in patients with diabetes or ischemia: a randomized, prospective, double-blind comparison of cefoxitin and ceftizoxime. *Clin Ther* 1987;10(suppl A):36–49.

23 Peterson LR, Lissack LM, Canter K, Fasching CE, Clabots C, Gerding DN. Therapy of lower extremity infections with ciprofloxacin in patients with diabetes mellitus, peripheral vascular disease or both. *Am J Med* 1989;86: 801–808.

24 Beam TR Jr, Gutierrez I, Powell S, et al. Prospective study of the efficacy and safety of oral intravenous ciprofloxacin in the treatment of diabetic foot infections. *Rev Infect Dis* 1989;11(suppl 5):S1163–S1164.

25 Nix DE, Cumbo TJ, Kuritzsky P, Devito JM, Schentag JJ. Oral ciprofloxacin in the treatment of serious soft tissue and bone infections: efficacy, safety and pharmacokinetics. *Am J Med* 1987;82(suppl 4A):146–153.

26 Jones EW, Edwards R, Finch R, Jaffcoate WJ. A microbiologic study of diabetic foot lesions. *Diabetes Med* 1984;2:213–215.

27 Pecoraro RE, Ahroni JH, Boyko EJ, Stensel VL. Chronology and determinants of tissue repair in diabetic lower extremity ulcers. *Diabetes* 1991;40:1305–1313.

28 Sapico FL, Bessman AN, Canawati HN. Bacteremia in diabetic patients with infected lower extremities. *Diabetes Care* 1982;5:101–104.

29 Cooper G, Platt R. *Staphylococcus aureus* bacteremia in diabetic patients: endocarditis and mortality. *Am J Med* 1982;73:658–662.

30 Gibbons GW. Diabetic foot sepsis. *Semin Vasc Surg* 1992;5:1–3.

31 Cronenwelt JL, McDaniel MD, Zwolak RM, et al. Limb salvage despite extensive tissue loss: free tissue transfer combined with distal revascularization. *Arch Surg* 1989;124:609–615.

32 McIntyre KE, Bailey SA, Malone JM, Goldstone J. Guillotine amputation in the treatment of nonsalvageable lower extremity infections. *Arch Surg* 1984;119:450–453.

33 Criado E, DeStefano AA, Keagy BA, Upchurch GR Jr, Johnson G Jr. The course of severe foot infection in patients with diabetes. *Surg Gynecol Obstet* 1992;175:135–140.

34 Gibbons GW, Wheelock FC Jr, Siembieda C, Hoar CS Jr, Persson AB. Noninvasive prediction of amputation level in diabetic patients. *Arch Surg* 1979;113:1253–1257.

35 Strandness DE Jr, Priest RE, Gibbon GE. Combined clinical and pathologic study of diabetic and non-diabetic peripheral arterial disease. *Diabetes* 1964;13:366–372.

36 Conrad MC. Large and small artery occlusion in diabetics and non-diabetics with severe vascular disease. *Circulation* 1967;36:83–91.

37 LoGerfo FW, Coffman JD. Vascular and microvascular disease of the foot in diabetics. *N Engl J Med* 1985;311:1615–1619.

38 Pomposelli FB, Jepsen SJ, Gibbons GW, et al. Efficacy of the dorsal pedal bypass for limb salvage in diabetic patients: short-term observations. *Diabetes Spectrum* 1992;5:338–342.

39 Pomposelli FB Jr, Jepsen SJ, Gibbons GW. A flexible approach to infrapopliteal vein grafts in patients with diabetes mellitus. *Arch Surg* 1991;126:724–729.

40 Tannenbaum GA, Pomposelli FB Jr, Marcaccio EJ, et al. Safety of vein bypass grafting to the dorsal pedal artery in diabetic patients with foot infections. *J Vasc Surg* 1992;15:982–990.

41 Hurley JJ, Auer AJ, Hershey FB, et al. Distal arterial reconstruction: patency and limb salvage in diabetics. *J Vasc Surg* 1987;5:796–802.

42 Clouse ME, Gramm HF, Legg M, Flood T. Diabetic osteoarthropathy: clinical and roentgenographic observations in 90 cases. *AJR* 1974;121:22–34.

43 Zlatkin MB, Pathria M, Sartoris DJ, Resnick D. The diabetic foot. *Radiol Clin North Am* 1987;25:1095–1105.

44 Seldin DW, Heiken JP, Feldman F, Alderson PO. Effect of soft-tissue pathology on detection of pedal osteomyelitis in diabetics. *J Nucl Med* 1985;26:988–993.

45 Newman LG, Waller J, Palestro CJ, et al. Unsuspected osteomyelitis in diabetic foot ulcers: diagnosis and monitoring by leukocyte scanning with indium In 111 oxyquinoline. *JAMA* 1991;266:1246–1251.

46 Park HM, Wheat J, Siddiqui AR, et al. Scintigraphic evaluation of diabetic osteomyelitis: concise communication. *J Nucl Med* 1982;23:569–573.

47 Yuh WTC, Corson JD, Baraniewski JM, et al. Osteomyelitis of the foot in diabetic patients: evaluation with plain film, 99mTc-MDP bone scintigraphy, and MR imaging. *AJR* 1989;152: 795–800.

48 Keenan AM, Tindel NL, Alavi A. Diagnosis of pedal osteomyelitis in diabetic patients using current scintigraphic techniques. *Arch Intern Med* 1989;149:2262–2266.

49 Schauwecker DS, Park HM, Burt RW, Mock BH, Wellman HN. Combined bone scintig-

raphy and indium-111 leukocyte scans in neuropathic foot disease. *J Nucl Med* 1988;29:1651–1655.

50 Maurer AH, Millmond SH, Knight LC, et al. Infection in diabetic osteoarthropathy: use of indium-labeled leukocytes for diagnosis. *Radiology* 1986;161:221–225.

51 Beltran J, Campanini S, Knight C, McCalla M. The diabetic foot: magnetic resonance imaging evaluation. *Skeletal Radiol* 1990;19:37–41.

52 Lipsky BA, Pecoraro RE, Wheat LJ. The diabetic foot: soft tissue and bone infection. *Infect Dis Clin North Am* 1990;4:409–432.

53 Grayson ML, Balogh K, Levin E, Karchmer AW. "Probing to bone": a useful clinical sign of osteomyelitis in diabetic fetid feet. Abstracts of the 30th Interscience Conference on Antimicrobial Agents and Chemotherapy, Atlanta, GA, October 1990; abstract no. 244.

54 Waldvogel FA, Medoff G, Swartz MN. Osteomyelitis: a review of clinical features, therapeutic considerations and unusual aspects. *N Engl J Med* 1970;282:198–206.

55 Bamberger DM, Daus GP, Gerding DN. Osteomyelitis in the feet of diabetic patients: long-term results, prognostic factors, and the role of antimicrobial and surgical therapy. *Am J Med* 1987;83:653–660.

56 Benton GS, Kerstein MD. Cost effectiveness of early digit amputation in the patient with diabetes. *Surg Gynecol Obstet* 1985;161:523–524.

57 LoGerfo FW, Gibbons GW, Pomposelli FB Jr, et al. Trends in the care of the diabetic foot: expanded role of arterial reconstruction. *Arch Surg* 1992;127:617–621.

58 Gibbons GW, Marcaccio EJ Jr, Burgess AM, et al. Improved quality of diabetic foot care, 1984 vs 1990: reduced length of stay and costs, insufficient reimbursement. *Arch Surg* 1993;128:576–581.

Splenic abscess: pathogenesis, clinical features, diagnosis, and treatment

J. DAVIS ALLAN

INTRODUCTION

Splenic abscess is a rare disease, often difficult to diagnose and treat. Without treatment it is usually fatal. In the preantibiotic era, it was most often reported as a complication of typhoid fever or malaria (1, 2). However, this is no longer the case, and numerous types of bacteria and other micro-organisms are now reported as causing abscesses in the spleen. Although it may occur as an isolated problem, often it is part of a more widely disseminated process involving multiple abscesses in the spleen and other organs. As is the case with many infections, the spectrum of clinical illness associated with splenic abscess is changing with advances in medical therapy. The increased numbers of patients with immunosuppression from chemotherapy, hematologic malignancies, organ transplantation, and human immunodeficiency virus type 1 (HIV-1) infection have resulted in an increased incidence of splenic abscess.

Thus far, the low incidence of splenic abscesses has made it a difficult problem to study. The centers with the greatest experience have only rarely reported information on more than 5 to 10 patients in a 20-year period. Comparing these different retrospective series over time is problematic given the enormous number of changes that have occurred in the underlying causes, efficiency of diagnosis as a result of newer imaging modalities such as computerized tomography (CT) and ultrasound, as well as changes in possible therapeutic approaches with the advent of guided percutaneous drainage techniques. This chapter reviews pathogenesis, microbiology, clinical manifestations, and therapeutic means potentially useful in the management of splenic abscess.

DEFINITIONS AND INCIDENCE

The spleen may be involved in many types of infections, either directly or indirectly, usually responding by hypertrophy. However, the term *splenic abscess* generally refers to those infections, usually pyogenic, that result in macroscopic focal processes within the body of the spleen and at least initially contained within the capsule of the spleen.

In a review published in 1976, Lawhorne and Zuidema (3) reported that only 23 cases of splenic abscess were identified among 16,199 (0.14%) autopsies performed from 1952 to 1974, and that the diagnosis was not made antemortem in any of the cases. In this same article, the authors were only able to identify 5 clinical cases in their hospital over this same period. Several other series have reported similar autopsy incidence rates of less than 0.5% (3–5) and clinical incidence by hospital discharge diagnoses of less than 1 case per 10,000 discharges (4, 5). However, higher incidence rates have been reported recently, particularly when case finding is by radiographic procedures; splenic abscesses account for 1.7% to 15% of all nontraumatic abnormalities in the spleen (6–8).

Despite the low incidence, splenic abscess remains an important clinical concern because it is a potential complication of many more common problems, notably endocarditis. In addition, the high mortality rate is markedly influenced by early diagnosis, which requires a high degree of suspicion on the part of clinicians (4, 9).

PATHOGENESIS

Anatomic considerations

In adults, the normal spleen is approximately $12 \times 7 \times 3$ to 4 cm and weighs between 100 and 250 gm (10). The left upper quadrant location is in close proximity to the diaphragm, the tail of the pancreas, the stomach, the colon, and the kidney. The spleen and the splenic vasculature may readily become secondarily involved by inflammatory processes in these adjacent structures. The blood supply of the spleen is from the splenic artery, which is derived from the celiac artery and terminates in 6 or more branches in the body of the spleen (10, 11). These branches are terminal arteries that do not have collateral arterial flow between the segments supplied by each branch (10,11). In addition, the nature of the microcirculation of the spleen results in a decreased rate of blood flow and increased viscosity as part of the "filtering" function (10, 12). These factors, in part, account for the susceptibility of the spleen to infarction, particularly in disease states characterized by splenic hypertrophy.

Animal models

There has been little experimental work regarding the pathogenesis of splenic abscesses. In 1937, Caldarera (13) published the results of an animal model study demonstrating that the spleen was refractory to abscess development following intravascular injection of *Staphylococcus aureus* unless the spleen had been previously traumatized or a branch of the splenic artery had been ligated. In contrast, abscesses in the liver and kidneys developed in essentially all the animals without requiring antecedent injury to those organs. These data are consistent with the clinical observations of trauma and infarction as predisposing conditions to abscess formation in the spleen, as well as the relative resistance to development of an abscess compared with other organs, and hence the clinical rarity of splenic abscess.

Predisposing conditions

In the preantibiotic era, malaria and typhoid fever were frequently listed as causes or predisposing conditions for the development of a splenic abscess (1, 2). However, 2 authors with extensive experience with malaria have reported very low frequencies for splenic abscess in this setting: 3 of 30,000 and 5 of 77,000 cases (2). Reports that span more recent periods do not list concurrent malaria (14, 15). Even accounting for geographic bias, malaria itself does not appear to be frequently associated with splenic abscess, and the rare reports of splenic abscess in patients with malaria may reflect coincident hemoglobinopathy and splenic infarct (16).

Table 2.1 lists conditions that have been reported to predispose to splenic abscess in several review articles (2, 5, 14, 17). Additional conditions that are cited include myeloproliferative disorders, infectious mononucleosis, alcoholism, cirrhosis, liver and other organ transplantation, hemodialysis, Felty's syndrome and other collagen vascular disorders, systemic corticosteroids, hypogammaglobulinemia, intravenous drug use, preexisting splenic cysts, therapeutic embolization, and diabetes mellitus (2–5, 9, 14, 15, 18–29). It should be noted that many of these conditions have as features in common increased susceptibility to splenic trauma or infarction and increased frequency of bacteremia or other infections with a propensity for bacteremia.

Table 2.1 Percentage of patients with specific conditions predisposing to the development of splenic abscess

	Chun (2)	Nelken (14)	Cohen (15)
Period of literature covered in report	1900–1977	1978–1986	1900–1988
Number of patients	173	171	277
Specific conditions (%)			
Infections*	73		69
Endocarditis	12	14	15
Urinary tract	6		7
Intraabdominal focus	8	22[†]	5
Respiratory tract[‡]	5		5
Noninfectious	32		31
Trauma	17	8	17
Hemoglobinopathy	12	7	12
Chemotherapy/Cancer		27	
Contiguous disease	2	6	3?
Unknown/none apparent		11	

*Other locations but less frequently cited include surgical wound, skin, otitis, urologic procedure, abdominal surgery, osteomyelitis, dental abscess/extraction (2, 4, 14, 174–177).
[†]Not differentiated, grouped as "metastatic infection."
[‡]Includes empyema, pneumonia, upper respiratory tract.

Concurrent infection at a distant site is consistently the most common condition predisposing to splenic abscess and is present in approximately 70% of patients. Of these infections, endocarditis is the most frequent single infection, accounting for 12% to 15% of all cases of splenic abscess. Obviously there may be significant overlap between endocarditis and intravenous drug use, and either can result in splenic infection as a consequence of embolic events and infarction, followed by hematogenous seeding (30–33). Recently published retrospective series addressing the complications of endocarditis give an incidence of 3% to 5% for splenic abscess (33–35). However, it is likely that these series underestimate the true incidence because CT or ultrasound would have been available for only a small portion of the patients reported. The incidence may be higher with some pathogens or types of endocarditis. In a series of cases of left-sided acute bacterial endocarditis due to *Pseudomonas aeruginosa*, 2 of 15 (13%) had concurrent splenic abscess (36). Given the occurrence of splenic infarction in endocarditis from either septic or bland emboli, determination of whether a splenic abscess is present or evolving may be difficult (30).

Of the noninfectious causes, antecedent traumatic injury to the spleen is the most common, occurring in 8% to 17% of patients. Generally, the trauma is reported to have occurred within 2 weeks to 4 months prior to development of the abscess (2, 15). In pediatric patients, noninfectious factors are more common; they account for almost 60% of all splenic abscesses in this age group. Leukemia (29%), hemoglobinopathy (14%), and trauma or torsion of the spleen (11%) are the most common (21).

A potentially misleading aspect of Table 2.1 should be emphasized. The frequency with which hematologic malignancy, organ transplantation, chemotherapy, HIV infection, and other immunosuppressed states are reported in these series that span the past century is certainly an underestimate of their current role in this condition. The reports by Nelken and colleagues (14) and Keidl and associates (21) begin to reflect these changes. Smaller series of more recent cases have a larger percentage of such patients, as high as 46% (22).

MICROBIOLOGY

Table 2.2 summarizes representative frequencies of various organisms reported from several reviews. Staphylococci (primarily S. *aureus*) and various streptococci are the most frequently reported organisms. Gram-negative aerobes are also common, and *Escherichia coli* is the most prominent among this group. More than 1 organism is isolated from at least 10% to 15% of all patients with splenic abscesses (2, 5, 21, 22). The frequency with which no growth is obtained from some samples of splenic abscess may reflect prior antibiotic therapy, failure to culture properly for anaerobes and other fastidious organisms, or perhaps sterile necrosis following infarction. At least 1 entity, Weber Christian disease, has been associated with sterile splenic abscesses (37).

The frequencies in Table 2.2 should be viewed as only broadly representative rather than precise. For example, both over time within each series and between series, specimens were obviously not handled uniformly, and the degree to which fastidious organisms, particularly anaerobes, were sought is impossible to determine. Many other

Table 2.2   Microbiology of splenic abscess*

	No. isolates/ patients[†] (%)	Range (%)
Sterile or only seen on smear	73/368 (20)	12–29
Aerobic	237/368 (64)	57–77
Staphylococci	68/368 (18)	15–28
Streptococci	20/368 (5)	7–22
Enterococci	13/239 (5)	0–8
Salmonella	37/368 (10)	0–11
Pseudomonas aeruginosa	3/239 (1)	0–8
Enterobacter	2/239 (1)	0–2
Escherichia coli	24/239 (10)	4–17
Anaerobic	46/368 (13)	1–39
Bacteroides	12/368 (3)	1–17
Propionibacterium	6/368 (2)	0–4
Clostridium	5/368 (2)	0–8
Fusobacteria	2/368 (1)	0–6
Peptostreptococci	5/368 (2)	0–6
Fungi	56/368 (15)	0–27
Candida spp.	45/368 (12)	0–27

*Derived from (2, 5, 14, 21, 86)
[†]Total number of given isolate/ number of patients with microbiology reported.

organisms have been the subject of case reports, including *Brucella spp.*; *Coryne-bacterium diphtheriae*; various *Pseudomonas spp.* other than *P. aeruginosa* (including *P. pseudomallei*); *Proteus mirabilis*; *Proteus vulgaris*; *Klebsiella pneumoniae*; *Morgan-ella morganii*; *Serratia marcescens*; *Shigella flexneri*; *Yersinia enterocolitica*; *Haemophi-lus influenzae*; *Eikenella corrodens*; *Lactobacillus spp.*; *Bacillus spp.*; *Clostridium difficile* and other *Clostridium spp.*; *Borrelia burgdorferi*; *Aspergillus spp.*; *Aureobassidium pullulans*; *Blastomyces dermatitidis*; specific *Candida spp.*; *Nocardia spp.*; *Mycobacterium tuberculosis*; *Mycobacterium-avium intracellulare*; other myco-bacteria; the agent of cat scratch disease; and *Entameba histolytica* (2, 14, 15, 21, 23, 30, 32–65). Of these, *Pseudomonas pseudomallei* may be a common cause of splenic abscess in those areas of the world where the organism occurs. One series from Thai-land found splenic abscess due to *Pseudomonas pseudomallei* in 19 of 34 (56%) of patients with a liver abscess caused by this same organism (66). The 34 cases repre-sented 8.7% of the cases of melioidosis seen at their hospital during the same period. This finding compared with a frequency of splenic abscess in 1 of 16 (6%) patients with pyogenic liver abscesses due to other bacteria.

In any given series, the particular spectrum of organisms reflects the nature of the predisposing factors or origin of the abscess. For example, series of cases with a predomi-nance of severely immunocompromised patients have a high rate of fungal splenic abscess, principally *Candida spp.* or of abscesses due to other unusual organisms. Those cases arising from an intra-abdominal focus via hematogenous spread or contiguous extension frequently contain bowel flora, including anaerobes, and often contain mixed bacterial species. Splenic abscesses in association with endocarditis tend to contain single isolates, and the microbiology is consistent with organisms characteristic of endocarditis. S. *aureus* is particularly prominent in such cases, perhaps in part a consequence of a high rate of concurrent intravenous drug use, but also a reflection of the propensity for S. *aureus* to produce metastatic infection in many sites (30–33, 66–68).

In general, although less frequently reported than in the past, Salmonella of various species, including S. *typhi*, have been prominent in most recent series and are still relatively common in splenic abscesses in some parts of the world (3, 4, 21, 22, 69–75). It is not clear whether this finding reflects the frequency of bacteremia associated with this organism or whether there is some special quality relative to its intracellular persistence in macrophages that may increase its propensity for causing splenic abscess (76). Although an increased incidence of bacteremic salmonella infection is associated with HIV infection (77), only a few cases of splenic abscess have been reported in this setting (78, 79).

CLINICAL MANIFESTATIONS

Many authors have commented on the nonspecific nature of symptoms and the difficulty of making a diagnosis of splenic abscess. However, the physical findings and symptoms are not particularly more occult than those of other intra-abdominal abscesses (80). It seems likely that these comments partly reflect the fact that, as a result of the rarity of splenic abscess, the diagnosis is often not considered, and that, in the past, imaging this area was difficult.

The presenting symptoms and signs reported in several reviews of splenic abscess are listed in Tables 2.3 and 2.4 (2, 5, 14, 17). Nearly all patients with splenic abscess complain of fever. Approximately 60% report abdominal pain, and approximately 30% to 40% report the pain as localized to the left upper quadrant. A smaller number have left thoracic discomfort that is usually pleuritic in quality, and some experience left shoulder pain. Other nonspecific symptoms of a systemic illness such as malaise and anorexia are sometimes noted. Prior to diagnosis, symptoms generally are present for 2 to 4 weeks, although symptoms of several months' duration are not uncommon.

On physical examination, fever is present in 90% to 100%, and leukocytosis is usually present, often accompanied by a left shift. In many series, abdominal tenderness can be demonstrated in more than half the cases, frequently left upper-quadrant tenderness. Splenomegaly is reported in 25% to 50% of patients and is often tender. A friction rub or tympany over the spleen are very helpful signs but are very rare (2–4, 81). Dullness to percussion, absence of normal diaphragmatic movement, or other auscultatory findings are frequently present at the left base on lung examination. In patients with multiple abscesses, the manifestations of splenic abscess may be more occult and overshadowed by the underlying disease or other manifestations of a disseminated infection (21, 82).

Approximately 40% to 75% of splenic abscesses are solitary lesions (2, 5, 21, 22). The proportion of single versus multiple abscesses in the spleen in any given series is

Table 2.3   Characteristics and symptoms reported by patients with splenic abscess

	Chun (2)	Nelken (14)	Westh (5)
Period of study	1900–1977	1978–1986	1982–1987
Number of patients in series*	173	189	20
Age (yr), mean/median	36.8 / –		– / 52
Range	0.5–83	0.5–82	22–90
Gender (%), male/ female	63 / 37	65 / 35	45 / 55
Duration of symptoms			
Mean / median	– / 22 d	– / –	–/33 d
Range	3 d–18 yr	2–28 d	5–270 d
Specific symptoms (%)[†]			
Fever	95	84	71
Abdominal pain (any)	60		69
Left upper quadrant pain	38	35	44
Diffuse abdominal pain	15	24	25
Left shoulder pain	10	4	
Anorexia	15		50
Nausea/vomiting	16	21	50
Weight loss	11		54

*Overall; however, the denominator for some symptoms may differ.
[†]Rounded to the nearest whole number.

Table 2.4   Signs reported in patients with splenic abscess

	Chun (2)	Nelken (14)	Westh (5)
Number of patients in series*	173	143	20
Fever (%)	95	88	89
Abdominal tenderness (any) (%)	59	46	
Left upper quadrant tenderness	42	39	61
Diffuse tenderness	17		18
Splenomegaly (%)	54	39	26
Chest examination abnormal at left base (%)	66	12	
Dullness	33		44
Rales	21		
Chest radiograph, abnormal at left base (%)	31	82	
Effusion	28		35
Infiltrate	18		20
Elevated leukocyte count (% with elevation)		84	
Mean (SD) × 10³/mm³	15.6	16.8 (8.5)	13.9
Range × 10³/mm³	2.4–41.0		4.8–46.0

*Overall; however, the denominator for some findings may differ.

dependent on the distribution of predisposing factors in the patients and often on the sensitivity of the predominant diagnostic method used. In patients whose risk factor for splenic abscess is endocarditis, splenic abscesses are solitary in approximately 60% to 85% (14, 67). In immunosuppressed patients, multiple abscesses are more common and also reflect the higher frequency of fungi (21, 22). Similarly, abscesses are present in other organs in approximately 23% of patients with splenic abscess overall: 15% of patients with solitary and 40% to 50% of patients with multiple splenic abscesses (2, 5, 21). The liver is the other organ most frequently affected.

COMPLICATIONS

The reported complications of splenic abscess include rupture of the abscess with development of peritonitis, erosion through the pleura with development of empyema (and in at least 1 reported case a bronchopleural fistula), rupture into the bowel, intestinal obstruction, and splenocutaneous fistula (2, 3, 14, 83–85). Many of these complications relate to delay in diagnosis, particularly in the preantibiotic era. The most frequently reported complication is rupture into the peritoneal cavity with development of peritonitis, and in most series this event is associated with a higher mortality rate (3, 14, 26).

DIAGNOSIS

Clinical presentation, symptoms, and physical findings are usually not specific enough to allow a diagnosis to be established on clinical grounds. However, the clinical presentation should raise sufficient suspicion about the possibility of a splenic abscess so that proper imaging studies are performed. The most useful tests for establishing a diagnosis of splenic abscess are CT and ultrasonography. As noted previously, the majority of series and reviews published to date contain relatively few patients in whom these modalities were employed. CT and ultrasound have been routinely available since the early 1980s, and the majority of the cases of splenic abscess reported in the literature antedate the use of CT. To date, there is not adequate experience reported with magnetic resonance imaging to evaluate a potential role in the diagnosis and management of splenic abscesses.

Plain radiography

Plain radiography of the chest appears to be surprisingly sensitive although not specific in these patients. Most reports indicate that 50% to 82% of patients have an abnormal chest radiograph (5, 14, 22, 86, 87). The most common findings are elevated left hemidiaphragm, left pleural effusion, and left basilar infiltrate or atelectasis. Plain radiography of the abdomen is also frequently abnormal (approximately 25–50%) but even less specific; findings include splenomegaly, ileus, and displaced bowel loops (2,

4, 5, 21, 70, 87). The most useful sign, extraintestinal gas in the left upper quadrant, is rarely seen; it is reported in less than 15% of patients (4, 5, 68, 86–88).

Barium sulfate and other contrast studies are generally not useful unless there is a contiguous disease process, such as gastric carcinoma, penetrating gastric or duodenal ulcer, or colonic carcinoma or diverticulitis at the splenic flexure, resulting in the development of a splenic abscess. Other nonspecific findings reported with contrast studies include spasm of the colon at the splenic flexure and displacement of the stomach by the splenic abscess or enlarged spleen (87).

Arteriography has been used in a small number of reported cases of splenic abscess, although the value of this procedure has been significantly diminished by the use of CT and ultrasound (82, 87, 89, 90). The findings on arteriogram are generally those of a mass lesion in the spleen. The mass may be avascular, with displacement and stretching of the splenic artery or branches, or vascular with tortuous vessels at the rim of the mass (57, 87, 90, 91). Arteriography may have value in complicated cases suspected of arising from or coincident with a mycotic aneurysm (90).

Radionuclide studies

Three types of radionuclide studies have been reported to be of some value in establishing the diagnosis of a splenic abscess. ^{99m}Tc liver-spleen scans, gallium scan, and indium (^{111}In)-labeled white blood cell scans have been used.

^{99m}Tc scans of the liver and spleen have been the most commonly reported radionuclide studies utilized in evaluating patients with splenic abscesses. On ^{99m}Tc scans, splenic abscesses appear as a photon-deficient area, or a "filling defect." However, tumors, particularly lymphoma, infarcts, cysts, and abscesses, can produce similar appearances on liver-spleen scan (87). These scans are generally unable to reliably detect lesions 2 cm in diameter or less. Because lesions are often not visualized except on specific views, multiple views, especially a posterior view, must be taken (9, 87). Overall, ^{99m}Tc scanning of the spleen is generally reported to have a sensitivity of 75% to 80% or less for detecting splenic abscesses (14, 87, 92). It is particularly less useful in detecting the multiple small abscesses more commonly seen in immunocompromised patients (21). Another limitation to ^{99m}Tc scanning is that it provides little or no information about adjacent structures, with the exception of the liver.

Gallium citrate scanning has been utilized in some patients with splenic abscesses. Because nearly all cases of its use in this setting appear to be highly selected, it is difficult to get a true estimate of the sensitivity of this imaging technique in detecting a splenic abscess. A significant drawback to these scans in evaluating the presence of an abscess in the spleen is that the normal spleen has a high level of background uptake, making it difficult to distinguish a focal lesion of increased uptake (4, 91, 93). In the setting of a systemic infection such as endocarditis, the spleen often has increased uptake above the already high baseline that may cause a false-positive result (4, 87). Lymphoma presents an additional problem because it is frequently included in the differential diagnosis of a focal splenic lesion but will concentrate gallium (4, 87, 91). Colonic uptake, particularly at the splenic flexure, may also present difficulty in interpretation. A false-negative rate of 28.6% for detecting splenic abscesses by gallium scan has been reported (87). A further limitation of gallium scanning is the time delay inherent in obtaining the result.

Some authors have commented on the value of combined use of gallium and ^{99m}Tc scanning, including subtraction methods, to enhance specificity (22, 87). However, this approach is obviously time-consuming, expensive, and is rarely of significant value since the advent of more sensitive techniques, such as CT.

A more limited experience has been reported with ^{111}In or ^{99m}Tc-hexamethylpropylene amineoxine (HMPAO)–labeled white blood cells for detection of intrasplenic abscess (86, 87, 94). The normal spleen concentrates labeled leukocytes, making interpretation difficult, similar to gallium scans (86, 87). The potential for confusion is illustrated by a case of a subphrenic abscess that mimicked the appearance of a normal spleen in uptake of ^{111}In-labeled white blood cells in a patient who had undergone splenectomy (95). Overall, at this point the relative value and limitations of labeled white cell studies in the diagnosis of splenic abscess appear similar to gallium scanning: the methodology is more problematic, and availability is more restricted (85–87).

Ultrasonography

Along with CT scanning, ultrasonography is now the most commonly employed and useful imaging technique for detection of focal lesions in the spleen, including splenic abscess (Figures 2.1–2.3). A relatively extensive clinical experience documenting its utility has been reported (5, 8, 14, 22, 49, 86, 91, 96–103). Ultrasound has also been used intraoperatively to localize an abscess in the spleen for drainage when the exact location was not readily apparent at surgery (104). On ultrasound, a splenic abscess appears as a focal, occasionally anechoic, but more commonly hypoechoic lesion with an irregular or poorly defined margin and variable internal echoes secondary to gas or debris (8, 22, 86, 87, 98, 100, 101). This pattern may be consistent with cysts, necrotic tumors, lymphoma, hematoma, and splenic infarct. The finding of intralesional gas is highly suggestive of an abscess (100). Simple cysts are fluid-filled structures that are anechoic with smooth, clearly defined borders and good through transmission of sound (105). Most abscesses do not show this appearance (8, 91, 105). With ultrasound alone, the distinction between lymphoma and abscess may be very difficult (7, 87). Similarly, differentiation between a fresh infarct and an abscess is also very difficult, although the evolution of the lesion over time usually allows the distinction to be made when the clinical situation permits this approach (7, 100, 106). The utility of ultrasound may be limited by the presence of gas-filled loops of bowel overlying the spleen, and the quality of the study is very operator-dependent (87, 107). Overall, the sensitivity of sonography for splenic abscess has been reported in several studies to be approximately 75% to 90% (5, 14, 21, 86).

Computerized tomography

Computerized tomography has been consistently reported to be the most sensitive and specific imaging technique for detecting splenic abscesses (14, 22) (see Figures 2.1–2.3). It has the additional advantage of providing anatomic detail regarding adjacent structures, as well as defining the presence of other intra-abdominal collections or contiguous

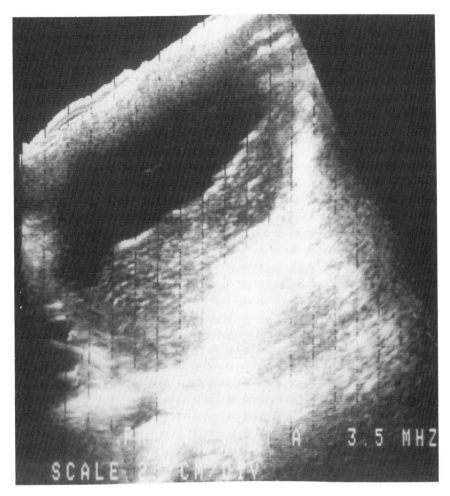

Figure 2.1 Splenic abscess due to *E. coli* in an 82-year-old man following cholecystectomy. **(a)** Ultrasound; longitudinal scan through the left upper quadrant of the abdomen demonstrating a large abscess essentially replacing the spleen with air and echogenic debris posteriorly.

processes that may be coincident with splenic abscess. The overall sensitivity for diagnosis of splenic abscess appears to be slightly better for CT than sonography: 86% to 100% (5, 7, 22, 97). In those few reports where both CT and ultrasound were employed, CT generally was more specific for abscess and able to detect lesions of smaller diameter (22, 86, 97, 107). The appearance of a splenic abscess on CT is usually a focal lesion of low attenuation that does not enhance with intravenous contrast (7, 89, 108–110). Fluid, gas, or internal septa can often be seen, and small amounts of gas appear to be more reliably detected with CT (111). If gas or an air fluid level is not present, the appearance of splenic abscess on CT may be similar to that of lymphoma, hematoma, infarct, cysts,

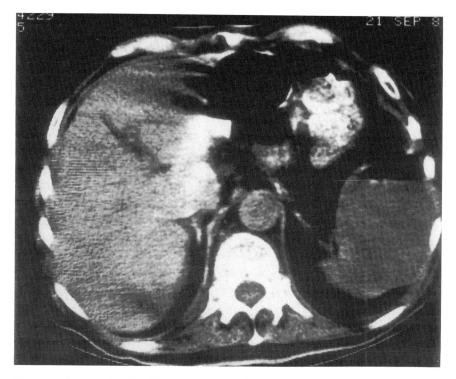

Figure 2.1 (cont.) **(b)** CT scan showing liquefaction of the entire spleen with an air-fluid level.

and pseudocysts (7, 87, 108, 109, 112). Hydatid cysts in the spleen are rare and can usually be distinguished from simple cysts on CT by the presence of calcification in the wall of the cyst or within the contents of the cyst (108).

The differentiation between infarct and abscess is most frequently a problem in the setting of endocarditis. Typically, splenic infarcts appear by CT to be well defined, peripheral, wedge-shaped defects, with the apex toward the hilus and extending to the capsule (7, 105, 108, 109, 113). Unfortunately, these findings are often not present, and the CT appearance may be consistent with that of an abscess (7, 114). In a series of 27 patients with endocarditis and splenic abscess, 4 abscesses were misdiagnosed as infarcts by CT (33). Given the likely pathogenesis of splenic abscess in the setting of endocarditis (i.e., septic embolism causing infarction that evolves into a frank abscess), such difficulties are to be expected, particularly early in the process. Over time, infarcts become better demarcated by CT and evolve to resolution without specific therapy, generally clarifying the nature of the lesion (7, 115). As discussed previously, abscess and infarct will both appear as filling defects on ^{99m}Tc scans; and gallium scanning and ^{111}In-tagged white cell scans are problematic in the setting of endocarditis. Often the clinical setting requires more direct differentiation of these processes, and percutaneous aspiration may be very helpful in establishing the diagnosis.

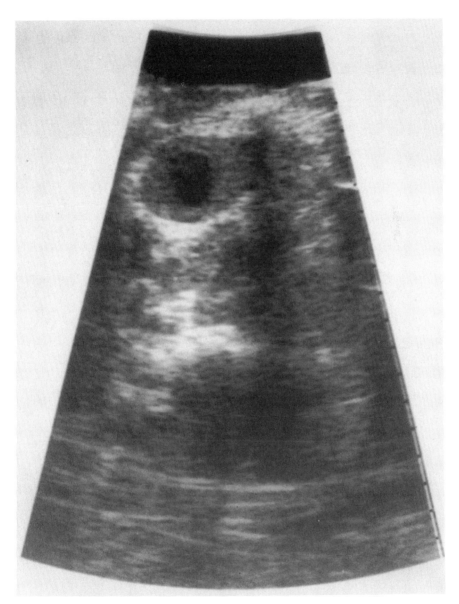

Figure 2.2 Splenic abscess in a 22-year-old woman with a history of inflammatory bowel disease. **(a)** Ultrasound; transverse scan through the tip of the spleen showing a hypoechoic area consistent with an abscess.

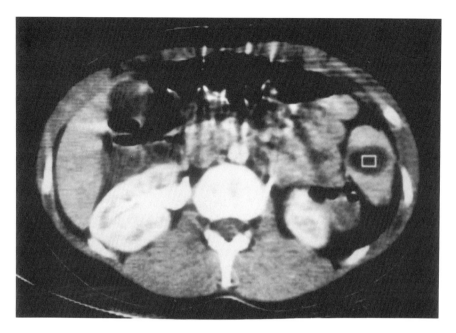

Figure 2.2 (cont.) **(b)** CT scan demonstrating a well-circumscribed, low-density area in the tip of the spleen.

Diagnostic microbiology

When the presence of a splenic lesion consistent with the diagnosis of splenic abscess is established, direct confirmation of the diagnosis is appropriate in most instances. The technique of needle aspiration has been very successful in confirming the diagnosis and identifying the organism with few complications (86, 96, 116). In a recent report, 12 of 14 cases had the specific microbiology established by this technique alone (86). If surgical intervention is imminent, it is reasonable to await confirmation and cultural data from surgery rather than subject patients to a second procedure. Any material obtained by fine-needle aspiration, catheter drainage, or surgery should be thoroughly evaluated given the range of organisms implicated. Specimens should be examined for aerobic and anaerobic bacteria, fungi, frequently mycobacteria, and, in rare instances, parasites.

Blood cultures are frequently positive in patients with a splenic abscess, particularly in the setting of endocarditis, but they have limitations. It is difficult to tell in most series how extensively patients were evaluated for bacteremia. In one review of patients who were not selected on the basis of predisposing factors, blood cultures were drawn in 72 and were positive in 42 (60%), although the same organism was obtained from the spleen in only 32 (44%) (2). In another series, 17 of 30 (57%) patients had positive blood cultures; 12 (71%) had the same isolate cultured from the spleen. However, in the subgroup of patients with a solitary abscess, only 1 of 7 had a positive blood culture. In this series, 10 of the 30 patients had endocarditis or intravenous drug use as a predisposing factor (82). In a third series of 13 patients, 4 of 7 (57%) patients had positive blood cultures (22). Obviously, blood cultures should be obtained in any

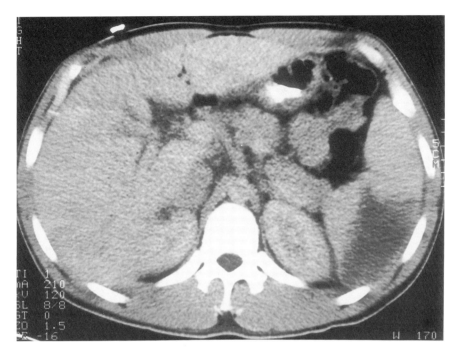

Figure 2.3 CT of a large splenic infarct in a patient with viridans streptococcal endocarditis. The "classic" wedge shape with apex toward the hilus extending to the capsule is seen.

patient with a splenic abscess, particularly because endocarditis is in the differential diagnosis in all such patients. However, even if positive, the blood culture isolate may not always accurately reflect the causative organism or all of the organisms present if the abscess is mixed.

TREATMENT

Although there have been a few reports of splenic abscesses treated successfully with medical therapy alone when surgery was believed to be contraindicated or was refused, these instances have been exceptional (14, 21, 72, 97, 117–121). Optimal therapy of pyogenic splenic abscesses requires both specific antimicrobial therapy as well as adequate drainage of the collection. More recently, evolving syndromes characterized by small, multifocal, splenic abscesses in immunocompromised patients may require a different approach and will be dealt with separately.

Surgical drainage

The most common methods of surgical drainage have been total splenectomy and splenotomy. Splenotomy, or external drainage established with a surgical procedure, is rarely used in the current management of splenic abscesses. It has been associated with a higher complication rate, a lower success rate, and slower convalescence than splenectomy (2, 3). Consequently, splenectomy is the most commonly advised method in the literature for draining splenic abscesses (3, 4, 5, 14, 17, 50, 57, 69, 71, 81, 121–124). Reported mortality rates in patients treated with splenectomy and antibiotics are 0% to 14% (5, 14, 17, 21, 22, 26, 71, 82), with a complication or morbidity rate of approximately 10% to 30% (14, 71, 73). Complications include intraoperative rupture of the abscess requiring postoperative drains, wound infection, subphrenic abscess, sepsis, empyema, and arterial bleeding (14, 17, 71, 86).

With the growing understanding of the important immunologic and other vital roles of the spleen, a great deal of interest has developed in preserving splenic function whenever possible in the treatment of many different conditions. The major concern has been the frequency of postsplenectomy sepsis syndrome, which occurs in both children and adults who undergo splenectomy (125–127). In an effort to preserve splenic function, at least one instance of a splenic abscess has been treated with partial splenectomy (128). More importantly, this line of reasoning has stimulated development of nonsurgical approaches to draining splenic abscesses.

Percutaneous drainage

Over the past 10 to 15 years, percutaneous drainage of intra-abdominal abscesses has emerged as an effective alternative to operative drainage (129–134). In many types of intra-abdominal abscess, percutaneous drainage under CT or ultrasound visualization is often utilized first; surgical drainage is reserved for patients who are inadequately treated with this technique or for whom surgical drainage is deemed more appropriate for other reasons. Although there has been much interest in efforts to avoid total splenectomy, use of this technique for the therapy of splenic abscess was uncommon in initial reports of percutaneous drainage of abscesses (130, 131, 133–135). Several reasons for this finding include the infrequency of splenic abscesses, concern regarding the vascular nature of the organ, and the difficult location of the spleen in proximity to the colon, lung, and pleura (136).

Over the last 5 to 10 years, however, increasing numbers of patients have been reported that were successfully treated with percutaneous drainage. Although 2 recent reviews suggested that the experience with percutaneous drainage was still too limited to replace splenectomy as the initial choice for drainage (133, 137), one was more positive (138). Table 2.5 summarizes the experience with percutaneous drainage of splenic abscess reported in the literature. In these studies, percutaneous drainage was achieved with single fine-needle aspirations with lavage, repeated aspirations, and, most commonly, by placement of a drainage catheter. The specific details of the techniques, including irrigation and catheter types, are summarized in several articles (86, 96, 129, 131). In general, the reported experience has indicated percutaneous drainage to have been very successful with few complications; overall, 75 of 90 (84%) abscesses were successfully drained with the initial or a subsequent percutaneous drainage. However, the potential selection bias of these reports needs to be kept in mind. In the least successful series, 3 of the 8 cases were complex abscesses with contiguous

Table 2.5   Reported experience with percutaneous drainage of splenic abscess

	No. drained*	No. failed	Required splenectomy[†]
Berkman et al (184)	2	0	
Bozkurt et al (187)	4	1	1
Cheesbrough et al (72)	2	1	1
Chou et al (96)	12	0	
Dwyer et al (180)	4	0	
Faught et al (17)	3	0	
Gerzof et al (130)	2	1[‡]	1[‡]
Gerzof et al (139)	8	3	3
Gleich et al (138)	1	0	
Goerg et al (8)	7	1	1
Hadas-Halpren et al (140)	8	0	
Handrick et al (178)	1	0	
Herman et al (188)	4	1	0
Kreel et al (181)	1	0	
Lambiase et al (186)	4	1[§]	1
Lerner et al (183)	4	1	1
Quinn et al (136)	9	2	
Ramakrishnan et al (179)	1	0	
Sclafani et al (185)	1	0	
Teich et al (50)	1	1	1
Tikkakoski et al (86)	4	0	0
van der Laan et al (111)	1	0	
Wernicke et al (182)	1	0	
Westh et al (5)	5	2	1
Total	90	15	11

*In some cases of percutaneous drainage, either repeat aspiration or a second percutaneous drainage procedure was required (in approximately 12 patients reported in this table).
[†]In some reports, subsequent management of the "failures" was not explicitly stated.
[‡]During the subsequent splenectomy, the abscess was shown to have already been adequately drained.
[§]One additional case termed *palliative*, but no subsequent splenectomy or drainage performed.

disease processes that required specific surgical therapy (139). Splenectomy was performed after initial percutaneous drainage in these cases. Five cases were solitary abscesses, 3 of which were successfully treated by percutaneous drainage, and 2 were successfully drained but were listed as failures because of dislodgment of the catheter in 1 and subsequent splenectomy in the second, although apparently some controversy existed as to whether it was required.

It is important to note that none of these reports represent randomized, prospective studies comparing this approach to splenectomy. Given the rarity, at least reported to date, of splenic abscesses and the complexity of the clinical situations in which they occur, it seems unlikely that such a direct comparison will be performed. Many of these reports provide little detail of the clinical severity of the illness at the initiation of therapy, the duration and nature of antibiotic therapy, or the duration of follow-up, all of which render them difficult to evaluate. However, it should be noted that most of the published experience of any one institution with splenectomy is also usually small and has similar limitations.

Neither the optimal nor even the average duration of percutaneous drainage required for adequate therapy of splenic abscess is defined by this experience. Reported durations have ranged from 1 to 28 days, with most less than 14 days (111, 139–141). One recurrence was reported after removal of a catheter that had been in place for 11 days despite continued antibiotic therapy but which responded to redrainage by a second catheter (86). Some authors have suggested the following guidelines for timing of catheter removal in percutaneous drainage of an abscess in any location: (1) improvement or resolution of clinical criteria, such as fever and leukocytosis; (2) decrease or resolution of the collection; and (3) decrease or clearing of the drainage in the catheter; most emphasize clinical improvement (131, 138).

Requirements for considering percutaneous drainage of a splenic abscess under CT or ultrasound guidance include absence or correction of a bleeding diathesis prior to the procedure, a well-defined abscess (as opposed to a phlegmon), and availability of a radiologist experienced with the technique. One author also lists location of the abscess in the hilus of the spleen as a contraindication for this procedure (136). Suspected hydatid splenic cysts should be avoided (142). Factors that have been associated with splenic abscesses less likely to be successfully drained by this technique include thick fluid in the abscess, multiple septations in the abscess, an abscess that is a result of contiguous disease, and the presence of multiple abscesses (134). Potential complications of percutaneous drainage include fistula, bacteremia, sterile pleural effusion, empyema, bowel perforation, intra-abdominal leakage of abscess contents, and bleeding (136–139). However, there have been very few complications reported in the cases of splenic abscess listed in Table 2.5, primarily sterile pleural effusion.

Antibiotic therapy

The published literature provides little guidance with regard to antibiotic therapy in the treatment of pyogenic splenic abscesses. Most of the studies do not indicate the specific agents used, dose, duration, or rationale for the specific choice. In selecting antibiotic therapy for splenic abscess, cultural and histopathologic data are critical given the wide spectrum of organisms that have been implicated. The best data are from fluid or material obtained directly from the abscess. Obviously, when the specific etiology is known, antibiotic therapy may be tailored to the causative agent. Given the severity of this infection, it is usually appropriate to initiate antibiotic therapy in advance of specific microbiology. However, both for purposes of drainage, as well as for clarifying the microbiology, there should be little delay in obtaining appropriate specimens. In selecting empirical antibiotic therapy in this setting, the choice should initially be based on the bacteriology of the known or suspected source of the abscess (e.g., endocarditis, intraabdominal infection). If no apparent predisposing illness is present, a regimen with a broad spectrum of activity emphasizing *Staphylococcus aureus* (which will cover most other gram-positive cocci except possibly enterococci, which are rarely isolated) as well as gram-negative aerobes is reasonable as initial therapy given the frequency with which these organisms are reported. If a bowel source is suspected, it is appropriate to also include an agent with good activity against bowel anaerobes.

Similarly, there is very little documentation in the literature regarding optimal duration of antibiotic therapy in this setting following drainage either by splenectomy or percutaneous drainage. Reported durations of antibiotic therapy range from a few days to 3 months, most between 1 and 6 weeks (2, 4). When it can be determined from published reports, the longer courses are usually in complicated situations often requiring several drainage procedures or in patients with endocarditis. In "uncomplicated" situations, where antimicrobial therapy of the splenic abscess is the only consideration, some authors advise approximately 10 to 14 days of therapy after splenectomy (2).

Overall approach

In the past, splenectomy combined with antibiotic therapy has been the standard approach to therapy of pyogenic splenic abscesses. This remains the most frequently published recommendation. However, it is important to recognize the marked limitations of the published literature on which many of these recommendations are based. Much of the experience included in large reviews antedate the antibiotic era. More importantly, very few cases of splenic abscess have been reported in adequate detail during the period when CT and ultrasound have been available for routine use. This point is critical because these modalities have an enormous impact on the timeliness of diagnosis, and, perhaps more importantly, they allow reliable, frequent evaluations of individual response to whatever therapeutic interventions have been made. Serial imaging by CT or ultrasound should allow changes in approach to be implemented before clinical deterioration has occurred. It is clear that significant effort to preserve splenic function is worthwhile. In this light, the debate should not necessarily be whether splenectomy or percutaneous drainage is superior in most patients, but rather how to judiciously employ each therapy to maximize the likelihood of preserving the spleen while treating the splenic abscess in a manner that minimizes mortality and morbidity.

On diagnosis, surgical consultation should be obtained, and surgical guidance and input should be maintained throughout the course of management. If an experienced interventional radiologist is promptly available, and if there are no apparent contraindications to the procedure and the number of abscesses is small, percutaneous aspiration for diagnosis and establishment of adequate drainage should be performed in most instances. Any empirical antimicrobial therapy that was instituted should then be modified based on the results of the percutaneous aspirate. If response to therapy is adequate, the patient can continue to be followed closely by clinical criteria and repeated imaging studies. In this regard, the relative simplicity and low cost of ultrasound are a distinct advantage over CT. When patients have responded clinically and the abscess is reduced in size, percutaneous drainage can be discontinued followed by periodic follow-up imaging to assure that reaccumulation of purulent material has not occurred. It is difficult to make specific recommendations regarding duration of antibiotic therapy in this setting, but a minimum of 10 to 14 days after drainage of the abscess is reasonable. The duration of antibiotic therapy should be extended if the clinical response is slow or if some undrained material remains. In individual patients, it is important to recognize as early as possible when such an approach is not working adequately and to move ahead with definitive surgical drainage rather than repeated replacement of percutaneous drains. This is obviously an extremely difficult clinical judgment to make, and experienced surgical advice is invaluable.

Approach to therapy of splenic abscess in the setting of endocarditis

The management of a splenic abscess in the setting of endocarditis warrants special consideration for a number of reasons, but most importantly because it is the setting in which it will be encountered by most internists. An abscess in this setting is most likely to be detected by CT or ultrasound during evaluation of a patient on therapy with symptoms or findings suggestive of a splenic process, or in a patient on therapy with persistent fever or leukocytosis during evaluation for undrained foci of metastatic infection. In the latter situation, clinicians try to make the difficult judgment as to whether the patient is failing medical therapy and valve replacement is necessary. Unfortunately, splenic infarction is a common complication of endocarditis; it occurs in 44% of autopsy cases and at similar rates of 24% to 38% in asymptomatic patients with endocarditis undergoing routine CT screening of the abdomen (30, 114, 143).

As discussed previously, splenic infarcts may be difficult to distinguish from abscess by CT or ultrasound. If the lesion is judged to be an infarct, no specific therapy is indicated in the majority of cases (30,33,115). If an abscess is suspected but the patient has defervesced and otherwise clinically does not appear to have uncontrolled infection, cautious observation with frequent reevaluation by ultrasound or CT may be reasonable, because most patients with endocarditis are likely to receive a prolonged course of intravenous therapy. Clearly, if this course is chosen, such patients are not appropriate candidates for short-course therapy of endocarditis. Of the cases of splenic abscess reported to have been treated successfully with antibiotics alone, the majority have been in patients with endocarditis. In contrast, if a patient has signs of uncontrolled infection, it is prudent to deal directly with the abscess and to drain it percutaneously, or, if unsuccessful, to perform splenectomy. Due to the implications for valve replacement in patients with persistent fever or other signs of sepsis, it is obviously important to resolve early whether the splenic abscess is the source. Similarly, in patients who appear likely to require valve replacement for whatever reason, it is critical to have resolved any issue regarding a continued nidus of infection in the spleen, or, if feasible, to delay valve replacement until such issues are resolved.

PROGNOSIS

The mortality of untreated splenic abscess approaches 100% (2, 9, 14). Reported mortality rates for treated splenic abscesses have ranged between 40% to 70% (2, 4, 9, 26, 49); most are closer to 40% and reflect combined antibiotic and surgical drainage approaches. Recent series have reported more favorable outcomes, with mortality rates of 0% to 14% (5, 14, 17, 21, 22). These recent reports more accurately reflect current management options and the impact of more timely diagnosis as a result of newer imaging modalities, particularly CT and ultrasound. Factors that adversely affect outcome include the presence of significant underlying diseases, rupture of the abscess prior to drainage, and, in some series, advanced age and the presence of multiple abscesses (9, 22, 26, 49, 81).

EMERGING SYNDROMES

Hepatosplenic candidiasis

A growing number of patients are being reported with multiple, relatively small splenic abscesses as a manifestation of disseminated fungal infection. This syndrome has been reported primarily in patients with leukemia receiving chemotherapy or undergoing bone marrow transplantation, although there have been reports in patients with other malignancies and aplastic anemia (58, 144–149). The responsible organism is usually *Candida albicans*, although other *Candida spp.*, and, more rarely, other fungi such as *Aspergillus spp.*, have been reported (14, 148, 150). There is one report of coagulase-negative staphylococci causing a similar syndrome (151). Patients generally present with fever, particularly fever that is persistent after neutropenia has resolved, and occasionally hepatosplenomegaly. Typically, multiple low-density lesions that do not enhance are visualized on CT in the spleen, the liver, and, less commonly, the kidney (152–155). Extramedullary hematopoeisis has been reported in 1 patient with leukemia to have a similar appearance in the liver and the spleen on CT scan (156). Ultrasonography is also very useful and has been reported to show a characteristic hypoechoic lesion with a densely echoic center ("target" or "bulls-eye" lesion) in the liver and a homogeneous hypoechoic appearance to the spleen (152–154, 157). CT scanning appears to be more sensitive for detecting smaller lesions (150). Amphotericin B is the standard therapy for hepatosplenic candidiasis and other disseminated fungal infections with splenic abscess in this setting, with variable response to therapy. More recently, fluconazole has been shown to be effective in the therapy of hepatosplenic candidiasis (158, 159). Although a number of these patients have been treated with splenectomy as well as antifungal therapy and splenectomy as advised by some authors, this approach is controversial (144, 145, 150). Given the nature of the disseminated process, the role of drainage in general and splenectomy in particular should be limited.

HIV-associated syndromes

Several different organisms have now been reported to cause multiple splenic abscesses as part of a disseminated infection in patients with HIV infection, most often in those meeting the clinical definition of the acquired immunodeficiency syndrome. Among those reported most frequently are *Pneumocystis carinii*, *Mycobacterium tuberculosis*, *Mycobacterium avium-intracellulare* complex (MAC), and, very rarely, the agent of bacillary angiomatosis (160–162).

Disseminated pneumocystosis has been seen primarily in those individuals receiving aerosolized pentamidine for primary, or, more often, secondary prophylaxis of pneumocystis pneumonia. Many extrapulmonary sites of dissemination have been reported in this syndrome, including skin, eye, ear, bone marrow, lymph nodes, central nervous system, peritoneum, intestine, kidney, liver, and spleen. The CT appearance of the affected spleen usually demonstrates multiple, small, low-density lesions that are nonenhancing (162, 163) (Figure 2.4). Lesions are also frequently seen in the liver and the kidney. On ultrasound, multiple, densely echoic lesions are demonstrated (164). Although the experience is limited, when this syndrome is diagnosed premortem, it appears to respond to systemic therapy for *Pneumocystis carinii* (165, 166).

Mycobacterium tuberculosis has been reported as a cause of splenic abscess in at least 20 patients with HIV infection (167–170). In most instances, patients appear to respond to antituberculous therapy without therapeutic splenectomy. However, there is one report of a patient who appeared to require splenectomy following clinical relapse while taking appropriate antituberculous therapy (171). Although disseminated infection with MAC has been much more common than with *Mycobacterium tuberculosis* to

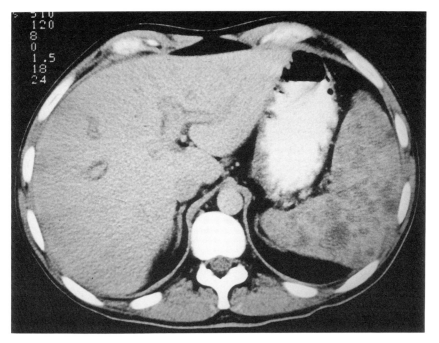

Figure 2.4 CT scan of a patient with HIV infection and disseminated *Pneumocystis carinii* infection involving the liver and spleen demonstrating mutiple small splenic abscesses. The patient had undergone splenectomy for suspicion of lymphoma to establish the diagnosis.

date, it appears to be much less likely to produce macroscopic lesions in the spleen that would appear as multiple abscesses on CT (161, 172, 173).

CONCLUSIONS

Splenic abscess remains an unusual condition, and no one center has extensive experience in the diagnosis and management of this problem. As a consequence, our understanding of this disease is based largely on retrospective analyses of a few cases at any given center and reviews of published case reports published over the last 50 to 100 years (only approximately 400 to 450 cases). Recently, our ability to diagnose and treat this disease has been radically altered with the advent of newer imaging modalities, primarily CT and ultrasound. It is clear that cases are being detected and reported at an increasing rate, in part as a result of these imaging techniques, but also as a consequence of other changes in medical care and the recognition of new diseases. Primarily these new cases represent larger numbers of severely immunosuppressed patients, either from the primary disease process, such as HIV infection, or as a consequence of therapy, such as organ transplantation and intensive chemotherapy. Percutaneous drainage will likely assume a more prominent role in the management of this condition and offers the possibility of preserving splenic function.

REFERENCES

1 **Billings AE**. Abscess of the spleen. *Ann Surg* 1928;88:416–428.

2 **Chun CH, Raff MJ, Contreras L, et al.** Splenic abscess. *Medicine* 1980;59:50–65.

3 **Lawhorne TW Jr, Zuidema GD**. Splenic abscess. *Surgery* 1976;79:686–689.

4 **Chulay JD, Lankerani MR**. Splenic abscess. Report of 10 cases and review of the literature. *Am J Med* 1976;61:513–522.

5 **Westh H, Reines E, Skibsted L**. Splenic abscesses: a review of 20 cases. *Scand J Infect Dis* 1990;22:569–573.

6 **Srp A, Bruna J**. Computed tomography of the spleen. *ACTA Universitatis Caroline Medica* 1989;35:11–30.

7 **Caslowitz PL, Labs JD, Fishman EK, Siegelman SS**. Nontraumatic focal lesions of the spleen: assessment of imaging and clinical evaluation. *Comp Med Imag Graph* 1990;14:133–141.

8 **Goerg C, Schwerk WB, Goerg K**. Splenic lesions: sonographic patterns, follow-up, differential diagnosis. *Eur J Radiol* 1991;13:59–66.

9 **Linos DA, Nagorney DM, McIlrath DC.** Splenic abscess. The importance of early diagnosis. *Mayo Clin Proc* 1983;58:261–264.

10 The lymphatic system. In: Clemente CD, ed. *Gray's Anatomy, 30th American ed*. Philadelphia: Lea & Febiger, 1985:867–932.

11 **McVay CB**. Abdominal cavity and contents. *Anson and McVay Surgical Anatomy, 6th ed*. Philadelphia: WB Saunders, 1984:585–777.

12 **Tavassoli M**. Structure and functions of the spleen. In: Williams WJ, Beutler E, Erslev AJ, Lichtman MA, eds. *Hematology, 4th ed*. New York: McGraw-Hill, 1990:54–62.

13 **Calderera E**. L'ascesso acuto della milza. *Ann Ital Clin* 1937;16:953–994.

14 **Nelken N, Ignatius J, Skinner M, Christensen N.** Changing clinical spectrum of splenic abscess. A multicenter study and review of the literature. *Am J Surg* 1987;154:27–34.

15 **Alonso-Cohen MA, Galera MJ, Ruiz M, et al.** Splenic abscess. *World J Surg* 1990;14:513–517.

16 **Cockshott WP, Weaver EJM**. Primary tropical splenic abscess: a misnomer. *Br J Surg* 1962;49:665–669.

17 Faught WE, Gilbertson JJ, Nelson EW. Splenic abscess: presentation, treatment options, and results. *Am J Surg* 1989;158:612–614.

18 Hammoudeh M, Siam AR. Salmonella peritonitis and splenic abscess in a patient with systemic lupus erythematosus (letter). *Ann Rheum Dis* 1992;51:140.

19 Nakamura T, Iwashima A, Honma T, Higuma N, Tamura K. Splenic abscess in a patient on hemodialysis (letter). *Nephron* 1992;60:255–256.

20 Fonseca V, Baillod R, Berger L, Fernando O, Moorhead J. Splenic abscess in patients on hemodialysis. *Am J Kidney Dis* 1990;15:273–275.

21 Keidl CM, Chusid MJ. Splenic abscesses in childhood. *Pediatr Infect Dis J* 1989;8:368–373.

22 Caslowitz PL, Labs JD, Fishman EK, Siegelman SS. The changing spectrum of splenic abscess. *Clin Imaging* 1989;13:201–207.

23 Kinnaird DW, Melo JC, McKeown JM. Splenic abscess due to Clostridium septicum in a patient with multiple myeloma. *South Med J* 1987;80:1318–1320.

24 Didlake RH, Miller RC. Epidermoid cyst of the spleen manifested as an abdominal abscess. *South Med J* 1986;79:635–637.

25 Jones KB, de Koos PT. Postembolization splenic abscess in a patient with pancreatitis and splenic vein thrombosis. *South Med J* 1984;77:390–393.

26 Simson JN. Solitary abscess of the spleen. *Br J Surg* 1980;67:106–110.

27 Vujic I, Lauver JW. Severe complications from partial splenic embolization in patients with liver failure. *Br J Radiol* 1981;54:492–495.

28 Dupuy D, Costello P, Lewis D, Jenkins R. Abdominal CT findings after liver transplantation in 66 patients. *AJR* 1991;156:1167–1170.

29 O'Dell KB, Gordon RS. Ruptured splenic abscess secondary to infectious mononucleosis. *Ann Emerg Med* 1992;21:1160–1162.

30 Ting W, Silverman NA, Arzouman DA, Levitsky S. Splenic septic emboli in endocarditis. *Circulation* 1990;82(suppl IV):105–109.

31 Fry DE, Richardson JD, Flint LM. Occult splenic abscess: an unrecognized complication of heroin abuse. *Surgery* 1978;84:650–654.

32 Nallathambi MN, Ivatury RR, Lankin DH, Wapnir IL, Stahl WM. Pyogenic splenic abscess in intravenous drug addiction. *Am Surg* 1987;53:342–346.

33 Robinson SL, Saxe JM, Lucas CE, Arbulu A, Ledgerwood AM, Lucas WF. Splenic abscess associated with endocarditis. *Surgery* 1992; 112:781–787.

34 de Gorgolas M, Fernandez-Giusti A, Azofra J, et al. Abscesos esplenicos: estudio clinicomicrobiologico de quince casos. *Rev Clin Esp* 1991;189:278–282.

35 Mansur AJ, Grinbert M, da Luz PL, Bellotti G. The complications of infective endocarditis: a reappraisal in the 1980's. *Arch Intern Med* 1992;152:2428–2432.

36 Komshian SV, Tablan OC, Palutke W, Reyes MP. Characteristics of left-sided endocarditis due to Pseudomonas aeruginosa in the Detroit Medical Center. *Rev Infect Dis* 1990;12: 693–702.

37 Lemley DE, Chun B, Cupps TR. Sterile splenic abscesses in systemic Weber Christian disease. Unique source of abdominal pain. *Am J Med* 1987;83:567–570.

38 Agarwala S, Bhatnagar V, Mitra DK, Gupta AK, Berry M. Primary tubercular abscess of the spleen. *J Pediatr Surg* 1992;27:1580–1581.

39 Tak PP, Visser LG, Hoogkamp-Korstanje JA, et al. Unusual manifestations of Yersinia enterocolitica infections diagnosed using novel methods. *Clin Infect Dis* 1992;15:645–649.

40 Perez-Pomata MT, Dominguez J, Horcajo P, Santidrian F, Bisquert J. Spleen abscess caused by Eikenella corrodens. *Eur J Clin Microbiol Infect Dis* 1992;11:162–163.

41 MacDonald HJ, Fong IW, Gardiner GW, Soutter DI. Splenic abscess caused by Blastomyces dermatitidis in association with peritoneal involvement: case report and review. *Clin Infect Dis* 1992;14:348–349.

42 Sastre J, Casas E, Sierra J, Puig JG, Gil A. Splenic abscess due to Fusobacterium necrophorum (letter). *Rev Infect Dis* 1991;13:1249–1250.

43 Wu CC, Chow KS, Lu TN, et al. Tuberculous splenic abscess: sonographic detection and follow-up. *J Clin Ultrasound* 1990;18:205–209.

44 Cox F, Perlman S, Sathyanarayana. Splenic abscesses in cat scratch disease: sonographic diagnosis and follow up. *J Clin Ultrasound* 1989;17:511–514.

45 Haber SW, Perlino CA. Splenic abscess from Fusobacterium nucleatum (letter). *Ann Intern Med* 1989;110:948.

46 Sherman ME, Albrecht M, DeGirolami PC, et al. An unusual case of splenic abscess and sepsis in an immunocompromised host. *Ann J Clin Pathol* 1987;88:659–662.

47 Rizkallah MF, Meyer L, Ayoub EM. Hepatic and splenic abscesses in cat scratch disease. *Pediatr Infect Dis J* 1988;7:191–195.

48 Studemeister AE, Beilke MA, Kirmani N. Splenic abscess due to *Clostridium difficile* and

Pseudomonas paucimobilis. Am J Gastroenterol 1987;82:389–390.

49 Pomerantz RA, Eckhauser FE, Thornton JW, Strodel WE, Knol JA, Zuidema GD. Covert splenic abscess: a continuing challenge. Am Surg 1986;52:386–390.

50 Teich S, Oliver GC, Canter JW. The early diagnosis of splenic abscess. Am Surg 1986; 52:303–307.

51 Walker GT, McRoyan DK, Luterman A, Dowling EA, Curreri PW. Splenic abscess caused by Blastomyces dermatitidis. South Med J 1986;79:773–776.

52 Salkin IF, Martinez JA, Kemna ME. Opportunistic infection of the spleen caused by Aureobasidium pullulans. J Clin Microbiol 1986;23:828–831.

53 Dunne WM Jr, Kurschenbaum HA, Deshur WR, et al. Propionibacterium avidum as the etiologic agent of splenic abscess. Diagn Microbiol Infect Dis 1986;5:87–92.

54 Drow DL, Mercer L, Peacock JB. Splenic abscess caused by Shigella flexneri and Bacteroides fragilis. J Clin Microbiol 1984;19:79–80.

55 Saginur R, Fogel R, Begin L, Cohen B, Mendelson J. Splenic abscess due to Clostridium difficile. J Infect Dis 1983;147:1105.

56 Dubuisson RL, Jones TB. Splenic abscess due to blastomycosis: scintigraphic, sonographic, and CT evaluation. AJR 1983;140:66–68.

57 Gangahar DM, Delany HM. Intrasplenic abscess: two case reports and review of the literature. Am Surg 1981;47:488–491.

58 Wald BR, Ortega JA, Ross L, Wald P, Laug WE, Williams KO. Candidal splenic abscesses complicating acute leukemia of childhood treated by splenectomy. Pediatrics 1981;67:296–299.

59 Squires RH, Keating JP, Rosenblum JL, Askin F, Ternberg JL. Splenic abscess and hepatic dysfunction caused by Shigella flexneri. J Pediatr 1981;98:429–430.

60 Levine S, Whelan TJ Jr. Melioidosis of the spleen. Am J Surg 1968;115:849–853.

61 Rabson AR, Koornhof HJ, Notman J, Maxwell WG. Hepatosplenic abscesses due to Yersinia enterocolitica. Br Med J 1972;4:341.

62 Rabson AR, Hallett AF, Koornhof HJ. Generalized Yersinia enterocolitica infection. J Infect Dis 1975;131:447–451.

63 Rank EL, Dias SM, Hasson J, et al. Human necrotizing splenitis caused by Borrelia burgdorferi. Am J Clin Pathol 1989;91:493–498.

64 Isaac-Renton JL, Boyko WJ, Chan R, Crichton E. Corynebacterium diphtheriae septicemia. Am J Clin Pathol 1981;75:631–634.

65 Margileth AM, Wear DJ, English CK. Systemic cat scratch disease: report of 23 patients with prolonged or recurrent severe bacterial infection. J Infect Dis 1987;155:390–402.

66 Vatcharapreechasakul T, Suputtamongkol Y, Dance DA, Chaowagul W, White NJ. Pseudomonas pseudomallei liver abscesses: a clinical, laboratory, and ultrasonographic study. Clin Infect Dis 1992;14:412–417.

67 Johnson JD, Raff MJ, Barnwell PA, Chun CH. Splenic abscess complicating infectious endocarditis. Arch Intern Med 1983;143:906–912.

68 Young SG, Davee T, Fierer J, Morey MK. Streptococcus sanguis II (viridans) prosthetic valve endocarditis with myocardial, splenic and cerebral abscesses. West J Med 1987;146:479–481.

69 Allal R, Kastler B, Gangi A, et al. Splenic abscesses in typhoid fever: US and CT studies. J Comput Assist Tomogr 1993;17:90–93.

70 Debeuckelaere S, Schoors DF, Buydens P, et al. Splenic abscess: a diagnostic challenge. Am J Gastroenterol 1991;86:1675–1678.

71 Sarr MG, Zuidema GD. Splenic abscess presentation, diagnosis, and treatment. Surgery 1982;92:480–485.

72 Cheesbrough JS, Jones EW, Finch RG. The management of splenic abscess. Q J Med 1985;57:653–657.

73 Grant CS, Al-Salem A, Khwaja MS, Sumer T, Al-Awamy B. Splenic abscess in children: aspects of management. J R Coll Surg Edinb 1987;32:342–345.

74 Rodan BA, Max RJ, Breiman RS, Rice RP. Splenic abscess due to Salmonella typhimurium bacteremia. South Med J 1981;74:382–383.

75 Fonollosa V, Bosch JA, Garcia-Bragado F, Vilardell M, Libenson C, Tornos J. Hemolytic anemia, splenic abscess, and pleural effusion caused by Salmonella typhi. J Infect Dis 1980;142:945.

76 Cohen JI, Bartlett JA, Corey GR. Extraintestinal manifestations of salmonella infections. Medicine 1987;66:349–388.

77 Sperber SJ, Schuelpner CJ. Salmonellosis during infection with human immunodeficiency virus. Rev Infect Dis 1987;9:925–934.

78 Torres JR, Rodriguez-Casas J, Balda E, Cebrian J. Multifocal Salmonella splenic abscess in an HIV infected patient. Trop Geogr Med 1992;44:66–68.

79 Drugas D, Duarte B, Robin A, Barrett J. Salmonella typhi splenic abscess in an intravenous drug abuser following splenorrhaphy: case report. J Trauma 1992;33:143–144.

80 Altemeier WA, Culbertson WR, Fullen WD, Shook CD. Intraabdominal abscesses. *Am J Surg* 1973;125:70–79.

81 Pickleman JR, Paloyan E, Block GE. The surgical significance of splenic abscess. *Surgery* 1970;68:287–293.

82 Gadacz T, Way LW, Dunphy JE. Changing clinical spectrum of splenic abscess. *Am J Surg* 1974;128:182–187.

83 Cowie MR, Hoffbrand BI, Grant DS. Lienocolonic fistula following splenic abscess. *J R Soc Med* 1992;85:636–637.

84 Neff CC. Splenobronchial fistula: interventional radiologic management. *Gastrointest Radiol* 1987;12:197–199.

85 Podgorny G. Splenic abscess causing obstruction of the large intestine: first reported case. *Am Surg* 1971;37:269–272.

86 Tikkakoski T, Siniluoto T, Paivansalo M, et al. Splenic abscess. Imaging and intervention. *Acta Radiol* 1992;33:561–565.

87 Johnson JD, Raff MJ, Drasin GF, Daffner RH. Radiology in the diagnosis of splenic abscess. *Rev Infect Dis* 1985;7:10–20.

88 Ooi LL, Nambiar R, Rauff A, Mack PO, Yap TL. Splenic abscess. *Aust N Z J Surg* 1992;62:780–784.

89 Grant E, Mertens MA, Mascatello VJ. Splenic abscess: comparison of four imaging methods. *AJR* 1979;132:465–466.

90 Miller FJ Jr, Rothermel FJ, O'Neil MJ, Shochat SJ. Clinical and roentgenographic findings in splenic abscess. *Arch Surg* 1976;111:1156–1159.

91 Hertzanu Y, Mendelsohn DB, Goudie E, Butterworth A. Splenic abscess: a review with the value of ultrasound. *Clin Radiol* 1983;34:661–667.

92 Zook EG, Bolivar JC, Epstein LI. The value of scintiscans in the diagnosis of splenic abscess. *Surg Gynecol Obstet* 1970;131:1125–1129.

93 Ammann W, Chiu BK, Wright JM. Subacute splenic abscess. Appearance on indium 111 leukocyte, gallium 67, and technetium 99m sulfur colloid imaging. *Clin Nucl Med* 1986;11:165–167.

94 O'Doherty MJ, Page C, Croft D. [111]In leukocyte imaging: intrasplenic abscesses. *Eur J Nucl Med* 1985;11:141–142.

95 Sklar DH, Marcus CS. Abscess mimicking normal spleen on In 111 WBC scan. *Clin Nucl Med* 1991;16:859.

96 Chou YH, Hsu CC, Tiu CM, Chang T. Splenic abscess: sonographic diagnosis and percutaneous drainage or aspiration. *Gastrointest Radiol* 1992;17:262–266.

97 Walia HS, Aman S, Walia HK. Rational approach to therapy in splenic abscess. *J R Coll Surg Edinb* 1990;35:154–158.

98 Ralls PW, Quinn MF, Colletti P, Lapin SA, Halls J. Sonography of pyogenic splenic abscess. *AJR* 1982;138:523–525.

99 Dubbins PA. Ultrasound in the diagnosis of splenic abscess. *Br J Radiol* 1980;53:488–489.

100 Pawar S, Kay CJ, Gonzalez R, Taylor KJ, Rosenfield AT. Sonography of splenic abscess. *AJR* 1982;138:259–262.

101 Goerg C, Schwerk WB, Goerg K. Sonography of focal lesions of the spleen. *AJR* 1991;156:949–953.

102 Knochel JQ, Koehler PR, Lee TG, Welch DM. Diagnosis of abdominal abscesses with computed tomography, ultrasound, and ^{111}In leukocyte scans. *Radiology* 1980;137:425–432.

103 Iko BO. Splenic abscess on ultrasonography. *Eur J Radiol* 1986;6:116–120.

104 Machi J, Sigel B, Beitler JC, et al. Ultrasonic examination during surgery for abdominal abscess. *World J Surg* 1983;7:409–415.

105 Brown JJ, Sumner TE, Crowe JE, Shaffner LD. Preoperative diagnosis of splenic abscess by ultrasonography and radionuclide scanning. *South Med J* 1979;72:575–580.

106 Merrick RD, Mehta JB, Cowan J, Donahue D, Young M. CT scan of the abdomen in the evaluation of splenic infarction. *J Tenn Med Assoc* 1990;83:77–78.

107 Baruch Y, Levy Y, Brook JG, Kleinhaus U, Hashmonai M. Splenic abscess diagnosed with the aid of abdominal computerized tomography: report of 2 cases. *Br J Surg* 1981;68:137–138.

108 Taylor AJ, Dodds WJ, Erickson SJ, Stewart ET. CT of acquired abnormalities of the spleen. *AJR* 1991;157:1213–1219.

109 Balthazar EJ, Hilton S, Naidich D, Megibow A, Levine R. CT of splenic and perisplenic abnormalities in septic patients. *AJR* 1985;144:53–56.

110 Moss ML, Kirschner LP, Peereboom G, Ferris RA. CT demonstration of a splenic abscess not evident at surgery. *AJR* 1980;135:159–160.

111 van der Laan RT, Verbeeten B Jr, Smits NJ, Lubbers MJ. Computed tomography in the diagnosis and treatment of solitary splenic abscesses. *J Comput Assist Tomogr* 1989;13:71–74.

112 Foster WL Jr, Heinsimer JA, Parrish DE. Left upper quadrant pain and intermittent bacteremia. *Invest Radiol* 1986;21:488–491.

113 Weingarten MJ, Fakhry J, McCarthy J, Freeman SJ, Bisker JS. Sonography after splenic embolization: the wedge-shaped acute infarct. *AJR* 1984;142:957–959.

114 Haft JI, Altieri J, Smith LG, Herskowitz M. Computed tomography of the abdomen in the diagnosis of splenic emboli. *Arch Intern Med* 1988;148:193–197.

115 Jaroch MT, Broughan TA, Hermann RE. The natural history of splenic infarction. *Surgery* 1986;100:743–750.

116 Freund R, Pichl J, Heyder N, Rodl W, Riemann JF. Splenic abscess clinical symptoms and diagnostic possibilities. *Am J Gastroenterol* 1982;77:35–38.

117 Genton A, Jacquat P. Abces spleniques: options therapeutiques. *Helv Chir Acta* 1992; 58:655–659.

118 Fernandes ET, Tavares PB, Garcette CB. Conservative management of splenic abscesses in children. *J Pediatr Surg* 1992;27: 1578–1579.

119 Jolobe OM, Melnick SC. Splenic abscess: successful non-surgical therapy. *Postgrad Med J* 1983;59:386–387.

120 Tooke MC. Medical treatment of splenic abscess. *South Med J* 1983;76:1572–1574.

121 Dylewski J, Portnoy J, Mendelson J. Antibiotic treatment of splenic abscess (letter). *Ann Intern Med* 1979;91:493–494.

122 Briggs RD, Davidson AI, Fletcher BR. Solitary abscesses of the spleen. *J R Coll Surg Edinb* 1977;22:345–347.

123 Gadacz TR. Splenic abscess. *World J Surg* 1985;9:410–415.

124 McSherry CK, Dineen P. The significance of splenic abscess. *Am J Surg* 1962;103:618–623.

125 Ellison EC, Fabri PJ. Complications of splenectomy. Etiology, prevention, and management. *Surg Clin North Am* 1983;63: 1313–1330.

126 Sekikawa T, Shatney CH. Septic sequelae after splenectomy for trauma in adults. *Am J Surg* 1983;145:667–673.

127 Green JB, Shackford SR, Sise MJ, Fridlund P. Late septic complications in adults following splenectomy for trauma: a prospective analysis in 144 patients. *J Trauma* 1986;26: 999–1004.

128 Bhattacharyya N, Ablin DS, Kosloske AM. Stapled partial splenectomy for splenic abscess in a child. *J Pediatr Surg* 1989;24:316–317.

129 Sones PJ. Percutaneous drainage of abdominal abscesses. *AJR* 1984;142:35–39.

130 Gerzof SG, Robbins AH, Johnson WC, Birkett DH, Nabseth DC. Percutaneous catheter drainage of abdominal abscesses. A five-year experience. *N Engl J Med* 1981; 305:653–657.

131 vanSonnenberg E, Ferrucci JT Jr, Mueller PR, Wittenberg J, Simeone JF. Percutaneous drainage of abscesses and fluid collections: technique, results and applications. *Radiology* 1982;142:1–10.

132 Mueller PR, vanSonnenberg E. Interventional radiology in the chest and abdomen. *N Engl J Med* 1990;322:1364–1374.

133 Levison MA. Percutaneous versus open operative drainage of intra-abdominal abscesses. *Infect Dis Clin North Am* 1992;6:525–544.

134 Haaga JR, Weistein AJ. CT-guided percutaneous drainage of abscesses. *AJR* 1980;135: 1187–1194.

135 Olak J, Christou NV, Stein LA, Casola G, Meakins JL. Operative vs. percutaneous drainage of intra-abdominal abscesses. *Arch Surgery* 1986;121:141–146.

136 Quinn SF, vanSonnenberg E, Casola G, Wittich GR, Neff CC. Interventional radiology in the spleen. *Radiology* 1986;161:289–291.

137 Haaga JR. Imaging intraabdominal abscesses and nonoperative drainage procedures. *World J Surg* 1990;14:204–209.

138 Gleich S, Wolin DA, Herbsman H. A review of percutaneous drainage in splenic abscess. *Surg Gynecol Obstet* 1988;167:211–216.

139 Gerzof SG, Johnson WC, Robbins AH, Nabseth DC. Expanded criteria for percutaneous abscess drainage. *Arch Surg* 1985; 120:227–232.

140 Hadas-Halpren I, Hiller N, Dolberg M. Percutaneous drainage of splenic abscesses: an effective and safe procedure. *Br J Radiol* 1992;65:968–970.

141 Stringel G, Anderson N, Martin D. Splenic abscess. *Can J Surg* 1985;28:269–270.

142 Franquet T, Cozcolluela R, Montes M, Sanchez J. Abscessed splenic hydatid cyst: sonographic and CT findings. *Clin Imaging* 1991;15:118–120.

143 von Eiff M, Essink M, Roos N, Hiddemann W, Buchner T, van de Loo J. Hepatosplenic candidiasis, a late manifestation of *Candida septicaemia* in neutropenic patients with haematologic malignancies. *Blut* 1990;60: 242–248.

144 Lerner PI, Weinstein L. Infective endocarditis in the antibiotic era. *N Engl J Med* 1966;274:199–206; 259–266.

145 Johnson JD, Raff MJ. Fungal splenic abscess. *Arch Intern Med* 1984;144:1987–1993.

146 Helton WS, Carrico CJ, Zaveruha PA, Schaller R. Diagnosis and treatment of splenic fungal abscesses in the immune suppressed patient. *Arch Surg* 1986;121:580–586.

147 Hatley RM, Donaldson JS, Raffensperger JG. Splenic microabscesses in the immune-compromised patient. *J Pediatr Surg* 1989; 24:697–699.

148 Haron E, Feld R, Tuffnell P, Patterson B, Hasselback R, Matlow A. Hepatic candidiasis: an increasing problem in immuno-compromised patients. *Am J Med* 1987; 83:17–26.

149 Tashjian LS, Abramson JS, Peacock JE Jr. Focal hepatic candidiasis: a distinct clinical variant of candidiasis in immunocompromised patients. *Rev Infect Dis* 1984;6:689–703.

150 Thaler M, Pastakia B, Shawker TH, O'Leary T, Pizzo PA. Hepatic candidiasis in cancer patients: the evolving picture of the syndrome. *Ann Intern Med* 1988;108:88–100.

151 Pagano L, Larocca LM, Marra R, Pizzigallo E, Leone G. A leukemic patient with hepato-splenic abscesses due to coagulase negative staphylococci (letter). *Clin Infect Dis* 1992; 14:364–365.

152 Fletcher BD, Magill HL. Wheel within a wheel patterns in hepatosplenic infections (letter). *Radiology* 1988;169:578–579.

153 Miller JH, Greenfield LD, Wald BR. Candidiasis of the liver and spleen in childhood. *Radiology* 1982;142:375–380.

154 Pastakia B, Shawker TH, Thaler M, O'Leary T, Pizzo PA. Hepatosplenic candidiasis: wheels within wheels. *Radiology* 1988;166: 417–421.

155 Shirkhoda A. CT findings in hepatosplenic and renal candidiasis. *J Comput Assist Tomogr* 1987;11:795–798.

156 Kopecky KK, Moriarty AT, Antony AC, Baker MK. Extramedullary hematopoiesis in acute lymphocytic leukemia masquerading as hepatic, renal, and splenic microabscesses. *AJR* 1986;147:846–847.

157 Bartley DL, Hughes WT, Parvey LS, Parham D. Computed tomography of hepatic and splenic fungal abscesses in leukemic children. *Pediatr Infect Dis* 1982;1:317–321.

158 Bodey AE, Kantarjian H, David C, et al. Fluconazole therapy for chronic disseminated candidiasis in patients with leukemia and prior amphotericin B therapy. *Am J Med* 1991;91:142–150.

159 Kauffman CA, Bradley SF, Ross SC, Weber DR. Hepatosplenic candidiasis: successful therapy with fluconazole. *Am J Med* 1991;91: 137–141.

160 Raviglione MC. Extrapulmonary pneumocystosis: the first 50 cases. *Rev Infect Dis* 1990;12:1127–1138.

161 Horsburgh CR Jr. *Mycobacterium avium* complex infection in the acquired immuno-deficiency syndrome. *N Engl J Med* 1991; 324:1332–1338.

162 Steeper TA, Rosenstein H, Weiser J, Inampudi S, Snover DC. Bacillary epithelioid angiomatosis involving the liver, spleen and skin in an AIDS patient with concurrent Kaposi's sarcoma. *Am J Clin Pathol* 1992; 97:713–718.

163 Lubat E, Megibow AJ, Balthazar EJ, Goldenberg AS, Birnbaum BA, Bsoniak MA. Extrapulmonary *Pneumocystis carinii* infection in AIDS: CT findings. *Radiology* 1990;174: 157–160.

164 Jeffrey RB Jr. Abdominal imaging in the immunocompromised patient. *Radiol Clin North Am* 1992;30:579–596.

165 Spouge AR, Wilson SR, Gopinath N, Sherman M, Biendis LM. Extrapulmonary *Pneumocystis carinii* in a patient with AIDS: sonographic findings. *AJR* 1990;155:76–78.

166 Northfelt DW, Clement MJ, Safrin S. Extrapulmonary pneumocystosis: clinical features in human immunodeficiency virus infection. *Medicine* 1990;69:392–398.

167 Pedro-Botet J, Maristany MT, Miralles R, Lopes-Colomes JL, Rubies-Prat J. Splenic tuberculosis in patients with AIDS. *Rev Infect Dis* 1991;13:1069–1071.

168 Khalil T, Uzoaru I, Nadimpalli V, Wurtz R. Splenic tuberculous abscess in patients positive for human immunodeficiency virus: report of two cases and review (letter). *Clin Infect Dis* 1992;14:1265–1266.

169 Wolff MJ, Bitran J, Northland RG, Levy IL. Splenic abscesses due to *Mycobacterium tuberculosis* in patients with AIDS. *Rev Infect Dis* 1991;13:373–375.

170 Soriano V, Tor J, Gabarre E, Gros T, Muga R. Multifocal splenic abscesses caused by Mycobacterium tuberculosis in HIV infected drug users (letter). *AIDS* 1991;5:901–902.

171 Giladi M, Ransohoff KN, Lovett MA. Splenic abscesses due to Mycobacterium tuberculosis in patients with AIDS: is splenectomy necessary? *Rev Infect Dis* 1991;13:1030–1301.

172 Nyberg DA, Federle MP, Jeffrey RB, Bottles K, Wofsy CB. Abdominal CT findings of

disseminated *Mycobacterium-avium intracellulare* in AIDS. *AJR* 1985;145:297–299.

173 Radin DR. Intra-abdominal *Mycobacterium tuberculosis* vs. *Mycobacterium avium-intracellulare* infections in patients with AIDS: distinction based on CT findings. *AJR* 1991;156:487–491.

174 Reese JH, Anderson RU, Friedland G. Splenic abscess arising by direct extension from a perinephric abscess. *Urol Radiol* 1990;12:91–93.

175 Reinberg Y, Moore LS, Lange PH. Splenic abscess as a complication of percutaneous nephrostomy. *Urology* 1989;34:274–276.

176 Reiber K, Leventhal I. Splenic abscess as complication of perinephric abscess. *Urology* 1987;30:269–271.

177 Abu-Dallo KI, Manny Y, Penchas S, Eyal Z. Clinical manifestations of splenic abscess. *Arch Surg* 1975;110:281–283.

178 Handrick W, Brettschneider D, Hormann D, Scholbach T. Ultraschallgezielte perkutane Punktion und Drainage eines Milzabszesses durch Salmonella heidelberg bei einem Kind. *Klin Padiatr* 1992;204:56–60.

179 Ramakrishnan MR, Sarathy TK, Balu M. Percutaneous drainage of splenic abscess: case report and review of literature. *Pediatrics* 1987;79:1029–1031.

180 Dwyer DE, Packham DR, Sorrell T. Aspiration drainage of splenic abscesses. *Aust N Z J Surg* 1986;56:689–692.

181 Kreel L. Splenic abscess. *Postgrad Med J* 1985;61:807–809.

182 Wernecke K, Heckemann R. Treatment of pyogenic splenic abscess by ultrasonically guided fine needle puncture. *Eur J Radiol* 1985;5:216–217.

183 Lerner RM, Spataro RF. Splenic abscess: percutaneous drainage. *Radiology* 1984;153:643–645.

184 Berkman WA, Harris SA Jr, Bernardino ME. Nonsurgical drainage of splenic abscess. *AJR* 1983;141:395–396.

185 Sclafani SJA, Goldstein AJ, Shaftan GW. Interventional radiology. *J Trauma* 1984;24:299–306.

186 Lambiase RE, Deyoe L, Cronan JJ, Dorfman GS. Percutaneous drainage of 335 consecutive abscesses: results of primary drainage with 1-year follow-up. *Radiology* 1992;184:167–179.

187 Bozkurt T, Butsch B, Langer M, Lux G. Perkutane, sonographisch gesteuerte Feinnadelpunktion und Drainage pyogener Abszesse. *Dtsch Med Wochenschr* 1991;116:1943–1947.

188 Herman P, de Oliveira e Silva A, Chaib E, et al. Abscesso esplenico: relato de oito casos e revisao da literatura. *Rev Hosp Clin Fac Med Sao Paulo* 1990;45:268–271.

Azithromycin and clarithromycin

ELLEN EISENBERG
MICHAEL BARZA

INTRODUCTION

Erythromycin has been widely used in pediatric and adult medical practice for many years. Its activity against gram-positive cocci and the agents of "atypical" pneumonia have made it a common choice for the treatment of infections of the upper and lower respiratory tract and for the treatment of soft-tissue infections in penicillin-allergic patients. It has also been found useful for *Campylobacter* diarrhea. Because erythromycin, especially given orally, frequently causes gastrointestinal upset, enteric-coated preparations have been developed. Problems have arisen with the bioavailability of some of these preparations.

Recently, 2 new macrolides were introduced to the market: clarithromycin (Biaxin) and azithromycin (Zithromax). Each is available only in an oral formulation. We compare the properties of the 2 new macrolides with those of erythromycin and suggest in what areas the new drugs may have particular clinical utility.

CHEMISTRY

Erythromycin is a 14-membered macrolide antibiotic. It has 2 side chains, the neutral cladinose and the amino-sugar desoamine. Slight structural differences between erythromycin and the 2 new agents result in important alterations of antimicrobial activity and, especially, pharmacologic behavior.

Clarithromycin differs from erythromycin in the methylation of the hydroxyl group at position 6. This alteration improves the antimicrobial activity of the drug and reduces the tendency of the macrolide ring to form inactive metabolites, including anhydroerythromycin, under acidic conditions. Formation of these metabolites contributes to erratic bioavailability and possibly to the gastrointestinal side effects that occur following oral administration of erythromycin (1). Clarithromycin is stable in an acidic environment and has better bioavailability than erythromycin (2,3).

Azithromycin differs from erythromycin in that it has a nitrogen molecule added to the 14-membered ring. The resulting 15-membered ring can be classified as an "azalide," but because of the close similarity of azithromycin to macrolides, we refer to it as a macrolide herein. The structural modification of azithromycin confers stability under acidic conditions, markedly enhances tissue penetration, and prolongs the half-life of the drug in the body. The change also increases the activity of the drug against gram-negative organisms but decreases activity against some gram-positive species (3).

IN VITRO ACTIVITY

Erythromycin, clarithromycin, and azithromycin are similar in their spectrum of activity, but differ in the extent of activity. In general, clarithromycin and erythromycin are more active than azithromycin against gram-positive cocci, whereas the reverse is true against gram-negative bacilli. Because of the unusual property of being accumulated in high concentration in phagocytic and other host cells, the activity of the macrolides in vivo may be markedly greater than would be expected from the activity in vivo. This issue will be discussed later. The data for in vitro susceptibility must be interpreted in light of the fact that the results with macrolides are highly dependent on the medium and the method used (4). Therefore, we have used data from studies in which at least 2 of the agents were included; in most instances, all 3 agents were examined.

Activity against bacterial pathogens, chlamydiae, and mycoplasma

Table 3.1 summarizes the activity of the 3 agents against common bacterial pathogens (2,5–9). Data also are shown for the 14-hydroxy metabolite of clarithromycin, which reaches appreciable concentrations in serum. Each value in Table 3.1 is based on studies of more than 10 strains except where indicated.

Approximately 80% of strains of *Staphylococcus aureus* are susceptible to the macrolides (7). Erythromycin and clarithromycin are approximately 4- to 8-fold more active than azithromycin against susceptible isolates, but strains resistant to erythromycin are resistant to the 2 newer drugs. Isolates of *S. aureus* resistant to methicillin are uniformly resistant to the macrolides (4). Coagulase-negative staphylococci are, like *S. aureus*, more susceptible to erythromycin and clarithromycin than to azithromycin, but are commonly resistant to all of the macrolides (4). All 3 drugs are highly active against streptococci, including *S. pneumoniae*, *S. pyogenes*, and *S. agalactiae*, but erythromycin and clarithromycin are several-fold more active than azithromycin against these species. Enterococci are generally resistant to all 3 drugs. The 14-hydroxy metabolite of clarithromycin has activity similar to that of the parent drug against gram-positive cocci.

Erythromycin, clarithromycin, and its metabolite have poor activity against *Haemophilus influenzae*; MIC_{90} (minimum inhibitory concentration for 90% of strains) values are in the range of 4 to 8 µg/mL (see Table 3.1). In contrast, the activity of azithromycin is several-fold greater than that of the other drugs. The combination of

Table 3.1   Macrolide activity against common bacterial pathogens*

Organism	Azithromycin	Erythromycin	Clarithromycin	14-OH Clarithromycin
S. aureus (methicillin-susceptible)	0.8–2.0	0.25	0.12	0.25
Coag-negative staphylococcus (methicillin-susceptible)	0.5–0.8	0.25		
S. pneumoniae	0.12	0.02–0.06	0.02	0.02
S. pyogenes	0.05–0.12	0.03	0.01–0.06	0.03
S. agalactiae	0.06–0.1	0.03–0.06	0.06	0.06
E. faecalis	>64	>64	>64[†]	
E. faecium	>64	>64		
L. monocytogenes	2	0.5	0.25	
H. influenzae	0.5–2.0	4.0–8.0	8	4
M. catarrhalis	0.06	0.25	0.25	
P. aeruginosa	>64[†]	>64[†]		
Anaerobic streptococci	2	4	4.0–8.0	
B. fragilis	2.0–6.25	1.56–8.0	2.0–4.0	
C. perfringens	0.25	1	0.5	

*Minimum inhibitory concentration for 90% of strains.
[†]<10 strains.
SOURCE: From References 2, 5–9, with permission.

clarithromycin and its metabolite have an additive effect against *H. influenzae* in vitro, with a 2- to 4-fold reduction in MIC and minimal bacteriocidal concentration (MBC) (2,5). The issue of activity of bactericidal against *H. influenzae* is of relevance in evaluating the utility of the drugs for certain respiratory infections. *Moraxella catarrhalis* is highly susceptible to all 3 drugs but especially azithromycin. Activity against *Pseudomonas aeruginosa* is negligible. Nevertheless, erythromycin has some activity against *P. aeruginosa* infections in vivo through mechanisms that are not clearly understood (10). Erythromycin and clarithromycin are more potent than azithromycin against *Listeria monocytogenes*.

All 3 macrolides have modest and roughly similar activity against anaerobic streptococci, *Bacteroides fragilis*, and *Clostridium perfringens*, with MIC_{90} values ranging from 0.25 to 8 μg/mL.

The activity of the macrolides against respiratory pathogens (2,4,9,11–16) is summarized in Table 3.2. The studies of *Legionella pneumophila* and *Chlamydia pneumoniae* were done in cell cultures. All 3 agents are exquisitely active against *Mycoplasma pneumoniae*. They are moderately active against *Legionella pneumophila*; clarithromycin is slightly more potent than the others. Clarithromycin is far more active than erythromycin or azithromycin against *C. pneumoniae* (15,16). All 3 drugs are highly potent against *Bordetella pertussis*.

Table 3.2   Macrolide activity against respiratory pathogens*

Organism	Azithromycin	Erythromycin	Clarithromycin	14-OH Clarithromycin
M. pneumoniae[†]	<0.01	0.004–0.01	0.03–0.5	
L. pneumophila	0.50–2.0	0.25–2.0	0.25	0.50
C. pneumoniae[†]	0.1–0.5	0.06–0.12	0.01–0.03	
B. pertussis	0.06	0.03	0.03	

*Minimum inhibitory concentration for 90% of strains.
[†]<10 strains.
Source: From References 2,4,9,11–16, with permission.

The macrolides are active against many enteric pathogens (Table 3.3) (4,9,17–19). All 3 agents are moderately active against *Campylobacter jejuni*; azithromycin is the most potent. They are highly active against *Helicobacter pylori*; clarithromycin is the most potent, with activity similar to that of ampicillin (19). Against salmonellae, shigellae, and *Escherichia coli*, only azithromycin generally has appreciable activity.

The activity of the drugs against selected sexually transmitted pathogens (2,4,13,14, 16,20,21) is summarized in Table 3.4. All 3 agents are moderately to highly active against the pathogens shown. Clarithromycin is the most active against *Chlamydia trachomatis* and *Ureaplasma urealyticum*, whereas azithromycin is the most active against *Neisseria gonorrheae*. There is little correlation between beta-lactamase production and the susceptibility of *N. gonorrheae* to macrolides. All 3 drugs are exquisitely active against *Haemophilus ducreyi*.

Activity against spirochetes, mycobacteria, and toxoplasma

The activity of the macrolides against *Borrelia burgdorferi*, *Treponema pallidum*, mycobacteria, and *Toxoplasma gondii* has been studied in vitro and in animal models.

In broth dilution tests in vitro, azithromycin (MBC, 0.04 µg/mL) was more active than erythromycin (MBC, 0.16 µg/mL) or tetracycline (MBC, 1.6 µg/mL) against *B. burgdorferi*. In the same study, the activity of the drugs in infected hamsters correlated with their activity in vitro except that erythromycin was less potent than expected (22). In another study, azithromycin and clarithromycin were slightly more potent (MIC$_{90}$, 0.015 µg/mL) than erythromycin (MIC$_{90}$, 0.06 µg/mL) in vitro, and azithromycin was more potent than clarithromycin in infected gerbils (23). These data suggest that azithromycin may be more potent than the other 2 macrolides against *B. burgdorferi* in vivo.

The susceptibility of 2 strains of *Treponema pallidum* to azithromycin was studied ex vivo. Protein synthesis was inhibited at the lowest concentration of azithromycin tested (2 µg/mL) (24). Erythromycin was of similar potency in this system. In rabbits infected intradermally with *T. pallidum*, the activity of azithromycin was similar to that of erythromycin and benzathine penicillin G, as determined by darkfield examination of aspirates from the chancres (25).

An in vitro study showed *Mycobacterium tuberculosis* to be more highly susceptible to the fluoroquinolones (MIC$_{90}$ range, 2.3–8.3 µg/mL) than to clarithromycin (MIC$_{90}$

Table 3.3   Macrolide activity against enteric pathogens*

Organism	Azithromycin	Erythromycin	Clarithromycin
C. jejuni	0.12–0.5	1.0–2.0	1.0–2.0
H. pylori	0.25	0.25	0.03
E. coli	4	64	
S. enteritidis	4	128	
S. typhi	8	>128	>128
S. sonnei	2	128	>128
S. flexneri[†]	1	16	>128

*Minimum inhibitory concentration from 90% of strains.
[†] < 10 strains.
SOURCE: From References 4,9,17–19, with permission.

Table 3.4   Macrolide activity against pathogens of sexually transmitted diseases

Organism	Azithromycin	Erythromycin	Clarithromycin
C. trachomatis[†]	0.25	0.06–0.128	0.016
N. gonorrheae	0.05–0.25	0.25–2.0	0.25–0.5
U. urealyticum	0.5–2.0	1.0–2.0	0.1–0.2
H. ducreyi	0.003	0.03–0.06	0.015

*Minimum inhibitory concentration for 90% of strains.
[†] < 10 strains.
SOURCE: From References 2,4,13,14,16,20,21, with permission.

> 10 µg/mL) (26). Another study of 10 strains of M. *tuberculosis* showed an MIC_{90} for clarithromycin of more than 32 µg/mL (data on file, Abbott Laboratories). Azithromycin also appears to have little activity against M. *tuberculosis*.

The activity of the macrolides against *Mycobacterium avium* complex (MAC) is better than against M. *tuberculosis*. Clarithromycin appears to be particularly potent in this regard. In a study of the activity of 12 macrolides and 28 strains of MAC from patients with the acquired immunodeficiency syndrome, the MIC_{90} of clarithromycin was 4 µg/mL, that of azithromycin was 32 µg/mL, and that of erythromycin was more than 64 µg/mL (27). In vivo, clarithromycin showed good activity in reducing the counts of bacteria in the spleen and liver in beige mice infected with MAC. Its activity was potentiated by the addition of clofazamine or rifabutin (28). In cultured macrophages infected by MAC, clarithromycin was more potent than erythromycin in eradicating the organisms (29). Despite its lesser activity in vitro, azithromycin has also been shown to reduce the counts of MAC in beige mice (30).

Clarithromycin has been found to be 10 to 50 times more active than erythromycin and 4 to 8 times more potent than azithromycin against M. *chelonae*, with an MIC_{90} of 0.25 to 0.5 µg/mL. Clarithromycin and azithromycin (MIC_{90} 0.5–2.0 µg/mL) are both more potent than erythromycin (MIC_{90} > 8.0 µg/mL) against M. *fortuitum* (31).

The new macrolides have some activity against *Toxoplasma gondii*, but there is evidence that they do not eradicate the infection. In cultures of infected macrophages, azithromycin and clarithromycin inhibited intracellular organisms, but doses adequate to inhibit the multiplication of organisms by 90% were toxic to macrophages (32). Furthermore, tachyzoites were still visible in monolayers even after exposure to concentrations 4-fold higher than the MIC_{90}. In mice infected by intraperitoneal inoculation of *T. gondii*, clarithromycin treatment was effective in preventing death, but organisms were visible in the brain of about approximately half the survivors (33). In another study, clarithromycin significantly reduced the parasitic burden in mice infected with *T. gondii* (34). In combination with minocycline, pyrimethamine, or sulfadiazine, clarithromycin prolonged the survival of infected mice, and the number of parasites was decreased (34,35). Azithromycin given to mice after intraperitoneal infection with *T. gondii* protected against death and appeared to eradicate organisms from the brain (36). Azithromycin protected against intraperitoneal and intracerebral toxoplasma infection in mice (34). These data suggest that the 2 new macrolides may have a role in the treatment of toxoplasma infections, possibly in combination with other agents.

Mechanisms of action and resistance to macrolides

The macrolides bind to the 50S component of the 70S ribosomal subunit and inhibit protein synthesis. Resistance to the macrolides is linked to resistance to lincosamides and streptogramin B and is therefore called "MLS resistance." At least 2 mechanisms of erythromycin resistance are found in staphylococci (37). One mechanism is by methylation of the ribosome, which impedes binding of the drug. This mechanism causes resistance to all macrolides, lincosamides, and type B streptogramins, and may be inducible or constitutive. The second mechanism occurs by an adenosine triphosphate–dependent efflux pump. This mechanism is inducible and extends only to 14- and 15-membered macrolides and type B streptogramins. The resistance genes are generally found on plasmids in staphylococci, streptococci, enterococci, and *Bacteroides* species but may be chromosomal in *S. pneumoniae* (2). The resistance can be inducible or constitutive in staphylococci but is usually constitutive in enterococci and streptococci. Strains resistant to erythromycin are generally resistant to the 2 newer macrolides although the MIC values may differ somewhat among the drugs.

The effect of serum, pH, and inoculum size

Studies of the effect of serum on the in vitro activity of the macrolides have yielded conflicting results. Whereas some studies have shown no effect of serum, others have shown that the presence of human serum *decreased* the MIC by up to 4-fold for clarithromycin and erythromycin and up to 64-fold for azithromycin (4). The mechanisms of the effect are not clear but could include buffering against decreases in the pH of the medium during incubation. Whether these changes have any significance for the in vivo activity of the macrolides is unclear. For most other antibiotics, if there is an effect of serum, it is to increase the MIC by binding the drug.

The activity of the macrolides is diminished in an acidic environment, possibly due to the fact that the macrolides, which are weak bases, are more highly ionized in an acidic milieu, and that the ionized form, being less lipid-soluble, is less able to penetrate the bacterial cell membrane than the nonionized molecule. The MIC values of erythromycin, clarithromycin, and azithromycin against a variety of species increased by approximately 5- to 10-fold, 5-fold, and 10- to 100-fold, respectively, as the pH decreased from 7.2 to 6 (38).

A moderate "inoculum effect" is observed for the macrolides. The MICs of clarithromycin for staphylococci and enterococci are unchanged as the inoculum is increased from 10^3 to 10^5 CFU/mL. With an increase to 10^7 CFU/mL, MICs increase 2- to 8-fold for staphylococci but are unchanged for enterococci (39).

Bactericidal and postantibiotic effects

Erythromycin is bacteriostatic for S. aureus but is bactericidal for species such as S. pyogenes and S. pneumoniae (2). Clarithromycin has bactericidal activity against S. pyogenes, S. pneumoniae, and M. catarrhalis (39). Azithromycin appears to have bactericidal activity against S. pyogenes and H. influenzae at concentrations equal to the MIC (40).

Both clarithromycin and azithromycin have an appreciable postantibiotic effect (i.e., they cause persistent suppression of bacterial growth after drug has disappeared from the medium). Applied at 4 times the MIC for S. aureus and S. pyogenes, clarithromycin had a postantibiotic effect that lasted for 6.25 and 3.5 hours, respectively, and was 3 times longer than the effect for erythromycin for both species (39). Azithromycin, applied at 4 to 8 times the MIC, produced a postantibiotic effect lasting for approximately 3 hours for S. pyogenes, S. pneumoniae, H. influenzae, and M. catarrhalis (40).

PHARMACOKINETIC PROPERTIES

The major difference between the newer macrolides and erythromycin is the pharmacokinetic profile. Table 3.5 provides data for the pharmacokinetic properties of the drugs (1,3,18,41–45). The data are in relation to a single oral dose of 500 mg, except where otherwise indicated.

Oral bioavailability

The oral bioavailability of erythromycin varies considerably with the preparation. The enteric-coated base and the estolate esters are better absorbed than the ethylsuccinate formulation. In general, the bioavailability of clarithromycin is more than twice that of erythromycin, and the bioavailability of azithromycin is 1.5 times that of erythromycin. Food somewhat enhances the rate and the extent of absorption of clarithromycin (41). In contrast, food decreases the rate and extent of absorption of azithromycin

Table 3.5   Pharmacokinetics after a single 500-mg dose given orally

	Azithromycin	Clarithromycin	14-hydroxy-clarithromycin	Erythromycin
Bioavailability %	37	55*	35	25
C_{max} (μg/mL)	0.4[†]	2.0–3.0[‡]	0.9	2.0–4.0
T_{max} (hr)	2.3	2.8	3.0	1.0–5.0
$T_{1/2}$ (hr)	11.0–14.0	4.0–7.0[‡]	7.2[‡]	1.5–3.0
Renal excretion (% of dose absorbed)	10	65[‡]	30	10
Biliary excretion (% of dose absorbed)	90			High
AUC ($\frac{μg}{mL} \cdot$ hr)	2.4–2.6	12.6	9.6	14.2
Protein binding (%)	12–50	65–75		70

*250 mg single-dose regimen.
[†]500 mg loading dose (day 1); then 250 mg daily.
[‡]Multiple 500 mg dose regimens.
Source: From References 1,3,18,41–45, with permission.

by approximately half (40). Peak serum concentrations (C_{max}) of all 3 drugs are attained 2 to 3 hours after an oral dose. The improved absorption of the new macrolides is related, at least in part, to increased acid stability. The serum concentrations of azithromycin are lower than those of the other 2 agents, a phenomenon related to the unusual distribution of azithromycin, which is heavily accumulated in various host cells (see Distribution section). Thus, the apparent volume of distribution (AVD) of erythromycin is 14.2 L/kg; it is 23 to 31 L/kg for azithromycin (3,45).

Metabolism and elimination

The macrolide antibiotics are metabolized (demethylated) by the cytochrome P450 microsomal enzyme system. Elimination of clarithromycin occurs mainly by the combination of hepatic metabolism (78%) and renal excretion. Only one of the metabolites, the 14-hydroxy moiety, has antibacterial activity. The half-life of clarithromycin after multiple doses, approximately 4 to 7 hours, is similar to that after a single dose (18). The result of the lower peak serum concentrations but the longer serum half-life of clarithromycin than of erythromycin results in a calculated "area under the curve" (AUC) that which is similar for the 2 drugs.

In the case of azithromycin, most of the dose absorbed is excreted either as the parent substance or as metabolites in the bile; the metabolites, which number as many as 10, are antibacterially inactive (40,42). The remainder is excreted mainly as the parent substance unchanged in the urine (40). The apparent serum half-life of azithromycin after a single dose is 11 to 14 hours, but after multiple doses it is approximately 48 to 72 hours (3,43). Azithromycin has a much longer half-life than clarithromycin, probably because clarithromycin undergoes more extensive hepatic metabolism (a rapid process) than azithromycin, and because azithromycin, especially after multiple doses, is accumulated in tissues from which it is slowly released. Despite its much longer serum half-life but because of its lower serum concentrations, the AUC of azithromycin is approximately one fifth to one sixth as great as that of clarithromycin and erythromycin. It must be emphasized that the AUC values apply to the serum: the situation will be quite different in the "periphery" (cells and tissues), in which the AUC might be greater for azithromycin than for the other drugs. Serum protein binding is of mild to moderate degree for all 3 macrolides; it is lowest for azithromycin (see Table 3.5). Unlike other antibiotics, which are bound almost exclusively to albumin, the macrolides are bound to alpha-1-glycoproteins.

The 14-hydroxy metabolite of clarithromycin reaches peak serum concentrations, which are approximately one quarter to one half as great as those of the parent drug and is eliminated more slowly than the parent drug (see Table 3.5). Approximately 30 percent of the metabolite is excreted unchanged in the urine.

The effect of renal impairment on elimination has been studied for clarithromycin (2,46). As the creatinine clearance decreases from normal to 30 to 80 mL/min and to less than 30 mL/min, the half-life of clarithromycin increases from 4 to 7 hours to 12 hours and to 32 hours, respectively (2). The half-life of the 14-hydroxy metabolite also increases correspondingly (46). Thus, the dosing interval must be extended by several-fold in patients with renal impairment. No data are available for the effects of renal impairment on the pharmacokinetics of azithromycin. Overall, hepatic failure has little effect on the half-life of clarithromycin (44); no data are available in this regard for azithromycin (45).

Distribution in tissues and extravascular fluids

The macrolides have the unusual property of being highly concentrated in host cells and tissues (Table 3.6) (47). This attribute probably results from the fact that these basic molecules are concentrated in lysosomes. The drugs are accumulated not only in phagocytic cells (48,49), but also in fibroblasts, liver, and other cells (50). After accumulation, azithromycin is slowly released into extracellular fluid (48,49). Thus, host cells can serve as a reservoir for slow release of the drug after serum concentrations have

Table 3.6   Peak macrolide concentrations in body tissues of healthy adults

Tissue (mg/kg)	Azithromycin (500 mg p.o.)	Clarithromycin (250 mg p.o.)	Erythromycin (1,000 mg p.o. b.i.d.)
Lung	1–9	17.4*	4.2
Tonsil	1–9	6.7	1.4
Nasal mucosa		8.3	1.8
Prostate	1–9		
Macrophages	23		

*500 mg p.o.
SOURCE: From References 3,43,47, with permission.

declined. Moreover, loaded phagocytic cells may carry drug to sites of infection (48). These phenomena seem to be most prominent and have been most extensively studied with azithromycin. However, the clinical significance of these processes is not clear, as will be discussed.

Concentrations of azithromycin in prostate, tonsil, lung (see Table 3.6), kidney, and gastric mucosa reach 10 to 100 times the serum concentration (43). The peak concentrations of azithromycin in alveolar macrophages and bronchial mucosa were reported as 23 and 3.9 µg/gm, respectively; these concentrations were at least 30 times as great as the 12-hour serum concentration (3). Drug concentrations in endothelial lining fluid and sputum were also in excess of the serum concentration (3). The half-life of azithromycin in prostatic, tonsillar, and lung tissues is 2 to 4 days (3,42).

Clarithromycin, like azithromycin, is accumulated in various tissues including lung, tonsil, and nasal mucosa, although the ratio of tissue:serum concentrations is not as great as for azithromycin (see Table 3.6). Clarithromycin is also accumulated in neutrophils and macrophages (2,3). The accumulation of clarithromycin is much greater than of erythromycin in relation to serum concentrations. Studies in animals show accumulation of clarithromycin in gastrointestinal tract, liver, spleen, lung, and kidney (3).

Although it would seem an attractive hypothesis that the high and persisting tissue concentrations of the macrolides, especially azithromycin, should produce an enhanced effect against microbes in tissues, this effect has not been proved, especially with regard to intracellular pathogens (51,52). For example, the drug could be sequestered in an intracellular compartment separate from that of the microbe (53), or the pH of the intracellular milieu might be unfavorable to the action of the drug. In contrast, it seems likely that the "reservoir" effect, with slow release of drug into extracellular fluids, should confer a benefit on the highly accumulated drugs for activity against extracellular pathogens.

In animals, the concentrations of azithromycin in brain tissue are much higher than in the cerebrospinal fluid (40). Concentrations in the cerebrospinal fluid of humans without meningeal irritation are less than 0.01 µg/mL (45). The activity of azithromycin in mice with cerebral toxoplasmosis support the evidence that appreciable concentrations are reached in brain tissue. The peak concentrations of clarithromycin in the cerebrospinal fluid of dogs were less than 1% of the peak serum concentrations (data on file; Abbott Laboratories). No data are available on the penetration of clarithromycin into the cerebrospinal fluid of humans.

Transfer of macrolides to fetus and into milk

We found no data for the excretion of clarithromycin or azithromycin into human breast milk. However, it should be presumed that the drugs are present in the milk of humans because they are present in the milk of lactating animals and because other macrolide antibiotics are excreted into human milk. We found no data for the transport of clarithromycin or azithromycin across the placenta, but some degree of transport is certain to occur.

Pharmacokinetics in pediatric patients

The pharmacokinetic properties of azithromycin in pediatric populations appear to be similar to those in adults (54). We found no data for the pharmacokinetics of clarithromycin in pediatric patients.

ADVERSE REACTIONS, DRUG INTERACTIONS, AND USE IN PREGNANCY

Adverse reactions

Both clarithromycin and azithromycin are well tolerated. The most prominent side effect of the macrolides—gastrointestinal upset—is less frequent with the new drugs than with erythromycin. Interestingly, laboratory studies have shown that the binding of clarithromycin to the putative motilin receptor of animals is less than that of other macrolides (55), but the clinical significance of this finding is uncertain.

Adverse effects related to clarithromycin have been studied in 3,768 patients in comparative Phase II and Phase III trials. Adverse effects were reported in 19.7% of patients given clarithromycin as opposed to 32.5% of those given erythromycin; 26.7% of those given ampicillin; and 25.2% of those given cefadroxil (18). In individual studies, the incidence of gastrointestinal side effects has been higher with clarithromycin than with pencillin V (56,57) or ampicillin (58). The most frequent side effects with clarithromycin have been nausea, dyspepsia, diarrhea, abdominal pain, and headache. Fewer than 3% of the 3,768 patients given clarithromycin withdrew from studies because of adverse effects (usually gastrointestinal intolerance), and fewer than 1% had severe adverse effects. Abnormalities of laboratory tests possibly related to clarithromycin are rare and include decreased white blood cell counts in fewer than 1% of adult patients and elevated liver function test results; these abnormalities disappeared after cessation of the drug. We are aware of no data regarding the incidence of adverse effects in pediatric patients.

Adverse reactions to azithromycin have been studied in 3,995 patients. Overall, side effects were recorded in 12%, resulting in discontinuation of the drug in 0.7%. There were 13 deaths, none of them attributable to the drug. The incidence of side effects with azithromycin was less than that with erythromycin (20.4%) and cefaclor (16.7%), but higher than that with ampicillin (4.7%) (59). The most common side effects of azithromycin, occurring in 9.6% of recipients, were gastrointestinal, including nausea, diarrhea, and abdominal pain. Headache and dizziness occurred in 1.3%, and rash occurred in 0.6% of azithromycin-treated patients. The only abnormalities in laboratory tests occurring in more than 1% of recipients were an increase (less than 2-fold) in alanine aminotransferase or aspartate aminotransferase levels and mild increases or decreases in leukocyte counts. These effects were all transient. Limited data in children suggest that azithromycin is also well tolerated in this age group (59).

Pseudomembranous colitis has not been reported with azithromycin. One case has been attributed to treatment with clarithromycin.

Drug interactions

Clarithromycin, like erythromycin, undergoes extensive oxidation by the cytochrome P450 system in the liver. Accordingly, clarithromycin increases the serum concentrations and AUC of drugs metabolized by this system. For example, given with a sustained-release theophylline preparation, clarithromycin increases the AUC of theophylline by 20% (44). Clarithromycin also causes an increase in the serum concentrations of carbamazepine (44). Because erythromycin can increase the effects of any drug metabolized by the cytochrome P450 system, including digoxin, oral anticoagulants, ergotamine, triazolam, cyclosporine, hexobarbital, and phenytoin, there should be concern that the same kind of interaction could occur with clarithromycin. In contrast, azithromycin does not appear to form complexes with the cytochrome P450 system and has not been shown to interfere with the pharmacologic behavior of drugs metabolized by this system.

Use in pregnancy

Preclinical studies of the effects of the macrolides in pregnancy have been conducted. Administration of clarithromycin to pregnant animals produced fetal growth retardation in monkeys, cleft palate in mice, and cardiovascular abnormalities in rats. The dosage given to mice in those studies was extremely high. Because of these findings, clarithromycin is listed in pregnancy category C (i.e., it should be used only if there is no alternative). Azithromycin did not produce abnormalities in pregnant animals and has been placed in pregnancy category B (i.e., it should be used only if clearly needed).

CLINICAL USES

The various clinical uses for which clarithromycin and azithromycin have been studied are summarized. We have tried to focus on comparative trials but have included a few informative but noncomparative studies. In only a few instances was erythromycin included in the comparison. In the trials of azithromycin, the course of treatment was generally shorter than with comparative agents, reflecting the unusual pharmacokinetic properties of azithromycin.

Upper respiratory tract infections

Several randomized studies have been done comparing the new macrolides with penicillin V for streptococcal pharyngitis in adults (Table 3.7) (56,60,61). The incidence of clinical and microbiologic cure for both the macrolide and penicillin V were high in all the studies, and differences between the 2 agents were not statistically significant. In the trial involving azithromycin, the drug was given for only 5 days, whereas penicillin V was given for a standard 10-day course. In that trial, 2.2% of isolates of *Streptococcus pyogenes* were resistant to azithromycin (61), suggesting that attention should be paid to the possibility that macrolide-resistant strains may be increasing in prevalence. In the

Table 3.7 Treatment of streptococcal pharyngitis

Regimens compared	No. assessable patients	Clinical cure (%)	Bacteriological cure (%)* (recurrence)[†]	Adverse effects (%)	Reference
Clarithromycin (250 mg b.i.d., 8–10 days)	67	96	100 (2)	6	Levenstein (56)
Penicillin VK (250 mg q.i.d., 10–14 days)	58	98	97 (2)	9	
Clarithromycin (250 mg b.i.d., 7–11 days)	43	86	88 (6)	43	Bachand (60)
Penicillin VK (250 mg q.i.d., 7–11 days)	47	77	91 (8)	27	
Azithromycin (500 mg day 1; 250 mg q.d. 2–5)	152	87	91 (9.6)	17	Hooton (61)
Penicillin VK (250 mg q.i.d., 10 days)	90	78	96 (11.9)	2	

*Cure = eradication at the end of treatment.
[†]Recurrence = positive culture in follow-up after negative culture at the end of treatment.

second trial shown in Table 3.7, a significantly higher proportion of clarithromycin-treated than penicillin-treated patients reported gastrointestinal side effects (60). In the azithromycin trial, the incidence of all side effects, most of which were gastrointestinal, was markedly and statistically significantly higher in the azithromycin group than in the penicillin V group (61).

Acute bacterial sinusitis in adults is most often caused by *S. pneumoniae, H. influenzae,* and anaerobic species, and less often by *S. aureus, S. pyogenes, M. catarrhalis,* and gram-negative bacilli (62). Table 3.8 summarizes studies in which newer macrolides were compared with other agents for this infection. Clarithromycin was compared to amoxicillin; both drugs were given for approximately 10 days. The incidence of clinical cure or improvement (only cure is shown in the table) and of microbiologic response (defined by the authors as the eradication of organisms) were approximately 90% in each instance. *H. influenzae* was eradicated from 78% of patients treated with clarithromycin and 90% of patients treated with amoxicillin. Adverse events occurred in 16% of patients given clarithromycin and 26% given amoxicillin. Diarrhea and abdominal pain were the most common side effects in both groups (63). None of the differences was statistically significant.

Azithromycin has also been compared with amoxicillin for maxillary sinusitis (see Table 3.8). The incidence of combined clinical cure or improvement (only cure is

Table 3.8   Treatment of maxillary sinusitis

Regimens compared	No. assessable patients	Clinical cure (%)	Bacteriological cure (%)	Adverse effects (%)	Reference
Amoxicillin (500 mg t.i.d., 9–11 days)	35	74	92	26	Karma (63)
Clarithromycin (500 mg b.i.d., 9–11 days)	33	59	89	16	
Amoxicillin (500 mg t.i.d., 10 days)	37	73	100	8	Casiano (6)
Azithromycin (500 mg day 1; 250 mg day 2–5)	41	74	100	5	

shown in the table) and of bacteriologic cure was 100% in the 2 groups. However, the microbiologic findings were unusual in that coagulase-negative and coagulase-positive staphylococci and *S. viridans* were predominant isolates; there were no isolates of *H. influenzae*. Side effects were infrequent and mild in both groups and were mainly gastrointestinal (64).

These studies indicate that the 2 new macrolides are similar in efficacy to penicillin V for streptococcal pharyngitis and to amoxicillin for acute maxillary sinusitis. The new drugs are generally well tolerated, but in 2 studies of streptococcal pharyngitis, the rates of adverse effects were significantly higher with the new macrolide than with penicillin V.

Bronchitis

The new macrolides are active in vitro against the major pathogens of community-acquired lower respiratory tract infections, including *S. pneumoniae, H. influenzae, M. catarrhalis, M. pneumoniae, L. pneumophila,* and *C. pneumoniae.* They have been compared to beta-lactam drugs in the treatment of acute exacerbations of chronic bronchitis and pneumonia.

The clinical and microbiologic efficacy of clarithromycin and ampicillin for acute exacerbations of chronic bronchitis have been compared in 2 studies (Table 3.9) (57,58). The efficacy of the 2 drugs was similar even though, in one study, almost one third of the bacterial isolates were resistant to ampicillin in vitro (57). In the other study, patients with β-lactamase–producing isolates were excluded from evaluation (58). Because of concern about the activity of the macrolides against *H. influenzae* and *S. pneumoniae,* it is of interest to examine the microbiological efficacy against these species. The incidences of eradication of *H. influenzae* with clarithromycin and ampicillin were 64% and 86%, respectively, in the first study (57) and 95% and 100% in the

Table 3.9   Treatment of acute bronchitis

Regimens compared	No. assessable patients	Clinical cure (%)	Bacteriological cure (%)	Adverse effects (%)	Reference
Clarithromycin (250 mg b.i.d., 6–15 days)	29	79	79	31	Bachand (57)
Ampicillin (250 mg q.i.d., 6–15 days)	34	68	85	32	
Clarithromycin (250 mg b.i.d., 7–14 days)	29	96	97	12	Aldons (58)
Ampicillin (250 mg q.i.d., 7–14 days)	24	91	100	2	
Clarithromycin (250 mg b.i.d.)	203	99*	94		Wettengel (65)
Cefaclor (500 mg t.i.d.)	195	98*	91		
Azithromycin (500 mg day 1; 250 mg days 2–5)	191[†]	36	94	22	Dark (66)
Cefaclor (500 mg t.i.d., 10 days)	81[†]	31	100	18	

*Clinical response (cure or improvement).
[†]Pooled data: 93% of patients receiving azithromycin had bronchitis, and 7% had pneumonia; 92% of patients receiving cefaclor had bronchitis, and 8% had pneumonia.

second (58). *S. pneumoniae* was eradicated in all patients in both studies. There was a significantly higher incidence of adverse effects with clarithromycin (11.7%) than with ampicillin (1.5%; $p < 0.05$) in the second study (58) but not in the first. Most of the adverse effects were gastrointestinal and mild. A third study, reported in abstract form (65), compared clarithromycin with cefaclor, for bronchitis (see Table 3.9). Overall, the drugs were similar in both clinical (combined cure and improvement) and microbiologic efficacy. The incidence of microbiologic cure of *H. influenzae* infection was 88% with clarithromycin and 90% with cefaclor. For *S. pneumoniae*, these values were 100% and 95%, respectively. The incidence of adverse effects was not stated.

Azithromycin has been compared with cefaclor in the treatment of lower respiratory infections (see Table 3.9). In a large trial, with a confusing scheme of "randomization," a 5-day course of azithromycin was compared to a 10-day course of cefaclor; most patients had bronchitis but 7% to 8% had pneumonia (see Table 3.9). Of 552 patients enrolled, 274 were excluded from the analysis, mainly because of resistant pathogens, lack of a baseline pathogen, or absence of assessment at the end of treatment. The most common pathogens were *H. influenzae, S. pneumoniae, S. aureus, M. catarrhalis,* and *H. parainfluenzae.* The incidences of clinical and microbiologic response in bronchitis were similar for the 2 drugs. The reason for the low clinical cure rate is not clear. The rate of eradication of *H. influenzae* was significantly higher with azithromycin (94%) than with cefaclor (61%; $p < 0.001$). For *S. pneumoniae,* these values were 97% and 95%, respectively. Adverse events were of similar frequency in the 2 groups and were mild.

Community-acquired pneumonia

Clarithromycin has been compared with erythromycin for the treatment of community-acquired pneumonia in a double-blind, randomized trial (Table 3.10) (67). Of 208 patients entered into the trial, only 108 were assessable for clinical response. The most common reason for nonassessability was a failure to confirm the radiographic diagnosis of pneumonia. Bacterial pathogens were isolated in only 14 patients assessable for efficacy, and a serological diagnosis was made in another 9 patients. The most common pathogens in these patients were *H. influenzae* and *S. pneumoniae.* The incidences of clinical cure and improvement were not statistically significant between the drugs. Nevertheless, an intention-to-treat analysis showed a significant superiority of clarithromycin in the combined categories of clinical cure or improvement. The incidences of eradication of specific pathogens were not given. Adverse events occurred in 19% of clarithromycin-treated and 35% of erythromycin-treated patients ($p = 0.01$). The most common side effects were diarrhea in the clarithromycin group and nausea in the erythromycin group.

A randomized, double-blind study compared azithromycin and cefaclor for community-acquired bacterial pneumonia (see Table 3-10) (68). Forty percent of

Table 3.10   Treatment of community-acquired pneumonia

Regimens compared	No. assessable patients	Clinical cure (%)	Improvement (%)	Bacteriological cure (%)	Adverse effects (%)	Reference
Clarithromycin (250 mg b.i.d., 14 days)	64	52	43	89	19	Anderson (67)
Erythromycin (500 mg q.i.d., 14 days)	44	40	51	100	35	
Azithromycin (500 mg day 1; 250 mg days 2–5)	32	47	59	80	19	Kinasewitz (68)
Cefaclor (500 mg t.i.d., 10 days)	39	41	47	93	12	

patients enrolled were excluded from the analysis, mainly because of lack of an identifiable pathogen. The most common pathogens were S. *pneumoniae*, H. *influenzae*, and S. *aureus*. The incidences of favorable clinical responses for the 2 drugs were similar. The incidence of bacteriologic cure was 80% for azithromycin and 93% for cefaclor ($p = 0.08$). The incidences of eradication of specific pathogens were not stated. Adverse events, mainly mild gastrointestinal symptoms, were reported in 19% of azithromycin recipients and 12% of cefaclor recipients.

Azithromycin, in a 5-day course, has been compared with erythromycin, in a 10-day course, for the treatment of "atypical" pneumonias (Table 3.11) caused by M. *pneumoniae* and C. *psittaci* in an unblinded study conducted in Yugoslavia (69). The diagnosis was proven by a 4-fold or greater increase in antibody titer. Symptoms resolved within 48 hours in 82% of azithromycin recipients and 84% of erythromycin recipients, and within 5 days in 18% and 16% of patients, respectively. Adverse effects occurred in 1.8% of patients in the azithromycin group and in 13.6% in the erythromycin group. The side effects were all gastrointestinal, except that a rash developed in 1 patient treated with erythromycin.

Because of the ability of azithromycin to persist in tissues in appreciable concentrations for days, the same authors conducted a clinical trial of short-course treatment in patients with a clinical, serologic, and radiographic diagnosis of "atypical" pneumonia (70). Efficacy could be assessed in 84 patients. One group received azithromycin (500 mg once daily for 3 days); the other group received 250 mg twice on the first day, then once daily for 4 days. The pathogens were M. *pneumoniae*, *Chlamydia* spp., and *Coxiella burnetii* (data for Coxiella were not furnished in the article). The severity of illness was not stated. All patients were cured clinically. Side effects, all gastrointestinal, were minimal.

We found only 1 study that deals with the new macrolides in the treatment of L. *pneumophila* infections (70a). Clarithromycin, usually in a dosage of 500 mg twice daily by mouth, was given for a mean of 27 days to 46 Pakistani patients with "moderate to severe" Legionnaire's disease, confirmed by culture (13 patients), direct fluorescent antigen staining of secretions (40 patients), or a 4-fold increase in antibody titer (41 patients). One patient was improved and the rest were cured in this open-label trial.

Table 3.11   Treatment of atypical pneumonia

| Regimens compared | No. assessable patients | Clinical cure (%) | Causative Pathogen | | Adverse effects (%) | Reference |
			M. pneumoniae, C. psittaci (% cure)			
Azithromycin (500 mg day 1; 250 mg days 2–5)	39	82	87	62	2	Schonwald (69)
Erythromycin (500 mg q.i.d., 10 days)	32	84	92	62	14	

These studies indicate that in the treatment of community-acquired pneumonia, clarithromycin and azithromycin have efficacy similar to that of erythromycin and cefaclor. The incidence of side effects with the newer macrolides is substantially lower than with erythromycin. Azithromycin appears to work well for atypical pneumonias, presumably mild in severity, when given in as short a course as 3 to 5 days.

Skin and soft-tissue infections

Clarithromycin has been compared to erythromycin and cefadroxil in the treatment of skin and skin-structure infections, including impetigo, folliculitis, cellulitis, abscess, and wound infection in 3 blinded trials, of which the combined results, as presented in a summary report (71), are shown in the top panel of Table 3.12. The most common infecting species was S. *aureus*. High rates of clinical cure and improvement, and of bacteriological cure, were noted with both regimens.

In a double-blind, randomized trial (72), azithromycin, in a 5-day course, was compared with cephalexin, in a 10-day course, for the treatment of infections of the skin and skin structures (see Table 3.12). The major pathogens were S. *aureus*, S. *pyogenes*, and S. *agalactiae*. As with the clarithromycin trials, the incidences of cure and improvement

Table 3.12   Treatment of skin and soft-tissue infections

Regimens compared	No. assessable patients	Clinical cure (%)	Bacterio- logical cure (%)	Adverse effects (%)	Reference
Clarithromycin (250 mg b.i.d., 7–14 days) Erythromycin (250 mg q.i.d., 7–14 days)	266	95	92		Gupta (71)
OR Cefadroxil (500 mg b.i.d., 7–14 days)	267	96	92		
Azithromycin (500 mg day 1; 250 mg days 2–5)	83	94	94	16	Kiani (72)
Cephalexin (500 mg b.i.d., 10 days)	96	96	90	11	
Azithromycin (500 mg day 1; 250 mg days 2–5)	102	99	99	11	Mallory (73)
Cephalexin (500 mg b.i.d., 10 days)	46	96	98	5	

and of bacteriologic eradication were high with both agents. Patients from whom a resistant pathogen was isolated were excluded from the efficacy analysis. A single-blinded study comparing azithromycin with cephalexin (see Table 3.12) yielded similar results (73). In both these studies, adverse effects were mild and mainly gastrointestinal.

In summary, the studies of skin and skin-structure infections show high incidences of efficacy for both clarithromycin and azithromycin. However, such trials tend not to be very informative because efficacy rates are high with virtually all agents studied.

Genital chlamydial infections

Azithromycin, given in short-course regimens, appears to be highly effective for the treatment of genital chlamydial infections. Steingrimsson and colleagues (74) compared 3 dosing regimens—a single 1-gram dose, 500 mg twice daily for 2 doses, and 500 mg on day 1 followed by 250 mg on days 2 and 3—with a standard regimen of doxycycline (100 mg b.i.d. for 7 days) in the treatment of patients with genital infections. The infections in 168 assessable patients were caused by *C. trachomatis* (138 patients), *N. gonorrheae* (43 patients), and *U. urealyticum* (45 patients). All but 1 patient were men. *C. trachomatis* was eradicated in 98% of patients given doxycycline, 98% of patients given a single dose of azithromycin, and 88% to 96% of patients given the multiple-dose regimens of azithromycin. *N. gonorrheae* was eradicated in 100% of patients given doxycycline, 92% given a single dose of azithromycin, and 88% to 100% given multiple doses of azithromycin. *U. urealyticum* was eradicated in 75% given doxycycline, 79% given a single dose of azithromycin, and 75% to 100% given other regimens of azithromycin.

Stamm and colleagues (75) reviewed studies comparing a single 1-gm dose of azithromycin with a 7-day course of doxycycline for uncomplicated chlamydial infections in 184 patients. The bacteriologic cure rates were 91% and 94%, respectively. The clinical cure rates were 77% versus 63%, respectively. Nilsen and associates (75a) treated men with uncomplicated chlamydial urethritis with either a single 1-gm dose of azithromycin (44 patients) or doxycycline (100 mg twice daily for 7 days) (42 patients). All recipients of either regimen were cured.

Azithromycin given in a single 1-gm dose has been compared with ciprofloxacin (500 mg b.i.d. for 7 days) for chlamydial infections of the urethra or cervix. Bacteriologic eradication occurred in 95% of patients treated with azithromycin and in 61% of patients treated with ciprofloxacin (75).

We have found no data for clarithromycin in the treatment of genital infections.

Gastrointestinal infections

Twelve patients with gastritis caused by *Helicobacter pylori* were treated with azithromycin for 7 days; 2 also received an H_2-blocker. The organisms were eliminated at the end of treatment in only 2 patients, and relapse occurred in these 2 patients within 3 months (76). Comparison of isolates obtained before and after therapy showed a sharp rise in resistance to the macrolide at the end of treatment.

Mycobacterium avium complex infection

Clarithromycin has been studied in several trials for the treatment of disseminated MAC infection in patients with the acquired immunodeficiency syndrome (AIDS). In a multicenter, randomized, double-blind study, 108 patients were allocated to receive clarithromycin (500, 1,000, or 2,000 mg b.i.d. for 12 weeks) (77). The response was monitored by quantitative blood cultures for mycobacteria. An interim analysis of the first 72 patients after 12 weeks of treatment showed reductions in mycobacterial counts of over 2 logarithms. The mean times to eradication of organisms (sterile blood cultures) in the 3 groups were 55 days (500 mg), 43 days (1,000 mg), and and 27 days (2,000 mg). The quality of life improved significantly during the study, and the symptoms of fevers and night-sweats improved in 76%, 47%, and 75% in the 3 groups, respectively. Adverse events requiring discontinuation of the drug occurred in 3 of 24 (12.5%), 2 of 24 (8%), and 11 of 24 (49%), respectively. The major adverse events were gastrointestinal. All isolates were initially susceptible to clarithromycin, but resistance developed in 16 of 72 (22%) patients.

In a small, randomized, double-blind, placebo-controlled trial, a group of 8 patients received clarithromycin alone for 6 weeks, then rifampin, isoniazid, ethambutal, and clofazimine for 6 weeks. Another group of 7 patients received placebo for 6 weeks, then clarithromycin together with the other 4 drugs (78). During treatment with clarithromycin alone, mycobacterial counts in blood cultures declined sharply in each of the 8 patients; cultures became sterile in 6. In contrast, counts slowly increased in the placebo group. Among patients crossed over from clarithromycin to the 4-drug regimen, mycobacterial counts increased during administration of the 4-drug regimen. Among patients crossed over from placebo to the 5-drug regimen, which included clarithromycin, mycobacterial counts decreased.

In a study to assess the efficacy of clarithromycin over a longer period of treatment, 77 patients with MAC bacteremia received clarithromycin in doses ranging from 500 to 2,000 mg daily for up to 8 months (79). Some of these patients may have been reported in other trials cited herein. Of 64 patients who could be evaluated, failure (i.e., continued positive blood cultures on treatment) occurred in 6 patients. Five of the 6 failures occurred in patients receiving less than 1,000 mg/day. Among patients initially responding, relapse during treatment occurred in 12 of 56 (21%) after 2 to 8 months of treatment. The incidence of relapse was higher among patients whose treatment had been interrupted for periods of 1 week or more. Among 6 patients with bacteriologic relapse, the MIC of clarithromycin increased from 0.5 to 2 µg/mL at baseline to 1,024 µg/mL. Increased liver enzyme measurements were noted in 20 patients, and hearing impairment occurred in 3. It was not stated if the adverse effects were dose-related.

In a noncomparative study, 17 patients with MAC infection and AIDS were given clarithromycin (500 or 1,000 mg b.i.d.) (80). Only 9 patients completed 10 weeks of treatment. The results are difficult to interpret, but, in general, the treatment appeared to be of benefit in reducing symptoms and mycobacterial blood counts in many of the patients.

In another small, noncomparative study, azithromycin (500 mg/day) was given for short periods to patients with AIDS who had MAC bacteremia. Among 21 patients, blood counts declined from a mean of 2,208 CFU at entry to 136 CFU after 20 or 30 days of treatment. Fifteen of 21 patients with fever and 12 of 18 with night sweats reported resolution of these symptoms during treatment (81).

In summary, these data suggest a benefit of clarithromycin for patients with AIDS and MAC bacteremia in reducing mycobacterial counts in blood cultures and in reducing symptoms. It appears that a dosage below 1,000 mg/day is relatively ineffective, but that higher dosages produce gastrointestinal intolerance. The incidence of the development of resistance during single-drug treatment is appreciable. Data for azithromycin are currently sparse.

INDICATIONS AND USUAL DOSAGE

The indications (44,45,82) and usual dosage of erythromycin, clarithromycin, and azithromycin are shown in Table 3.13. The indications are for mild to moderate, but not severe, infections. As shown in the table, the list of indications is greater for erythromycin than for the newer agents. In most instances, the macrolides are an alternative, but not an agent of choice, except in patients allergic to beta-lactam agents. Erythromycin is an agent of choice for only a few infections (i.e., Legionnaire's disease, diphtheria, and pertussis); the utility of the new macrolides for these infections is not proved. The primary indications for the new macrolides are in the treatment of upper and lower respiratory tract infections and skin and skin-structure infections. Azithromycin is also approved in a single-dose regimen for chlamydial genital infections. There are some differences among the drugs in the specific pathogenic agents of respiratory tract infection for which they are approved.

USE IN CLINICAL PRACTICE

The most common areas in which macrolides are a preferred treatment in adult medicine are: (1) streptococcal and staphylococcal infections in penicillin-allergic patients; (2) atypical pneumonia; and (3) certain sexually transmitted diseases. There are also a few uncommon infections, as discussed, in which erythromycin, but not the newer macrolides, is a drug of choice (i.e., Legionnaire's disease, diphtheria and pertussis).

The most obvious advantages of the newer macrolides over erythromycin are their better pharmacologic attributes and tolerance. The 2 new agents differ from one another in this regard (Table 3.14). Whereas erythromycin is given 3 or 4 times daily, clarithromycin is given twice daily and azithromycin once daily. Moreover, azithromycin is given in a much shorter course, usually 5 days, as opposed to 7 to 14 days for the other agents. The advantages of less frequent dosing should not be underestimated; busy patients have low compliance rates for taking drugs given more than twice daily. The absorption of azithromycin is impaired by food, but it should be easy to warn patients to take the drug before breakfast. Of great value in practice, the new agents produce less gastrointestinal upset, perhaps half as much, as erythromycin. A subtler, but important advantage is that azithromycin is essentially free of drug interactions. For these advantages, the consumer pays dearly (see Table 3.14). A 10-day course of

Table 3.13 Indications (abbreviated) and usual dosages of the macrolides*

	Erythromycin	Clarithromycin	Azithromycin
Usual dosage in adults	250 (up to 500) mg four times daily, or 333 mg three times daily for 7–14 days	250 (up to 500) mg q12 h for 7–14 days	250 mg tablets, 2 tablets at once on day 1; one tablet daily days 2–5
Streptococcal pharyngitis	10-day course	10-day course	5-day course (test susceptibility in vitro)
Sinusitis	S. pneumoniae; H. influenzae (with a sulfonamide); S. pyogenes	S. pneumoniae	
Bronchitis (acute exacerbation)	S. pneumoniae; M. pneumoniae; S. pyogenes	S. pneumoniae; H. influenzae; M. catarrhalis	S. pneumoniae; H. influenzae; M. catarrhalis
Pneumonia	S. pneumoniae; M. pneumoniae; L. pneumophila‡; S. pyogenes	S. pneumoniae; M. pneumoniae	S. pneumoniae; H. influenzae (not high risk)†
Skin and skin structure	S. aureus; S. pyogenes	S. aureus; S. pyogenes	S. aureus; S. pyogenes; S. agalactiae
Sexually transmitted diseases	C. trachomatis (alternative to tetracycline)		C. trachomatis (single 1-gm dose) (may not cure gonorrhea or syphilis)
Miscellaneous	SBE prophylaxis; T. pallidum; N. gonorrheae; B. pertussis; L. monocytogenes; E. histolytica		

*All indications are for mild to moderate infection only.
†Elderly, debilitated, severe underlying disease, suspected bacteremia.
‡No controlled efficacy studies, but in vitro and limited clinical data suggest efficacy.

clarithromycin or a 5-day course of azithromycin costs approximately $40 to the retailer, whereas a 10-day course of generic erythromycin costs approximately 10 times less (manufacturers' list prices). For further comparison, a typical 10-day course of cefaclor (500 mg t.i.d.) costs $94, amoxicillin-clavulanic acid (500 mg amoxicillin t.i.d.) costs approximately $60, ciprofloxacin (500 mg b.i.d.) and ofloxacin (300 mg b.i.d.) cost approximately $50, but generic versions of cephalexin and dicloxacillin cost less than $15, and generic versions of amoxicillin and trimethoprim-sulfamethoxazole cost less than $4. The price to patients will be higher than these prices cited. It is

Table 3.14 Pharmacological considerations and costs of macrolides

	Erythromycin	*Clarithromycin*	*Azithromycin*
Dosing	3–4 doses daily	2 doses daily	1 dose daily; shorter course
Effect of meals	No effect with enteric coated	No effect	Food impairs absorption
Adverse effects (mainly GI)	Common	Less than with erythromycin	Less than with erythromycin
Drug interactions	Many (see text)	Many (see text)	Few or none
Cost per course*	10-day course, 3–4 doses per day generic: $3–7	10-day course, 500 mg b.i.d.: $43	5-day course, 500 mg day 1, then 250 mg/day: $41

*Manufacturer's list price.

important for physicians and patients to bear these financial considerations in mind. Indeed, if not for cost considerations, we would distinctly prefer the new macrolides over erythromycin for all indications by the oral route.

In the following paragraphs, we offer our personal views as to the potential role of the new macrolides, including their use in infections for which there is no approved indication. It is more difficult to predict efficacy from in vitro susceptibility data with the macrolides than with other classes of drugs, such as β-lactams, because of the unusual pharmacokinetic behavior of the macrolides: The high tissue concentrations *may* result in greater efficacy than would be predicted from in vitro data. However, it seems reasonable to draw some inferences by analogy to erythromycin. It should be stressed that we would not suggest any macrolide as a drug of choice for suspected severe infection (e.g., in patients with suspected bacteremia).

For streptococcal pharyngitis, penicillin should remain the drug of choice because of its low cost and good efficacy. If one were to choose an alternative, it should probably be a cephalosporin because, in meta-analyses, beta-lactamase–stable drugs have shown somewhat better efficacy than penicillin (83). In contrast, the macrolides are not apparently more effective than penicillin and they have significantly more side effects. Nevertheless, a macrolide would be a good choice in patients allergic to β-lactam drugs. Erythromycin would be the most cost-effective choice.

For bacterial sinusitis, there is no obvious advantage of either new macrolide over amoxicillin, the reference agent in clinical trials. Generic cephalexin or trimethoprim-sulfamethoxazole would be other inexpensive choices. For refractory infections, amoxicillin-clavulanic acid or a fluoroquinolone might be considered.

Acute exacerbations of chronic bronchitis have generally responded well to a variety of antibiotics in clinical trials. In comparative trials, clarithromycin was similar in efficacy to ampicillin and cefaclor, and azithromycin was similar to cefaclor. In one trial, there were significantly more side effects with clarithromycin than with ampicillin. In using a macrolide for this indication, the possibility of an interaction with theophylline must be borne in mind. Generic amoxicillin, ampicillin, trimethoprim-sulfamethoxazole, or cephalexin would be reasonable first choices for bronchitis. Refractory cases could be treated as for sinusitis.

Community-acquired pneumonia is an attractive indication for the macrolides because of their activity against the pathogens of "atypical" pneumonia. Tetracylines might also be a good choice for this indication. Unfortunately, for the most serious consideration—L. *pneumophila* infection—no agent, including erythromycin, has been demonstrated to be effective in controlled trials. Nevertheless, most infectious disease physicians would consider a macrolide the drug of choice for suspected atypical pneumonias. The incidence of atypical pneumonia in patients with community-acquired pneumonia has varied from study to study and it is impossible to know, other than by culture or serologic testing, the causative pathogen in community-acquired pneumonia. Although a variety of agents, such as amoxicillin, cephalexin, and trimethoprim-sulfamethoxazole, might be effective for community-acquired pneumonia, we favor a macrolide because of concern about atypical pathogens. We would not generally recommend a fluoroquinolone in this circumstance because of uncertain efficacy against atypical pathogens and the pneumococcus. For more severe community-acquired pneumonia, we generally favor the combination of a broad-spectrum β-lactam, given intravenously for ordinary bacterial infection, and a macrolide. As to the specific macrolide to be chosen, we tend to favor one of the new agents because the greater convenience and tolerance make compliance more likely. The greater cost may be warranted in this potentially serious infection. If severe Legionnaire's disease is suspected, intravenous erythromycin should generally be given.

The incidences of eradication of H. *influenzae* and S. *pneumoniae* in patients with respiratory tract infections treated with the macrolides are of interest. The incidence of eradication of H. *influenzae* was somewhat lower with clarithromycin (78%) than with amoxicillin (90%) in one study of sinusitis (62), and was lower with clarithromycin (64%) than with ampicillin (86%) in a study of bronchitis (57). In another study of bronchitis (68), the incidence of eradication of H. *influenzae* was higher with azithromycin (94%) than with cefaclor (61%; $p < 0.001$). These data suggest that azithromycin may be more effective than clarithromycin for H. *influenzae* infection. S. *pneumoniae* was generally eradicated by both of the new macrolides.

Many skin and skin-structure infections, presumably caused by S. *aureus* or S. *pyogenes*, barely require antimicrobial treatment. In most patients, cost considerations should weigh heavily. Erythromycin or generic dicloxacillin sodium would be good choices. If the infection is likely to be streptococcal (e.g., in a patient with recurrent cellulitis), penicillin V or amoxicillin would be good choices.

Azithromycin, in a single 1-gm dose, is highly effective for the treatment of chlamydial urethritis or cervicitis. The convenience of the regimen makes azithromycin a drug of choice for the indication. However, attention must be paid to the possibility of incompletely treated gonococcal or syphilitic infection.

The spectrum and minimal degree of urinary excretion of the macrolides makes them a poor choice for urinary tract infection. The minimal data so far available are not encouraging for the use of the macrolides for *Helicobacter pylori* infection. Although erythromycin has some utility in *Campylobacter* diarrhea, we are not aware of any data for the newer macrolides.

Clarithromycin, as a single agent, appears to have unusual efficacy for the control of MAC infection in patients with AIDS. Daily dosages have ranged from 500 to 4,000 mg. Although the extent of reduction in bacterial counts in the blood and the incidence of side effects were dose-related, the degree of improvement in symptoms was not dose-related in one study (77). For this reason, and because of the considerable expense of treatment, it might be prudent to start patients at a lower dosage (e.g., 1,000 mg/day) and to increase the dosage only if the response is not satisfactory. Development of resistance during treatment has been noted, especially in patients in whom treatment was interrupted for periods of 1 week or more. Whether the addition of a second agent would ameliorate this problem is not clear. Data for azithromycin in the treatment of MAC infections are sparse.

There are a number of other infections in which the new macrolides may have some potential but for which data are scanty and preliminary. These include *M. chelonae*, *M. fortuitum*, and *M. leprae* infections (clarithromycin is especially active), toxoplasmosis, and *Pneumocystis carinii* infection (clarithromycin has been studied in animals).

In conclusion, the new macrolides offer advantages of more convenient dosing regimens and much better tolerance over erythromycin but at a considerable increase in cost. The most compelling justifications for the new drugs are in the treatment of community-acquired pneumonia (either drug), chlamydial genital infection (azithromycin), and MAC infection in patients with AIDS (clarithromycin).

REFERENCES

1 Chu S, Wilson D, Guay D. Clarithromycin pharmacokinetics in healthy young and elderly volunteers. *J Clin Pharmacol* 1992;32: 1045–1049.

2 Neu HC. The development of macrolides: clarithromycin in perspective. *J Antimicrob Chemother* 1991;27(suppl A):1–9.

3 Piscitelli S, Danziger L, Rodvold K. Clarithromycin and azithromycin: new macrolide antibiotics. *Clin Pharm* 1992;11:137–152.

4 Hardy D, Hensey D, Beyer J, Voitko C, McDonald E, Fernandes P. Comparative in vitro activities of new 14-, 15-, and 16-membered macrolides. *Antimicrob Ag Chemother* 1988;32:1710–1719.

5 Olsson-Liljequist B, Hoffman BM. In vitro activity of clarithromycin combined with its 14-hydroxy metabolite A-62671 against *H. influenzae*. *J Antimicrob Chemother* 1991;27(suppl A):11–17.

6 Williams JD. Spectrum of activity of azithromycin. *Eur J Clin Microbiol Infect Dis* 1991;10:813–820.

7 Maskell JP, Sefton AM, Williams JD. Comparative in vitro activity of azithromycin and erythromycin against gram positive cocci, *H.*

influenzae, and anaerobes. *J Antimicrob Chemother* 1990;25(suppl A):19–24.

8 Fernandes P, Bailer R, Swanson R, et al. In vitro and in vivo evaluation of A-56268, a new macrolide. *Antimicrob Ag Chemother* 1986;30: 865–873.

9 Retsema J, Girard A. Spectrum and mode of action of azithromycin, a new 15-membered ring macrolide with improved potency against gram-negative organisms. *Antimicrob Ag Chemother* 1987;31:1939–1947.

10 Hirakata Y, Kaku M, Tomono K, et al. Efficacy of erythromycin lactobionate for treating *Pseudomonas aeruginosa* bacteremia in mice. *Antimicrob Ag Chemother* 1992;36:1198–1203.

11 Ridgway GL, Mumtaz G, Fenelon L. The in-vitro activity of clarithromycin and other macrolides in the type strain of *Chlamydia pneumoniae*. *J Antimicrob Chemother* 1991; 27(suppl A):43–47.

12 Cassell GH, Drnec J, Waites KB, et al. Efficacy of clarithromycin against *M. pneumoniae*. *J of Antimicrob Chemother* 1991;27(suppl A):47–61.

13 Rylander M, Hallander H. In vitro comparison of the activity of doxycycline, tetracycline,

erythromycin, and a new macrolide, CP 62993, against *Mycoplasma pneumoniae*, *Mycoplasma hominis*, and *Ureaplasma urealyticum*. *Scand J Infect Dis.* 1988;(suppl 53):12–17.

14 **Renaudin H, Bebear C.** Comparative in vitro activity of azithromycin, clarithromycin, erythromycin, and lomefloxacin against *Mycoplasma pneumoniae*, *Mycoplasma hominis* and *Ureaplasma urealyticum*. *Eur J Clin Microbiol Infect Dis* 1990;9:838–841.

15 **Hammerschlag MR, Qumei KK, Roblin PM.** In vitro activities of azithromycin, clarithromycin, L-ofloxacin, and other antibiotics against *Chlamydia pneumoniae*. *Antimicrob Ag Chemother* 1992;36:1573–1574.

16 **Slaney L, Chubb H, Ronald A, Brunham R.** In vitro activity of azithromycin, erythromycin, ciprofloxacin, and norfloxacin against *Neisseria gonorrhoeae*, *H. ducreyi*, and *Chlamydia trachomatis*. *J Antimicrob Chemother* 1990; 25(suppl A):1–5.

17 **Metchock B.** In-vitro activity of azithromycin compared with other macrolides and oral antibiotics against *Salmonella typhi*. *J Antimicrob Chemother* 1990;25(suppl A):29–31.

18 **Bahal N, Nahata M.** The new macrolide antibiotics: azithromycin, clarithromycin, dirithromycin, and roxithromycin. *Ann Pharmacother* 1992;26:46–55.

19 **McNulty CA, Dent JC.** Susceptibility of clinical isolates of *Campylobacter pylori* to twenty-one antimicrobial agents. *Eur J Clin Microbiol Infect Dis* 1988;7:566–569.

20 **Scieux C, Bianchi A, Chappey B, Vassias I, Perol Y.** In vitro activity of azithromycin against *C. trachomatis*. *J Antimicrob Chemother* 1990;25(suppl A):7–10.

21 **Dangor Y, Miller SD, Exposto da L, Koornhof H.** Antimicrobial susceptibilities of southern African isolates of *Haemophilus ducreyi*. *Antimicrob Ag Chemother* 1988;32:1458–1460.

22 **Johnson R, Kodner C, Russell M, Girard D.** In vitro and in vivo susceptibility of *Borrelia burgdorferi* to azithromycin. *J Antimicrob Ag Chemother* 1990;32:755–757.

23 **Preac-Mursic V, Wilske B, Schierz G, Sub E, Grob B.** Comparative antimicrobial activity of the new macrolides against *Borrelia burgdorferi*. *Eur. J Clin Microbiol Infect Dis* 1989; 8:651–653.

24 **Stamm LV, Parrish EA.** In vitro activity of azithromycin and CP-63,956 against *Treponema pallidum*. *J Antimicrob Chemother* 1990;25(suppl A):11–14.

25 **Lukehart S, Fohn M, Baker-Zander S.** Efficacy of azithromycin for therapy of active syphilis in the rabbit model. *J Antimicrob Chemother* 1990;25(suppl A):91–99.

26 **Gornyski E, Gutman S, Allen W.** Comparative antimycobacterial activities of difloxacin, temafloxacin, enoxacin, pefloxacin, reference fluoroquinolones, and a new macrolide, clarithromycin. *Antimicrob Ag Chemother* 1989;33: 591–592.

27 **Naik S, Ruck R.** In vitro activities of several new macrolide antibiotics against mycobacterium avium complex. *Antimicrob Ag Chemother* 1989;33:1614–1616.

28 **Klemens SP, DeStefano MS, Cynamon MH.** Activity of clarithromycin against *Mycobacterium avium* complex infection in beige mice. *Antimicrob Ag Chemother* 1992;36:2413–2417.

29 **Yajko D, Nassos P, Sanders C, Gonzalez P, Hadley W.** Comparison of the intracellular activities of clarithromycin and erythromycin against *Mycobacterium avium* complex strains in J774 cells and in alveolar macrophages from human immunodeficiency virus type 1-infected individuals. *Antimicrob Ag Chemother* 1992;36:1163–1165.

30 **Inderlied C.** In vitro and in vivo activity of azithromycin against the *Mycobacterium avium* complex. *J Infect Dis* 1989;159:994–997.

31 **Brown B, Wallace R, Onyi G, DeRosas V, Wallace R.** Activities of four macrolides, including clarithromycin, against *Mycobacterium fortuitum*, *Mycobacterium chelonae*, and *M. chelonae*-like organisms. *Antimicrob Ag Chemother* 1992;36:180–184.

32 **Chang H, Pechere J.** In vitro effects of four macrolides on *Toxoplasma gondii*. *Antimicrob Ag Chemother* 1988;32:524–529.

33 **Chang HR, Rudareanu FC, Pechere JC.** Activity of A-56268 (TE-031), a new macrolide, against *Toxoplasma gondii* in mice. *J Antimicrob Chemother* 1988;22:359–361.

34 **Araujo F, Prokocimer P, Lin T, Remington J.** Activity of clarithromycin alone or in combination with other drugs for treatment of murine toxoplasmosis. *Antimicrob Ag Chemother* 1992; 36:2454–2457.

35 **Derouin F, Caroff B, Chau F, Prokocimer P, Pocidalo J.** Synergistic activity of clarithromycin and minocycline in an animal model of acute experimental toxoplasmosis. *Antimicrob Ag Chemother* 1992;36:2852–2855.

36 **Araujo FG, Shepard RM, Remington JS.** In vivo activity of the macrolide antibiotics azithromycin, roxithromycin and spiramycin against *Toxoplasma gondii*. *Eur J Clin Microbiol Infect Dis* 1991;10:519–524.

37 **Eady E, Ross J, Tipper J, Walters C, Cove J, Noble W.** Distribution of genes encoding erythromycin ribosomal methylases and an

erythromycin efflux pump in epidemiologically distinct groups of staphylococci. *J Antimicrob Chemother* 1993;31:211–217.

38 **Barry AL, Jones RN, Thornsberry C.** In vitro activities of azithromycin (CP 63,993), clarithromycin (A-56268; TE-031), erythromycin, roxithromycin, and clindamycin. *Antimicrob Ag Chemother* 1988;32:752–754.

39 **Hardy D, Guay D, Jones R.** Clarithromycin, a unique macrolide. *Diag Microbiol Infect Dis* 1988;15:39–53.

40 **Drew R, Gallis H.** Azithromycin—spectrum of activity, pharmacokinetics and clinical applications. *Pharmacotherapy* 1992;12:161–173.

41 **Chu S, Park B, Locke C, Willson D, Cavanaugh JC.** Drug-food interaction potential of clarithromycin, a new macrolide antimicrobial. *J Clin Pharmacol* 1992;32:32–36.

42 **Schentag J, Ballow C.** Tissue directed pharmacokinetics. *Am J Med* 1991;91(suppl 3A):3–11.

43 **Foulds G, Shepard RM, Johnson RB.** The pharmacokinetics of azithromycin in human serum and tissues. *J Antimicrob Chemother* 1990;25(suppl A):73–82.

44 Biaxin Product Information (package insert).

45 Zithromax Product Information (package insert).

46 **Guay D.** Pharmacokinetics of new macrolides. *Infec Med* 1991 (suppl A) Vol 9:31–38.

47 **Fraschini F, Scaglione F, Pintucci G, Maccarinelli G, Dugnani S, Demartini G.** The diffusion of clarithromycin and roxithromycin into nasal mucosa, tonsil and lung in humans. *J Antimicrob Chemother* 1991;27(suppl A):61–68.

48 **Gladue RP, Bright GM, Isaacson RF, Newborg MF.** In vitro and in vivo uptake of azithromycin (CP-62,993) by phagocytic cells: possible mechanism of delivery and release at sites of infection. *Antimicrob Ag Chemother* 1989;33:277–282.

49 **Frank MO, Sullivan GW, Carper HT, Mandell GI.** In vitro demonstration of transport and delivery of antibiotics by polymorphonuclear leukocytes. *Antimicrob Ag Chemother* 1992;36:2584–2588.

50 **Gladue RP, Snider ME.** Intracellular accumulation of azithromycin by cultured human fibroblasts. *Antimicrob Ag Chemother* 1990;34:1056–1060.

51 **Watanabe Y, Craig W.** Bactericidal effect of antibiotics on non-growing intracellular *Staphylococcus aureus* (SA) in human pneumocytes. Program and Abstracts, 32nd Interscience Conference on Antimicrobial Agents and Chemo-

therapy, American Society for Microbiology, Anaheim, California, Oct 11–14 1992.

52 **Barza M.** Challenges to antibiotic activity in tissue. *Clin Infect Dis.*

53 **Schwab JC, Slowik MR, Cao Y, Joiner KA.** Azithromycin uptake and intracellular distribution in *Toxoplasma gondii* and infected CHO cells. Program and Abstracts, 32nd Interscience Conference on Antimicrobial Agents and Chemotherapy, American Society for Microbiology, Anaheim, California, 1992.

54 **Nahata MC, Koranyi KI, Gadgil SD, Hilligoss DM, Fouda HG, Gardner MJ.** Pharmacokinetics of azithromycin in pediatric patients after oral administration of multiple doses of suspension. *Antimicrob Ag Chemother* 1993;37:314–316.

55 **Nellans H, Petersen A, Peeters J.** Gastrointestinal side effects: clarithromycin superior to azithromycin in reduced smooth muscle contraction and binding. Abbott Laboratories. 1991 ICAAC.

56 **Levenstein J.** Clarithromycin versus penicillin in the treatment of streptococcal pharyngitis. *J Antimicrob Chemother* 1991;27(suppl A):67–74.

57 **Bachand R.** Comparative study of clarithromycin and ampicillin in the treatment of patients with acute bacterial exacerbations of chronic bronchitis. *J Antimicrob Chemother* 1991;27(suppl A):91–100.

58 **Aldons P.** A comparison of clarithromycin with ampicillin in the treatment of outpatients with acute bacterial exacerbation of chronic bronchitis. *J Antimicrob Chemother* 1991;27(suppl A):101–108.

59 **Hopkins S.** Clinical toleration and safety of azithromycin. *Am J Med* 1991;91(suppl 3A):40–45.

60 **Bachand R.** A comparative study of clarithromycin and penicillin in the treatment of outpatients with streptococcal pharyngitis. *J Antimicrob Chemother* 1991;27(suppl A):75–82.

61 **Hooton T.** A comparison of azithromycin and penicillin V for the treatment of streptococcal pharyngitis. *Am J Med* 1991;91(suppl 3A):23S–26S.

62 **Gwaltney J.** Sinusitis. In: Mandell G. *Principles and Practice of Infectious Diseases.* New York: Churchill Livingstone, 1990:510–514.

63 **Karma P, Pukander J, Penttila M, et al.** The comparative efficacy and safety of clarithromycin and amoxycillin in the treatment of outpatients with acute maxillary sinusitis. *J Antimicrob Chemother* 1990;27(suppl A):83–90.

64 **Casiano R.** Azithromycin and amixicillin in

the treatment of acute maxillary sinusitis. *Am J Med* 1991;91(suppl 3A):27–30.

65 **Wettengel R.** Comparison of clarithromycin and cefaclor in the treatment of mild to moderate bronchitis. The First International Conference on the Macrolides, Azalides and Streptogramins, Sante Fe, New Mexico, January, 1992.

66 **Dark D.** Multicenter evaluation of azithromycin and cefaclor in acute lower respiratory tract infections. *Am J Med* 1991;91(suppl 3A):31–35.

67 **Anderson G, Esmonde T, Coles S, Macklin J, Carnegie C.** A comparative safety and efficacy study of clarithromycin and erythromycin stearate in community-acquired pneumonia. *J Antimicrob Chemother* 1991;27(suppl A):117–124.

68 **Kinasewitz G, Wood RG.** Azithromycin versus cefaclor in the treatment of acute bacterial pneumonia. *Eur J Clin Microbiol Infect Dis* 1991;10:872–877.

69 **Schonwald S, Gunjaca M, Kolacny L, Car V, Gosev M.** Comparison of azithromycin and erythromycin in the treatment of atypical pneumonias. *J Antimicrob Chemother* 1990;25(suppl A):123–126.

70 **Schonwald S, Skerk V, Petricevic I, Car V, Majerus-Misic L, Gunjaca M.** Comparison of three-day and five-day courses of azithromycin in the treatment of atypical pneumonia. *Eur J Clin Microbiol Infect Dis* 1991;10:877–880.

70a **Hamedani P, Ali J, Hafeez S, et al.** The safety and efficacy of clarithromycin in patients with Legionella pneumonia. *Chest* 1991;100:1503–1506.

71 **Gupta S, Siepman H.** Comparative safety and efficacy of clarithromycin versus standard agents in the treatment of mild to moderate bacterial skin or skin structure infections. Presented at the First International Conference on the Macrolides Azalides and Streptogramins, Santa Fe, New Mexico, January 22–25 1992.

72 **Kiani R.** Double blind, double-dummy comparison of azithromycin and cephalexin in the treatment of skin and skin structure infections. *Eur J Clin Microbiol Infect Dis* 1991;10:880–884.

73 **Mallory S.** Azithromycin compared with cephalexin in the treatment of skin and skin structure infections. *Am J Med* 1991;91(suppl 3A):36–39.

74 **Steingrimsson O, Olafsson J, Thorarinsson H, Ryan R, Johnson R, Tilton R.** Azithromycin in the treatment of sexually transmitted disease. *J Antimicrob Chemother* 1990;25(suppl A):109–114.

75 **Stamm W.** Azithromycin in the treatment of uncomplicated genital chlamydial infections. *Am J Med* 1991;91(Suppl 3A):19–22.

75a **Nilsen A, Halsos A, Johansen A, et al.** A double blind study of single dose azithromycin and doxycycline in the treatment of chlamydial urethritis in males. *Genitourin Med* 1992;68:325–327.

76 **Glupczynski Y, Burette A.** Failure of azithromycin to eradicate *Campylobacter pylori* from the stomach because of acquired resistance during treatment. *Am J Gastroenterol* 1990;85:98–99.

77 **Chaisson RE, Benson C, Dube M, et al.** Clarithromycin therapy for disseminated *Mycobacterium avium*-complex in AIDS patients. Johns Hopkins University, Baltimore, Rush Medical College, Chicago, LAC-USC Medical Center, Los Angeles, NIAID, Bethesda, Abbott Lab, Abbott Park. [Abstract] 8th International Conference on AIDS III SPD World Conference, Amsterdam, Netherlands, July 19–24, 1992

78 **Dautzenberg B, Truffot C, Legris S, et al.** Activity of clarithromycin against *Mycobacterium avium* infection in patients with the acquired immune deficiency syndrome. *Am Rev Respir Dis* 1991;144:564–569.

79 **Dautzenberg B, Saint Marc T, Chauvin J-P, Hazebroucq J.** Clarithromycin in AIDS patients with disseminated *M. avium* infection. Presented at the First International Conference on the Macrolides, Azalides, and Streptogramins, Santa Fe, New Mexico, January 22–25 1992.

80 **Loss S, Watson D, Nightingale S, Peterson D, Cal S.** The safety and efficacy of clarithromycin in the therapy of disseminated *Mycobacterium Avium* complex infection in AIDS patients. Presented at the First International Conference on the Macrolides, Azalides, and Streptogramins, Santa Fe, New Mexico, January 22–25 1992.

81 **Young LS, Wiviott L, Wu M, Kolonoski P, Bolan R, Inderlied C.** Azithromycin for treatment of *Mycobacterium avium-intracellulare* complex infection in patients with AIDS. *Lancet* 1991;338:1107–1109.

82 Erythromycin Product Information (package insert).

83 **Pichichero M, Margolis P.** A comparison of cephalosporins and penicillins in the treatment of Group A beta-hemolytic streptococcal pharyngitis: a meta-analysis supporting the concept of microbial copathogenicity. *Pediatr Infect Dis J* 1991;10:275–281.

Biologic and geographic factors in prevention and treatment of malaria

GODFRED L. MASINDE
DONALD J. KROGSTAD

INTRODUCTION

Incidence of malaria

Approximately half the world's population lives in malaria-endemic areas. The world-wide incidence of malaria (estimated at 200–300 million cases per year) is difficult to calculate precisely because many cases are undiagnosed and therefore unreported. Whatever the precise figure, 200 to 300 million is likely a substantial underestimate. In Nigeria alone, there are 100 million people who typically have several episodes of malaria each year. However, a high incidence of malaria is not new. As evidenced by sickle-cell disease, the incidence of malaria has been great enough for millenia that malaria has been (and continues to be) a significant force in human evolution. Despite that fact that sickle homozygotes have a fitness (survival) close to zero, selection for the protection of sickle heterozygotes against malaria has been strong enough that prevalence of the sickle hemoglobin gene is 25% to 35% in many parts of sub-Saharan Africa.

Definitions

Hypoendemic Malaria. Areas where there is little malaria transmission with parasite rates less than 10% among children 2–9 years of age.
Mesoendemic Malaria. Variable transmission and variable effects in rural subtropical communities, with parasite rates of 11–50% among children 2–9 years of age.
Hyperendemic Malaria. Intense but seasonal transmission, with parasite rates consistently greater than 50% among children from 2–9. Immunity among the population is insufficient to prevent the occurrence of malaria and its morbidity among all age groups.
Holoendemic Malaria. Intense perennial transmission as evidenced by parasite rates greater than 75% among infants, with considerable immunity to infection (and infrequent disease) among adults.

Estimated malaria mortality

Most malaria mortality is due to *Plasmodium falciparum* infection among children less than 5 years old in sub-Saharan Africa. Recent estimates of this mortality range from 1 to 2 million children per year, with a minimum of 1 million (1). Thus, malaria is a disease with an overwhelming worldwide impact on health in the developing world, which also affects expatriate travelers to the tropics.

Effects of malaria on expatriate versus indigenous populations

This chapter is targeted primarily to physicians who care for expatriate travelers. Because the effects of malaria are markedly different in expatriate (vs indigenous) populations, an appreciation of these differences is essential to understand current strategies for malaria prevention and control.

Malaria in the nonimmune host   In nonimmune expatriates, malaria may be a rapidly lethal infection. Parasites (*P. falciparum*) that invade red cells of all ages can multiply from low to high life-threatening parasitemias (from 1,000 to $\geq 100,000$ parasites/μL blood) within 2 cycles of replication (96 hr). Therefore, the goal of chemoprophylaxis in expatriate travelers is to prevent bloodstream infection.

Prevention of disease in indigenous populations   In contrast, because parasite replication is slower in the semi-immune host, time is a less critical factor in the diagnosis and treatment of malaria among semi-immune indigenous populations. Prevention of infection is currently an unrealistic goal for indigenous populations, who are often exposed to more than 100 infective anopheline bites per person per year (2) and cannot receive chemoprophylaxis indefinitely. For these reasons, most malaria control programs concentrate on preventing complications and deaths by treating persons with symptomatic infection, and restrict chemoprophylaxis to persons at increased risk of complications and death, such as pregnant women and young children.

BIOLOGIC FACTORS

Life cycle

For a common disease, the malaria life cycle (Figure 4.1) is complicated and potentially vulnerable. Yet, despite its apparent vulnerability, malaria transmission persists and has been difficult or impossible to eradicate in most endemic areas.

Human reservoir   Infected persons with gametocytes in their peripheral blood are essential for transmission from humans to anopheline mosquitoes. In endemic areas, asymptomatic semi-immune persons often have low numbers of asexual parasites with similar or higher numbers of gametocytes. This observation may explain the intense malaria transmission observed in areas with large numbers of semi-immune persons who

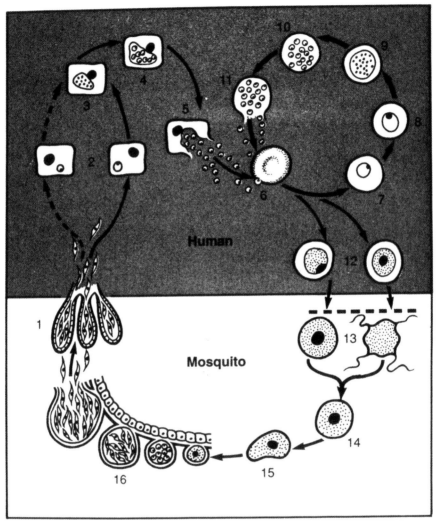

Figure 4.1 Malaria life cycle. Sporozoites released from the salivary gland of the female *Anopheles* mosquito are injected under the skin when the mosquito bites a human (*1*). They then travel through the bloodstream and enter the liver (*2*). Within liver cells, the parasites mature to tissue schizonts (*4*). They are then released into the bloodstream as merozoites (*5*) and produce symptomatic infection as they invade and destroy red blood cells (*RBCs*). However, some parasites remain dormant in the liver as hypnozoites (*2, dashed lines from 1–3*). These parasites (in *P. vivax, P. ovale*) cause relapsing malaria. Once within the bloodstream, merozoites (*5*) invade RBCs (*6*) and mature to the ring (*7, 8*), trophozoite (*9*), and schizont (*10*) asexual stages. Schizonts lyse their host RBCs as they complete their maturation and release the next generation of merozoites (*11*), which invade previously uninfected RBCs. Within RBCs, some parasites

have low or undetectable numbers of asexual parasites in their peripheral blood. This pattern contrasts markedly with infection in nonimmune hosts, who typically have large numbers of asexual parasites with few if any gametocytes because the time required to produce gametocytes (8–10 days) is considerably longer than the asexual cycle (2–3 days). As a result, most nonimmune expatriates become ill and seek medical attention before they have significant numbers of gametocytes in their peripheral blood. These observations suggest that 1) low-level bloodstream infection in asymptomatic semi-immune persons is an important factor in endemic malaria transmission, and 2) waiting for the appearance of characteristic banana-shaped gametocytes to diagnose *P. falciparum* infection is a potentially fatal mistake.

Meiotic (reduction) division in the mosquito　Malaria parasites that circulate in the bloodstream are haploid. In the mosquito, male and female (haploid) gametocytes mature to gametes and fuse to form a diploid ookinete, which undergoes meiosis and ultimately forms the haploid sporozoites, which migrate to the mosquito salivary gland and complete the cycle by infecting humans. Recent studies indicate that large numbers of crossovers occur during this reduction division (3) and suggest that these crossovers are essential in maintaining genetic variability, thus permitting the parasite to adapt to changing conditions.

Environmental factors　Parasite maturation from gametocyte to sporozoite in the mosquito proceeds more rapidly at higher temperatures, although mosquito survival paradoxically decreases under the same conditions. Thus, malaria transmission is a complex function that is simultaneously enhanced and inhibited by environmental factors such as temperature.

Entry and hepatocyte infection in the human host　Haploid sporozoites injected under the skin by female anopheline mosquitos travel through the lymphatics or the bloodstream to the liver, where they invade hepatocytes via a receptor that binds the predominant protein on the sporozoite surface (circumsporozoite protein [CSP]) (4). In the hepatocyte, most sporozoites mature to tissue schizonts containing 10,000 to

---

differentiate to sexual forms (male and female gametocytes, *12*). When these are taken up by a female *Anopheles* mosquito, the male gametocyte loses its flagellum to produce male gametes, which fertilize the female gamete (*13*) to produce a zygote (*14*). The zygote invades the gut of the mosquito (*15*) and develops into an oocyst (*16*). Mature oocysts produce sporozoites, which migrate to the salivary gland of the mosquito (*1*) and repeat the cycle. The *dashed line* between *12* and *13* indicates that absence of the mosquito vector precludes natural transmission via this cycle. Note that infection by the injection of infected blood bypasses this constraint and permits transmission of malaria among intravenous drug addicts and to persons who receive blood transfusions from infected donors.

30,000 merozoites, each of which is capable of invading a red cell and establishing the asexual erythrocytic cycle. In relapsing malarias, some of the sporozoites that invade hepatocytes become hypnozoites, which remain dormant for 6 to 11 months before they mature to tissue schizonts and release merozoites, which invade red cells and thus produce symptomatic asexual parasitemias. Hypnozoites cause relapse (or delayed primary infection in persons receiving chemoprophylaxis) (5). They are found in P. *vivax* and P. *ovale* infections (the relapsing human malarias) but not in either P. *falciparum* or P. *malariae* infections (nonrelapsing human malarias).

Asexual erythrocytic stages in the bloodstream Symptomatic human infection results from asexual erythrocytic parasites in the blood. Neither gametocytes nor sporozoites produce recognizable symptoms or signs. Particularly in nonimmune hosts, the magnitude of the asexual parasitemia is related to the risk of morbidity (e.g., cerebral malaria, renal failure) and death (6). In contrast, semi-immune persons with similar parasitemias may be either ambulatory or comatose. Thus, it is clear that there are important factors other than the magnitude of the parasitemia which determine clinical outcome. Although these factors have not yet been identified, cytokines such as tumor necrosis factor-alpha (INF-α) may have important roles in the pathogenesis of severe and complicated malaria (7).

Antigenic differences among parasite stages The differences among parasite stages in the life cycle (see Figure 4.1) are not restricted to morphology. The predominant surface antigens also vary among these stages (e.g., antibodies directed against CSP, which neutralize sporozoites have no effect on either asexual erythrocytic or gametocyte-stage parasites).

Parasite determinants of the outcome of infection

Species of the infecting parasite The ability of a parasite to invade red blood cells is determined by its species. P. *falciparum* merozoites invade red cells of all ages and can thus produce overwhelming parasitemias; P. *vivax* and P. *ovale* are restricted to invading young red cells (reticulocytes) and thus to parasitemias less than 50,000/μL in persons with normal numbers of reticulocytes; P. *malariae* preferentially invades older red cells and is thus restricted to parasitemias 10,000/μL or less (8). Because the risk of death is proportional to the magnitude of the asexual parasitemia (6), the ability to invade large numbers of red cells is a virulence factor. Although other virulence factors undoubtedly exist, they have not yet been identified, in part because there are no model systems with which to test for them.

Drug resistance The number of antimalarial drugs is limited, and alternatives to chloroquine are often expensive. Although semi-immune persons may clear infections due to resistant parasites after treatment with chloroquine alone, this response rarely if ever occurs in nonimmune expatriates. Thus, antimalarial resistance to chloroquine, pyrimethamine, Fansidar, and quinine has increased malaria morbidity and mortality among both expatriates and lifelong residents of endemic areas.

Mechanism of chloroquine resistance   Thus far, every chloroquine-resistant strain of *P. falciparum* examined has demonstrated rapid chloroquine efflux (i.e., an initial chloroquine efflux half-time of approximately 2 min vs $\geq$50–75 min for susceptible strains) (10–12). Studies of natural isolates and cloned progeny from a genetic cross indicate that rapid efflux and chloroquine resistance are produced by the same gene, or are so closely linked that they cannot be separated from one another in the genetic cross (3). On the basis of these observations, a rapid diagnostic test has been developed to determine whether a *P. falciparum* isolate is chloroquine-resistant within 2 to 3 hours (13). The efflux responsible for chloroquine resistance is an adenosine triphosphate–dependent process phenotypically similar to the efflux of carcinogens and mutagens associated with the mammalian multidrug-resistance (*mdr*) gene (14). Despite this phenotypic similarity, chloroquine resistance in *P. falciparum* is not linked genetically to either of the *mdr*-like genes present in the parasite (3).

Partial resistance to quinine and quinidine   For reasons that are not clear, *P. falciparum* strains resistant to quinine and quinidine *in vitro* (based on a high IC_{50}) are typically only partially resistant to quinine and quinidine *in vivo*. In contrast, virtually all strains resistance to chloroquine *in vitro* are also resistant to chloroquine *in vivo*. Although *P. falciparum* strains resistant to chloroquine on the basis of rapid chloroquine efflux also demonstrate rapid quinine and quinidine efflux (15), rapid quinine and quinidine efflux are not linked to quinine and quinidine resistance in the same way that rapid chloroquine efflux is linked to chloroquine resistance (Table 4.1). Parasites with rapid quinine and quinidine efflux half-times have a range of quinine and quinidine IC_{50}, as do parasites with prolonged quinine and quinidine efflux half-times. Thus, a minimum of 1 additional genetic locus (in addition to the locus responsible for chloroquine resistance) must be involved in quinine and quinidine resistance (15).

Pyrimethamine resistance   In contrast to chloroquine resistance, the mechanism responsible for pyrimethamine resistance is reduced drug binding by the enzyme target site (dihydrofolate reductase [DHFR]) (16). There is no evidence for enzymatic modification or rapid efflux of pyrimethamine from resistant parasites. Nucleic acid sequencing of DHFR genes from resistant *P. falciparum* has demonstrated several point mutations at the pyrimethamine binding site, which presumably interfere with the binding of pyrimethamine to the enzyme. Recent studies using the polymerase chain reaction (PCR) suggest that similar point mutations are associated with pyrimethamine resistance in malaria-endemic areas, such as the Amazon River basin of Brazil (17).

***Chloroquine resistance in* Plasmodium vivax**   *P. vivax* is the most common cause of malaria worldwide, but, in contrast to *P. falciparum*, it has always been susceptible to chloroquine. However, in the last several years, there have been several reports of *P. vivax* infections resistant to chloroquine (18–20). These reports from Papua, New Guinea, Indonesia, and Brazil suggest that *P. vivax* infection may develop in persons receiving chloroquine chemoprophylaxis in those areas. Thus far, these infections have responded to treatment with oral mefloquine. The biologic basis of this resistance is not

Table 4.1 Drug efflux and drug resistance in *Plasmodium falciparum*

Chloroquine	
Short efflux half-time (approximately 2 min)	Chloroquine–resistant
Prolonged efflux half-times ($\geq$ 50–70 min)	Chloroquine-susceptible
Quinine*	
Short efflux half-times (1–3 min)	Variable susceptibility
Prolonged efflux half-times ($\geq$ 30 min)	Variable susceptibility

*Similar patterns were observed with quinidine.

clear (i.e., it is not clear whether these parasites have a chloroquine efflux mechanism similar to that observed in resistant *P. falciparum*).

Resistance to other antimalarials The mechanisms responsible for resistance to mefloquine and halofantrine have not been defined. However, recent experience in Thailand suggests that most strains resistant to mefloquine *in vivo* are also resistant to halofantrine; thus, their mechanisms of resistance may be similar. Limited studies with radiolabeled mefloquine have not revealed evidence of efflux in mefloquine-resistant strains of *P. falciparum*.

Intrinsic host factors that affect the outcome of infection

Plasmodium falciparum Genetic and epidemiologic studies have shown that genes which protect against severe *P. falciparum* infection are more common in areas where *P. falciparum* infection is endemic. Sickle-cell disease, as noted, protects against complications and death from *P. falciparum* infection and is common in the malarious regions of sub-Saharan Africa. Sickle-cell hemoglobin restricts parasite replication under conditions of low oxygenation, such as those found in the peripheral capillaries and venules, where mature *P. falciparum* parasites sequester *in vivo* (21). Glucose-6-phosphate dehydrogenase (G6PD) deficiency also protects against severe *P. falciparum* infection by restricting parasite replication (22,23).

   P. vivax is a less powerful selective force than *P. falciparum* because it produces fewer deaths and less morbidity. Nevertheless, there are important genetic factors in its distribution. Duffy factor is an antigenic determinant on the red blood cells of Caucasians that is absent from the red cells of most Africans, and correlates with red cell susceptibility to invasion by *P. vivax* (24,25). For this reason, *P. vivax* infection is extremely rare in African populations. In sub-Saharan Africa, the most common relapsing malaria is *P. ovale*, which does not require Duffy factor for red cell invasion.

Acquired host factors that affect the outcome of infection

Although several acquired host factors affect the outcome of malaria, repeated natural infections do not produce immunity (i.e., protection against infection and disease).

Thus, it is not yet clear what factors are required for protective immunity against malaria or whether those factors can be produced by either natural infection or immunization (i.e., a malaria vaccine).

Humoral immune response   Natural infection produces antibodies against many parasite antigens, including potentially protective antibodies directed against antigens such as CSP, merozoite surface protein-1 (MSP-1), and Pfs25, a gametocyte antigen (26). Thus far, protective humoral immunity has been produced in humans only by immunization with irradiated sporozoites, which is not practical for large numbers of persons in malaria-endemic areas.

Cellular immunity   Although helper (CD4+) and cytotoxic (CD8+) T cells are produced during natural infection, it is not yet clear whether T cells reactive against species-specific or strain-specific antigens can produce protective immunity in humans. Because the development of reactive T cells against some parasite antigens is immune-restricted, and thus dependent on the human leukocyte antigen type of the host, the ability of such antigens (including CSP) to protect against malaria may vary within and among populations (27).

The spleen   In malaria, the spleen provides a significant reservoir of sensitized lymphocytes. It also removes parasitized red cells because of their reduced deformability (which does not permit them to pass through the red pulp) and because of macrophages in the white pulp. The uncontrolled *P. falciparum* parasitemias observed in splenectomized persons provide *in vivo* support for the critical role of the spleen in protection against malaria.

Effects of cytokines   Cytokines such as TNF-α, interferon-gamma (IFN-γ) and interleukin-6 (IL-6) are increased in malaria. These cytokines may increase the number of receptors available for cytoadherence by parasitized red cells and may also exacerbate the consequences of malaria infection (e.g., via the known hypotensive effects of TNF-α). However, the significance of these observations is currently unclear. For example, it is not clear whether monoclonal antibodies to TNF-α will prevent complications or death due to *P. falciparum* infection.

GEOGRAPHIC FACTORS

Distribution of malaria parasite species

In this section, we consider the current status of malaria and its local (national) and regional (international) distribution (Table 4.2). The 4 malaria parasites that infect humans are *P. falciparum, P. vivax, P. ovale,* and *P. malariae. P. vivax* is the predominant malaria parasite in most parts of the world. It is found virtually everywhere malaria is endemic and is the only human malaria parasite with a range that extends into the temperate regions. *P. falciparum* is limited to the tropics and the subtropics. *P. ovale* is

Table 4.2 Distribution of plasmodial species infecting humans

Species	Distribution
Plasmodium vivax	Cosmopolitan (most common malaria), extending into temperate zones
Plasmodium falciparum	Cosmopolitan, mainly tropical and subtropical
Plasmodium ovale	Worldwide with a patchy distribution, primarily in West Africa
Plasmodium malariae	Cosmopolitan with a patchy distribution

widely distributed in tropical Africa and supplants *P. vivax* almost entirely in West Africa because that population is Duffy factor–negative. *P. ovale* also occurs in Southeast Asia and in South America (28,29). *P. malariae* occurs primarily in subtropical and temperate areas, where other species of malaria are also found, but is less prevalent than *P. vivax* or *P. falciparum*.

Africa The most intense transmission and the greatest prevalence of malaria in the world occur in sub-Saharan Africa. Although transmission occurs throughout the year in most malaria-endemic areas of Africa, seasonal rains and years with heavy rainfall markedly increase malaria transmission in sub-Saharan countries such as Burundi, Botswana, Kenya, Madagasgar, Rwanda, Swaziland, Zaire, and Zambia (30).

Northern Africa In Morocco, transmission of *P. vivax* occurs primarily in the provinces of Kenitra and Sidi Kasem, near Rabat. In Algeria, the foci of transmission and disease are in rural areas on the Mediterranean coast and in the Wilaya of Adrar Oasis in southern Algeria (31). The number of cases reported has remained stable in recent years, with 839 in 1990 and 830 in 1989 (32).

Tunisia and Libya are almost free of malaria, although *P. falciparum* transmission has been reported at the Oasis of Ghat in southern Libya. In Egypt, malaria is more widespread; *P. vivax* malaria transmission has been reported in the Nile Delta, in El Faiyum on the banks of the Nile, in Bitter Lake areas of the Suez Canal, and in some oases in southern Egypt (33). The overall incidence of malaria in Egypt may be decreasing; 192 cases were reported in 1989 and 75 in 1990 (32).

The Horn of Africa Malaria transmission is spotty in the horn of Africa. Most transmission occurs in Djibouti, in eastern Ethiopia, and in Somalia, east of Brava. In these areas, malaria is usually caused by *P. falciparum*, although *P. malariae* and *P. vivax* also occur (34).

Southern Africa There is no known malaria transmission in southern Africa, except for Swaziland and the northern Transvaal. Although malaria had been eradicated from the Indian Ocean islands of Reunion and Mauritius, *P. vivax* transmission has been reestablished recently in Mauritius and is now present throughout the main island. There were 700 malaria cases reported in 1982 and 296 in 1983, with a scattered distribution (33).

Malaria has been eradicated from most of the Cape Verde Islands, although transmission persists on Maio and Santiago in the Sotavento Islands. On the islands of Sao Tome e Principe, malaria is mesoendemic to hyperendemic. Although P. *falciparum* is predominant, all 4 species of human plasmodia are present (28).

Tropical (sub-Saharan) Africa   Tropical (sub-Saharan) Africa is the area most affected by malaria. Transmission typically occurs throughout the year, and the prevalence of infection exceeds 50% among children 0 to 5 years of age in many regions. Malaria transmission is hyperendemic or holoendemic in most of sub-Saharan Africa. One major reason for the intensity of transmission in sub-Saharan Africa is the efficient anopheline vectors that are present: *Anopheles arabiensis*, A. *funestus*, and A. *gambiae*. Malaria is the principal cause of death among infants and small children in sub-Saharan Africa; it kills up to 25% of live-born children before age 5.

West Africa   Although transmission occurs throughout the year, malaria transmission is less intense in West Africa during the dry season in Mauritania, Senegal, The Gambia, Mali, Guinea-Bissau, Cote d'Ivoire (Ivory Coast), Burkina Faso, Niger, and Chad. Year-round transmission occurs in Ghana, Togo, Benin, and Nigeria, although transmission may also be seasonal in these countries. Most malaria in West Africa is due to P. *falciparum*, although P. *malariae* and P. *ovale* are also present (34).

Central Africa   Malaria transmission is holoendemic with transmission throughout the year in Cameroon, Equatorial Guinea, Gabon, Angola, Congo, Zaire, and the Central African Republic. In order of importance, the human malaria parasites in this region are P. *falciparum*, P. *malariae*, P. *vivax*, and P. *ovale* (35).

Central Southern Africa   Malaria transmission is typically hyperendemic in central southern Africa, which includes Namibia, Botswana, Zimbabwe, and Mozambique. In Botswana, hyperendemic transmission is restricted to the Okavango River basin. In other areas of Botswana and Namibia, epidemics may occur because transmission is mesoendemic or hypoendemic (28).

East Africa   Malaria is mesoendemic to hyperendemic with year-round transmission in the East African countries of Zambia, Malawi, Tanzania, Kenya, Uganda, Sudan, Rwanda, Burundi, Madagascar, and Comoros. In descending order of importance, the parasites responsible for human malaria in this region are P. *falciparum*, P. *malariae*, and P. *ovale* (36).

The Americas   In 1974, there were only 26,900 malaria cases reported from the Americas, for an annual incidence of 1.34 per 1,000 population in the malarious areas of the Americas. Since that time, the number of cases has been increasing steadily: 111,400 cases were reported in 1989 and 1,057,000 in 1990. Although more than half the cases have been reported from Brazil, where P. *falciparum* infection is common (30), P. *vivax* predominates in the rest of the Americas (67% of infections).

Central America   The 7 countries that make up Central America are Belize, Guatemala, El Salvador, Honduras, Panama, Nicaragua, and Costa Rica. In Belize and Guatemala, malaria incidence is high. The prevalence of malaria has decreased in Nicaragua, Honduras, and El Salvador, although transmission persists. Panama has reported the lowest number of malaria cases, and most cases in Costa Rica are imported. *P. vivax* causes most malaria in Central America, although *P. falciparum* infection also occurs (32).

The Caribbean   In the Caribbean, malaria is now endemic only on the Island of Hispaniola, although transmission occurred previously on most Caribbean Islands except the Bahamas and the Netherlands Antilles. Malaria transmission occurs at varying intensities in different areas of the Dominican Republic and Haiti. *P. falciparum* is the predominant species in both countries, although *P. malariae* also occurs in Haiti (28).

Northern South America, including the Amazon Basin   On the northern coast of South America, Venezuela and Guyana have eradicated malaria. Although French Guiana had eradicated malaria, transmission has now returned and has become endemic again. Suriname has reduced the prevalence of malaria. Although *P. falciparum* has been the predominant species in this region, *P. vivax* is also present and is increasing (37). From 1986 to 1990, the proportion of malaria cases due to *P. falciparum* decreased from 55% to 45%. Approximately 99% of *P. falciparum* cases are from the Amazon region (particularly Brazil), where there are frontier settlements associated with economic development such as forest clearing followed by subsistence agriculture and mining in previously inaccessible areas (30). Of the original 7 million km^2 of malarious areas in Brazil, 5 million are in the Amazon region.

East Central South America   Malaria transmission remains endemic in most of Brazil, except the coastal areas and the states of Sergipe, Espirito Santo, and Rio de Janeiro, where it has been eliminated or greatly reduced. Similar progress has been made in parts of Maranhão, Piani, Goiàs, and the Federal District of Brasilia. Transmission occurs throughout the year in Brazil. *P. vivax* predominates in eastern Brazil, and *P. falciparum* predominates in western Brazil (32).

South America (southern cone or tip)   In this region, which contains Argentina, Chile, Paraguay, and Uruguay, malaria is endemic only in Paraguay and in northern Argentina. All 4 species of human malaria parasites are found, although *P. ovale* is least common. The immigration of infected persons from southern Brazil into Paraguay is a major factor in this region. In Argentina, the incidence of malaria has remained stable; 1,660 cases were reported in 1990, and 1,620 in 1989. In Paraguay, vector control measures reduced the incidence of malaria from 5,200 cases in 1989 to 1,700 in 1990 (32).

Asia   All 4 human malaria species are present in Asia, although *P. ovale* transmission is restricted to isolated foci.

Near East (Southwestern Asia)   In Turkey, malaria has been eliminated from all but a few areas. Although *P. falciparum* was the predominant parasite before the onset of control activities, *P. vivax* malaria is now the only parasite found in indigenous patients. In Iraq, most malaria transmission is now due to *P. vivax* in the north. Malaria control activities have significantly reduced the transmission of *P. falciparum* in the region around Basra in the south.

In the United Arab Emirates, low malaria risk zones extend from the Al Ain District of Abu Dhabi to Oman and along the coast from Abu Dhabi to Umm Al Qawain. There are high malaria risk zones in the Emirates of Ras Al Khaimah and Fujeirah, the eastern region on the Gulf of Oman and the foothills of the central plateau. Most malaria cases are due to *P. vivax*; *P. falciparum* accounts for only 24% of cases (33).

In Saudi Arabia, *P. falciparum* is the dominant species; it accounts for 65% to 100% of infections, *P. malariae* for up to 31.5%, and *P. vivax* for up to 17% (28).

In the Yemen Arab Republic, malaria transmission is year-round, although there is marked variability in the intensity of transmission, with hypoendemic, mesoendemic, and hyperendemic areas. *P. falciparum* is the predominant species, although *P. malariae* and *P. vivax* are also present (30). In Democratic Yemen, the prevalence of infection may be as high as 18%. Most infections (>90%) are due to *P. falciparum*; approximately 4% are due to *P. malariae*, and approximately 1% are due to *P. vivax* (28).

Middle South Asia   The northwestern border of this region is Iran, the southeastern border is Burma. In Iran, the reported number of malaria cases increased from 53,000 to 77,000 between 1988 and 1990. *P. vivax* is the predominant species in the north, and *P. falciparum* is the predominant species in the south (28,32).

Malaria transmission occurs in all parts of Afghanistan and may be hyperendemic. *P. malariae* and *P. vivax* are the predominant species; *P. falciparum* is uncommon (<1%) (28,30).

In Pakistan, malaria epidemics often occur at 8-year intervals. The predominant species in Pakistan are *P. falciparum* (which has been increasing) and *P. vivax* (32).

Most of the 1.8 to 2.0 million malaria cases reported annually in India are indigenous, although some are imported. *P. vivax* is the predominant species, although *P. falciparum* also occurs (28). Significant *P. falciparum* transmission occurs in eastern India along the border with Myanmar (Burma).

There is malaria transmission in Nepal, especially along its border with India. Transmission occurs almost entirely below 1,400 m and is due to *P. vivax* (92%), *P. falciparum* (approximately 6%), and *P. malariae* (approximately 2%). The malaria situation in Nepal has remained relatively stable; 23,000 cases were reported annually in 1989 and 1990. However, the incidence of *P. falciparum* infections has declined, from 7,500 (1985) to 2,300 (1989) and 1,500 (1990) (32). In Bhutan, east of Nepal, malaria transmission is limited to the subtropical southern part of the country. The most prevalent parasites are *P. falciparum* and *P. vivax* (32).

Malaria transmission occurs year round and throughout the country in Bangladesh. The predominant parasites are *P. falciparum* (approximately 65%) and *P. vivax* (approximately 35%), with rare *P. malariae* infections (28,32).

Southeast Asia   Malaria is endemic in Myanmar. The predominant species is *P. falciparum*; *P. vivax* and *P. malariae* are significantly less common (33).

In Thailand, the number of malaria cases has decreased consistently during the last 10 to 20 years. Most cases now occur in refugee camps or other areas where nonimmune persons (e.g., refugees from nonendemic areas) come into contact with the sylvatic vector *Anopheles dirus* for the first time. The predominant species in Thailand is *P. falciparum*; the other major species is *P. vivax*, and *P. malariae* infection is rare (<1%) (32).

In Vietnam, malaria transmission is hypoendemic; the predominant parasite species is *P. falciparum*, followed in order of importance by *P. vivax* and *P. malariae* (28).

In Indonesia, there are 25,000 to 32,000 reported cases per year. The predominant parasite species are *P. vivax* and *P. falciparum*; few cases are caused by *P. malariae* (28,32).

In China, malaria is transmitted in many areas of the country. Although limited data are available, most infections are due to *P. vivax* or *P. falciparum*; relatively few are due to *P. malariae* (28). Drug-resistant *P. falciparum* infections are endemic in the southern region of China, which borders Myanmar, Thailand, Laos, and Vietnam.

In the Philippines, most malaria is caused by either *P. falciparum* (which is predominant) or *P. vivax* (32).

Intensity of malaria transmission

Female mosquitoes inadvertently ingest malaria parasites when they take blood meals required for maturation of their eggs. Subsequent transmission of malaria from these infected mosquitoes to humans depends on the sporozoite rate: the proportion of female anopheline mosquitoes with infectious sporozoites in their salivary glands. Factors that affect the sporozoite rate include susceptibility of the vector to parasite infection and replication, vector population density, feeding habits, longevity, and the duration of the extrinsic incubation period (temperature) (38). For example, warm weather shortens the extrinsic incubation period required for parasite maturation in the mosquito. Paradoxically, warm weather also shortens the mosquito lifespan, thus decreasing the probability that an infected mosquito will live long enough to take a second blood meal with infectious sporozoites in her salivary gland and transmit malaria.

Anopheles gambiae complex mosquitoes are the most efficient vectors of malaria known and have been studied in considerable detail. In Cameroon, densities of the principal vector *Anopheles nili Theobald* are related to the river level (i.e., vector populations increase with flooding, which creates many mosquito breeding sites). In Cameroon, the malaria innoculation rate due to A. *nili* is approximately 104 infective bites/person/year. On the basis of these criteria, *Anopheles gambiae Giles* is a less important vector (39). Sporozoite rates and the intensity of transmission have also been studied in Madagascar, where mosquitoes of the *Anopheles gambiae* complex are the principal vectors. Those studies have shown that *Anopheles gambiae* is highly anthropophilic (i.e., preferentially bites humans rather than animals) and exophilic (i.e., preferentially bites outside of houses) (40). The malaria inoculation rate is approximately 100 infective bites/person/year. In Kenya, the majority of anopheline vectors transmitting malaria are from the *Anopheles gambiae* complex (38). Sporozoite rates range from 4% to 18%, and malaria inoculation rates range from 10 to 100 infective bites/person/year.

Distribution of drug resistance

Drug resistance is the ability of a parasite to grow and multiply in the presence of antimalarial concentrations that normally inhibit parasite growth *in vivo*. Resistance is best demonstrated *in vitro* with parasites that grow in the culture system developed by Trager and Jensen for *P. falciparum* (41).

Chloroquine-resistant strains of *P. falciparum* have been identified in most countries with *P. falciparum* transmission except Haiti, the Dominican Republic, Central America north of the Panama Canal, and the Middle East and Egypt. Resistance to chloroquine and Fansidar is widespread in Thailand, Myanmar, Cambodia, sub-Saharan Africa, and the Amazon River basin in South America (42–46).

Chloroquine-resistant *P. falciparum*
South America   Chloroquine-resistant strains of *P. falciparum* were first reported from Venezuela in 1960. They subsequently spread to other countries in the Americas, including Bolivia, Brazil, Colombia, Ecuador, French Guiana, Guiana, Peru, and Suriname.

Southeast Asia   Chloroquine-resistant *P. falciparum* appeared in Southeast Asia at the beginning of the 1960s and were first reported from Thailand (47). Asian countries now known to have chloroquine-resistant *P. falciparum* include Afghanistan, Bangladesh, Bhutan, Cambodia, China, India, Indonesia, Iran, Laos, Malaysia, Myanmar (Burma), Nepal, Oman, Pakistan, Papua New Guinea, the Philippines, the Solomon Islands, Sri Lanka, Thailand, Vanuatu, Vietnam, and Yemen.

Africa   Chloroquine-resistant strains of *P. falciparum* were first reported from Africa 10 to 20 years later in 1977. African countries now affected include Angola, Benin, Botswana, Burkina Faso, Burundi, Cameroon, the Central African Republic, Chad, Comoros, Congo, Cote d'Ivoire, Djibouti, Equatorial Guinea, Ethiopia, Gabon, The Gambia, Ghana, Guinea, Guinea Bissau, Kenya, Liberia, Madagascar, Malawi, Mali, Mozambique, Namibia, Niger, Nigeria, Rwanda, Senegal, Siera Leone, Somalia, South Africa, Sudan, Swaziland, Tanzania, Togo, Uganda, Zaire, Zambia, and Zimbabwe (48).

Patterns in the development of chloroquine resistance
There are several important differences between the spread of chloroquine resistance (CQ^r) in South America versus Southeast Asia and Africa (49). In South America, chloroquine-resistant *P. falciparum* were reported simultaneously from several different sites. Conversely, in Southeast Asia, chloroquine-resistant *P. falciparum* strains were initially confined to a small area of the Indian subcontinent (Thailand, Vietnam, Laos, Kampuchea). Subsequently, chloroquine-resistant strains of *P. falciparum* spread east and west, reaching

their present distribution in approximately 1985. In Africa, chloroquine resistance spread from east to west contiguously similar to that observed in Southeast Asia (43).

The similarity in the spread of chloroquine resistance between South America and Southeast Asia is that resistance appeared on both continents during massive chloroquine distribution programs that were part of the unsuccessful global effort to eradicate malaria. Although massive malaria eradication programs were not present in Africa during the 1970s and 1980s, large-scale chloroquine chemoprophylaxis was being used to reduce maternal and child mortality in several countries.

Sulfadoxine/pyrimethamine (fansidar) resistance   Resistance to the sulfadoxine/pyrimethamine combination (Fansidar) has been reported in areas where this combination was used on a large scale for either chemoprophylaxis or treatment. Fansidar resistance was first reported from the Thai-Cambodian border in the 1980s (50,51) and has been an important limiting factor in the prevention and treatment of *P. falciparum* infections since that time. Currently, the majority of *P. falciparum* infections on the Indian subcontinent are Fansidar-resistant. The situation is similar in many areas of South America, where chloroquine-resistant *P. falciparum* are often also Fansidar-resistant. This is a particularly severe problem in the Amazon River basin regions of Brazil and Colombia, although it developed less rapidly there than in Southeast Asia (52). (This association is consistent with drug selection *in vivo* in areas where CQ^r and Fansidar-resistant strains of *P. falciparum* are present. It does not require that CQ^r and Fansidar resistance be genetically linked to one another, for which there is no experimental evidence.) In contrast, there are only a few reported cases of Fansidar resistance from sub-Saharan African countries. Although some of these cases were due to abnormalities in drug absorption, metabolism, or elimination rather than intrinsic drug resistance (43), *in vitro* evidence for pyrimethamine resistance (Pyr^r) has now been reported from several African countries that had previously reported *P. falciparum* strains resistant to Fansidar *in vivo*.

Quinine (Qn^r) and quinidine (Qd^r) resistance   Quinine (and quinidine) resistance first received widespread attention when quinine was used to treat CQ^r and Fansidar-resistant *P. falciparum* infections in Laos and Vietnam. Quinine resistance was subsequently confirmed in Thailand in 1984 (44), and 82% or more of *P. falciparum* infections in Vietnam (52) and Cambodia (53,54) have been reported to be Qn^r or Qd^r. Qn^r has also been reported from the Solomon islands and Vanuatu (55,56). Thus far, Qn^r and Qd^r have been limited to Indochina and to islands in the western Pacific. There have not yet been reports of Qn^r or Qd^r from sub-Saharan Africa.

Mefloquine resistance   Resistance of *P. falciparum* to treatment with mefloquine at the recommended dosage was first reported from Thailand in 1982. The current situation in Thailand is that mefloquine failures are common (43). Work by Oduola and colleagues (45) has shown relatively low sensitivity of natural *P. falciparum* isolates to mefloquine as judged by the IC_{50} values for inhibition of parasite growth *in vitro*. Despite the fact that mefloquine resistance is a major problem in Thailand, where 50%

of *P. falciparum* infections no longer respond in many areas, mefloquine remains an important drug for CQ^r *P. falciparum* malaria in other areas of the world.

PREVENTION OF MALARIA

All individuals traveling to endemic areas should be counseled about malaria. Recommendations for prevention of malaria, including chemoprophylaxis regimens, should be individualized after reviewing each traveler's medical history for allergies and other drug reactions. All travelers should be informed that they will be at risk for malaria, regardless of the drugs employed, and that symptoms of malaria may develop as soon as 8 days after exposure, or as long as months after their return. Travelers to areas with *P. falciparum* should be informed that malaria can be treated effectively early in the course of the disease but may have serious or fatal complications if diagnosis and treatment are delayed.

Malaria chemoprophylaxis should begin 1 to 2 weeks before travel to malaria-endemic areas to allow for detection of side effects and for development of alternative regimens before departure, if necessary. This strategy also ensures adequate drug levels in the blood at the time of arrival. Chemoprophylaxis should continue during exposure in the endemic area and for 4 weeks after leaving the endemic area to ensure adequate drug blood levels for chemoprophylaxis of infections acquired near the time of departure (Table 4.3) (42, 57–61).

Chemoprophylaxis regimens for areas without chloroquine resistance

Chloroquine is a synthetic 4-aminoquinolone that is rapidly absorbed after oral administration and is active against the asexual stages of *P. vivax*, *P. malariae*, *P. ovale*, and chloroquine-susceptible *P. falciparum*. Because it has a serum half-life of 7 to 10 days, chloroquine is taken weekly. Oral chloroquine is usually well tolerated at the recommended dosage, even when taken for long periods, and is the only

Table 4.3 Prophylaxis of malaria

Areas without chloroquine-resistant *Plasmodium falciparum*	
Chloroquine phosphate (Aralen)	500 mg (300-mg base) orally per week
Areas with chloroquine-resistant *Plasmodium falciparum*	
Mefloquine (Lariam)	250 mg orally weekly
OR	
Doxycycline (Vibramycin)	100 mg orally daily
OR	
Proguanil (Paludrine)	200 mg orally daily
PLUS	
Chloroquine phosphate	500 mg (300-mg base) orally weekly

antimalarial known to be safe for pregnant women and young children. The nausea reported by some persons receiving chloroquine chemoprophylaxis can usually be eliminated by taking the drug with meals. Ocular symptoms and headache, which are also reported by a small number of persons, can usually be reduced or eliminated by taking half the recommended dose twice weekly rather than the full dose once weekly. Long-term, high-dose treatment of patients with autoimmune disorders may produce an irreversible retinopathy and blindness (500–1,000 mg daily vs 500 mg weekly). This retinopathy rarely if ever occurs at the dosages used for chemoprophylaxis.

Hydroxychloroquine is a congener of chloroquine that has similar antiplasmodial and pharmacokinetic properties. It may be used when chloroquine is not available.

Amodiaquine is a 4-aminoquinoline related to chloroquine. Although it is effective, it should not be used for chemoprophylaxis because it may also cause agranulocytosis and hepatitis.

Chemoprophylaxis regimens for areas with chloroquine resistance

Mefloquine is a synthetic quinoline methanol developed for its schizonticidal activity against chloroquine-resistant P. falciparum. Although mefloquine rarely causes serious side effects at the dosages recommended for prophylaxis, there have been neurologic reactions such as dizziness, hallucinations, seizures, and psychoses. Gastrointestinal disturbances are reported more frequently. Contraindications to the use of mefloquine include the use of β-blockers or other drugs that prolong cardiac conduction times and the need to perform tasks that require fine coordination and spatial discrimination (e.g., airline pilots) (42,58,59).

Doxycycline is active against the blood stages of Plasmodium species, but probably does not act on the primary hepatic stage (tissue schizont). Because of its short serum half-life, doxycycline must be taken daily. Doxycycline is effective for the prevention of P. vivax infections and for multidrug-resistant P. falciparum. Although doxycycline is well tolerated by most people, side effects include yeast vaginitis and photosensitivity. Photosensitivity may present as a severe sunburn on the exposed skin. This risk may be reduced by taking the drug in the evening and avoiding prolonged direct exposure to the sun. Pregnant women and children under the age of 8 should not use doxycycline because it is concentrated in growing bones and teeth.

Fansidar may be effective in preventing infections due to chloroquine-resistant P. falciparum, although it is less effective against P. vivax. Fansidar chemoprophylaxis is no longer recommended because a severe and potentially fatal adverse reaction, such as the Stevens-Johnson syndrome, develops in 1 in 10,000 to 20,000 persons. In addition, the prevalence of Fansidar-resistant P. falciparum infections is increasing, thus reducing its efficacy. The most marked increases in Fansidar resistance have been in Thailand and other neighboring countries in southeast Asia (58).

Proguanil is a prodrug that is metabolized to the dihydrofolate reductase inhibitor cycloguanil in vivo and has little known toxicity. Although it has not been effective in West Africa, it may prevent P. falciparum infection in East Africa when combined with chloroquine (see Table 4.3). When taken with daily doses of sulfisozole, it may prevent multidrug-resistant *P. falciparum* infection in Thailand (59).

Chemoprophylaxis regimen for the prevention of relapse

Because primaquine is effective against hypnozoite stages of *P. vivax* and *P. ovale*, it prevents relapses (or delayed primary attacks in persons initially receiving chemoprophylaxis) in persons with those infections. Because primaquine may cause hemolysis in persons with G6PD deficiency, patients should be tested for that defect before prescribing primaquine. Although G6PD deficiency is more common among Africans, it is most severe in Mediterranean populations. Because some persons with *P. vivax* infections acquired in southeast Asia or Oceania have relapsed after the usual 14-day course of primaquine, longer durations of treatment (21–28 days) have been used for persons who were exposed in those regions (42,58).

Limiting vector-human contact

Because the *Anopheline* mosquitoes that transmit malaria bite primarily at dawn and dusk, measures to reduce vector-human contact should concentrate on those times. Appropriate measures include use of screens, mosquito nets, clothing that covers the arms and legs, and effective insect repellents such as N,N-diethylmetatoluamide (DEET). Repellents should be applied sparingly to exposed skin or clothing. They should not be applied to the hands of children, which are likely to come in contact with the eyes or mouth, or to wounds or irritated skin (58).

Bednets (or curtains) impregnated with permethrin are highly effective and are currently available in most countries. They are nontoxic, easy to use, long-lasting, and also offer protection from other biting nocturnal insects (42,59).

Pyrethroid-based insect sprays may be employed in addition to the previously described measures or when there is no other protection. Sleeping quarters should be sprayed approximately 30 minutes before bedtime, including walls, ceilings, and spaces under beds and furniture where anophelines rest (58). Mosquito coils and other preparations of vaporized pyrethrum for night-time use have limited effectiveness as single agents in reducing the frequency of mosquito bites (58,59).

TREATMENT OF MALARIA

For nonimmune persons infected with *P. falciparum*, there is a limited period (window of opportunity) in which to begin effective treatment before the risk of complications and death increases. Chloroquine should be used for persons who were infected in areas without chloroquine-resistant *P. falciparum*. Conversely, persons who acquired *P. falciparum* infection in areas with chloroquine resistance should be treated with drugs effective against chloroquine-resistant *P. falciparum* unless the rapid *in vitro* test for chloroquine resistance is available and indicates that the parasite is susceptible (13).

Infections due to chloroquine-susceptible parasites

Infections due to chloroquine-susceptible parasites (including *P. falciparum*) should be treated with chloroquine (Table 4.4). There is no evidence that quinine, quinidine, or other antimalarials are more effective than chloroquine in the treatment of *P. vivax, P. ovale, P. malariae,* or chloroquine-susceptible *P. falciparum* infections (including complications such as cerebral malaria) (9,59,60).

Infections due to chloroquine-resistant parasites

P. falciparum infections that recur after treatment with chloroquine, *P. falciparum* infections acquired while receiving chloroquine chemoprophylaxis, and *P. falciparum* infections resistant to chloroquine *in vivo* or by the rapid *in vitro* test for chloroquine resistance should be treated with alternative regimens known to be effective against chloroquine-resistant *P. falciparum* (see Table 4.4).

Table 4.4   Treatment of malaria

Persons with *P. vivax, P. ovale, P. malariae,* or chloroquine-susceptible *P. falciparum*	
Chloroquine	
Oral	600-mg base (10 mg base/kg) (or 1,000 mg salt), followed by additional doses of 300-mg base after 6 hours, and again on days 2 and 3.
Intramuscular	2.5-mg base/kg every 4 hours or 3.5 mg/kg/6 hours (total dose not to exceed 25-mg base/kg).
Intravenous	10-mg base/kg over 4 hours, followed by 5-mg base/kg every 12 hours (in a 12-hour infusion) (total dose ≤ 25-mg/kg base).
Persons who may have chloroquine-resistant *P. falciparum*	
Mefloquine	
Oral	750 mg (10–12 mg/kg) as a single dose.
Quinine (Qn)	
Oral	650 mg quinine sulfate salt (540-mg base) every 8 hours for 10 days if given alone; for 3 days, or until improvement occurs if given with Fansidar or tetracycline.
Qn + Fansidar	3 tablets in a single dose (25/500 mg apiece).
Qn + Tetracycline	250 mg every 6 hours × 7–10 days.
Intravenous	16.7-mg base/kg quinine dihydrochloride loading dose over 4 hours, followed by 8.3-mg base/kg over 2–4 hours every 8 hours.
Intramuscular	8.3-mg base/kg of quinine dihydrochloride (10 mg salt/kg) every 8 hours (maximum of 1,800-mg salt [1,500-mg base] per day).
Quinidine	
Intravenous	6.25-mg base/kg quinidine (10 mg quinidine gluconate) IV over 1–2 hours, followed by constant IV infusion of 0.0125-mg base/kg/min (0.02 mg quinidine gluconate) until parasitemia is <1% or patient can take oral medications.

Treatment of severe or complicated malaria

Hyperparasitemia ($\geq$ 100,000 parasites/μL blood) is associated with an increased risk of complications and death in *P. falciparum* infection and with complications such as cerebral malaria, renal failure, massive hemolysis, and pulmonary edema (9). Hyperparasitemia and specific complications must be addressed for effective treatment (Table 4.5). Patients with hyperparasitemia may fail to respond to treatment with drugs effective *in vitro* against the parasites causing the patient's infection. Especially with parasitemias more than $4 \times 10^5/\mu$L (>10% of the patient's red cells), the usual recommended drug dosages may be inadequate for the number of parasites present. Strategies that may be helpful in this situation include exchange transfusion (to remove 80%–90% of the red cell mass and thus 80%–90% of parasitized red cells) and constant drug infusion, with monitoring of plasma drug levels to allow for the fact that most drug will be taken up by parasitized red cells (62).

Patients with an altered neurologic status (especially those with seizures) should be given 50% dextrose intravenously if the blood glucose level cannot be determined rapidly because 20% to 30% of patients with cerebral malaria may have hypoglycemia as the cause of their altered neurologic function (63). Steroids should not be used because they prolong the duration of coma (64).

FUTURE STRATEGIES

Novel antimalarials

The most effective antimalarials currently available (i.e., chloroquine, quinine, mefloquine, qinghaosu) act on the parasite food vacuole, which is the unique parasite organelle responsible for digesting the hemoglobin internalized by the parasite from its host red cell. Alternative interesting antimalarials include drugs that act on other unique parasite organelles, such as the mitochondrion (5-fluoro-orotic acid analogues and atovaquone inhibit the mitochondrial enzyme, dihydro-orotic acid dehydrogenase), or on other pathways, such as the polyamine or purine salvage pathways.

Table 4.5 Treatment of hyperparasitemia and complicated malaria

Hyperparasitemia
   Drug infusion with measurement of plasma drug levels
   Exchange transfusion
Cerebral malaria
   Intravenous 50% dextrose for symptomatic hypoglycemia
   Avoid treatment with dexamethasone
Massive hemolysis
   Red cell replacement
Pulmonary edema
   Positive pressure ventilation

Antidisease strategies

Even in malaria-endemic areas, it is not clear why one person remains well with the same parasitemia that incapacitates another. Until this question has been answered, it will be impossible to devise effective antidisease strategies. However, once these questions have been answered, there will be a number of potentially useful strategies. For example, if cytokines are found to be important in the pathogenesis of complicated malaria, one could theoretically decrease complications and deaths by reducing circulating cytokine levels or by inhibiting the actions of those cytokines on their target cells (7).

Potential vaccine-disease interactions

In addition to the antidisease strategies discussed, there are at least 2 ways in which vaccines could provide protection against malaria: (1) the ideal result—effective immunity resulting from immunization alone (especially for nonimmune expatriate tourists); and (2) a less ideal, but still worthwhile result—incomplete or short-term immunity that required frequent *in vivo* boosting from natural infection. This result would be helpful for semi-immune residents of endemic areas but not for most expatriates.

Manipulation of the anopheline vector

When the biology of vector capacity is understood, it may be possible to alter the genes that make anophelines effective vectors of malaria. Because it is now possible to transfect mosquito eggs and obtain transient expression of those exogenous genes, it may be possible in the future to use constructs that reduce vector capacity and simultaneously provide a selective advantage for that mosquito over its competitors in nature.

SUMMARY

More effective prevention and treatment of malaria will require a better understanding of drug action and resistance. Development of an effective malaria vaccine will require information we do not yet have about immunity to malaria. Reducing malaria mortality will require new information about the mechanisms responsible for malaria complications and deaths.

REFERENCES

1 **Bremen JG, Campbell CC.** Combating severe malaria in African children. *Bull WHO* 1988;66:611–620.

2 **Beier JC.** Characterization of malaria transmission by *Anopheles* in western Kenya in preparation for malaria vaccine trials. *J Med Entomol* 1990;27:570–577.

3 **Wellems TE, Panton LJ, Gluzman IY, et al.** Chloroquine resistance not linked to mdr-like genes of *Plasmodium falciparum*. *Nature* 1990;345:253–255.

4 **Ceremi C, Frevert U, Sinnis P, et al.** The basolateral domain of the hepatocyte plasma membrane bears receptors for the circum-

sporohzoite protein of *Plasmodium falciparum* sporozoites. *Cell* 1992;70:1021–1033.

5   **Krotoski WA, Collins WE, Bray RS, et al.** Demonstration of hypnozoites in sporozoite-transmitted *Plasmodium vivax* infections. *Am J Trop Med Hyg* 1982;31:1291–1293.

6   **Field JW.** Blood examination and prognosis in acute falciparum malaria. *Trans R Soc Trop Med Hyg* 1949;43:33–48.

7   **Playfair JH, Taverne T, Bate CA, et al.** The malaria vaccine: anti-parasite or anti-disease? *Immunol Today* 1990;11:25–27.

8   **Neva FA.** Looking back for a view of the future: observations on immunity to induced malaria. *Am J Trop Med Hyg* 1977;26(suppl):210–215.

9   **Warrell DA, Molyneux ME, Beales PF (editors), et al.** Severe and complicated malaria. *Trans R Soc Trop Med Hyg* 1990;84(suppl 2):1–65.

10   **Krogstad DJ, Gluzman IY, Kyle DE, et al.** Efflux of chloroquine from *Plasmodium falciparum*: mechanism of chloroquine resistance. *Science* 1987;238:1283–1285.

11   **Krogstad DJ, Schlesinger PH, Herwaldt BL, et al.** Antimalarial agents: mechanism of chloroquine resistance. *Antimicrob Agents Chemother* 1988;32:799–801.

12   **Krogstad DJ, Gluzman IY, Wellems TE, et al.** Characterization of chloroquine resistance in *Plasmodium falciparum*. In: Peregrine AS, ed. *Proceedings of a Symposium on the Chemotherapy of Trypanosomiasis*. Nairobi, Kenya; ILRAD, 1990:85–90.

13   **Gluzman, Krogstad DJ, Orjih AU, et al.** A rapid *in vitro* test for chloroquine-resistant *Plasmodium falciparum*. *Am J Trop Med Hyg* 1990;42:521–526.

14   **Krogstad DJ, Herwaldt BL, Schlesinger PH, Wellems TE, et al.** Energy dependence of chloroquine accumulation and chloroquine efflux in *Plasmodium falciparum*. *Biochem Pharmacol* 1992;43:57–62.

15   **Krogstad DJ, Gluzman IY, Panton LJ, et al.** Genetic studies of quinine and quinidine resistance in *P. falciparum*: partial linkage to chloroquine resistance. American Society of Tropical Medicine and Hygiene, New Orleans, LA, 1990.

16   **Peterson DS, Milhous WK, Wellems TF, et al.** Molecular basis of differential resistance to cycloguanil and pyrimethamine in *Plasmodium falciparum* malaria. *Proc Natl Acad Sci USA* 1990;87:3018–3022.

17   **Peterson DS, Di Santi SM, Povoa M, et al.** Prevalence of the dihydrofolate reductase Asn-108 mutation as the basis for pyrimethamine-resistant *Plasmodium falciparum* malaria in the Brazilian Amazon. *Am J Trop Med Hyg* 1991;45:492–497.

18   **Rieckmann KH.** *Plasmodium vivax* resistant to chloroquine? *Lancet* 1989;2:1183–1184.

19   **Schwartz IK, Lackritz EM, Patchen LC, et al.** Chloroquine-resistant *Plasmodium vivax* from Indonesia (letter). *N Engl J Med* 1991;324:927.

20   **Schuurkamp GJ, Spicer PE, Kereu RK, et al.** Chloroquine-resistant *Plasmodium vivax* in Papua New Guinea. *Trans R Soc Trop Med Hyg* 1992;86:121–122.

21   **Friedman MJ.** Erythrocytic mechanism of sickle cell resistance to malaria. *Proc Natl Acad Sci USA* 1978;75:1994–1997.

22   **Luzzatto L, Usanga EA, Reddy S, et al.** Glucose-6-phosphate dehydrogenase deficient red cells: resistance to infection by malarial parasites. *Science* 1969;164:939–941.

23   **Vulliamy T, Mason P, Luzzatto L, et al.** The molecular basis of glucose-6-phosphate dehydrogenase deficiency. *Trends Genet* 1992;8:138–143.

24   **Fang XD, Kaslow DC, Adams JH, et al.** Cloning of the *Plasmodium vivax* Duffy receptor. *Mol Biochem Parasitol* 1991;44:125–132.

25   **Adams JH, Sim BK, Dolan SA, et al.** A family of erythrocyte binding proteins of malaria parasites. *Proc Natl Acad Sci USA* 1992;89:7085–7089.

26   **Day KP, Marsh K.** Naturally acquired immunity to *Plasmodium falciparum*. *Immunol Today* 1991;12:A68–A71.

27   **Good MF.** A malaria vaccine strategy based on the introduction of cellular immunity. *Immunol Today* 1992;13:126–129.

28   **Haworth J.** The global distribution of malaria and the present control effort. In: Wernsdorfer WH, MacGregor IA, eds. *Malaria: Principles and Practice of Malariology*. Edinburgh; Churchill-Livingstone, 1988;1379–1420.

29   **Cox FEG.** Malaria parasites. In Cox FEG, ed. *Modern Parasitology*. London: Blackwell Scientific, 1982:22–26.

30   **World Health Organization.** Malaria situation in 1990. *WHO Weekly Epidemiol Rec* 1992;67:161–168.

31   **Naji M, Omari M, El Mellouki, W, et al.** Le paludisme d'importation au Maroc. *Rev Int Serv Sane Armées Terre* 1985;58:241–243.

32   **World Health Organization.** World malaria situation in 1990. *Bull WHO* 1992;70:801–807.

33   **World Health Organization.** World malaria situation, 1983. *WHO Stat Q* 1985;40:142–170.

34   **World Health Organization.** World malaria situation in 1985. *WHO Stat Q* 1987;40:142–170.

35 Ngimbi NP, Beckers A, Wery M, et al. Apercu de la situation epidemiologique du paludisme a Kinshasa (Republique du Zaire) en 1980. *Ann Soc Belg Med Trop* 1982;62:121–137.

36 Coosemans MH, Wery M, Storme B, et al. Epidémologie du paludisme dans la plaine de la Ruizi, Burundi. *Ann Soc Belg Med Trop* 1984;64:135–158.

37 Juminer B, Robin Y, Pajot FX, et al. Physionomia du paludine en Guyane. *Med Trop* 1981;41:135–146.

38 Beier JC, Copeland RS, Mtalib R, et al. Oökinete rates in Afrotropical mosquitoes as a measure of human malaria infectiousness. *Am J Trop Med Hyg* 1992;47:41–46.

39 Carnevale P, LeGoff G, Toto JC, et al. *Anopheles nili* as the main vector of human malaria in villages of southern Cameroon. *Med Vet Entomol* 1992;6:135–138.

40 Fonteneille D, Lepers JP, Colluzzi M, et al. Malaria transmission and vector biology on Sainte Marie Island, Madagascar. *J Med Entomol* 1992;29:197–202.

41 Trager W, Jensen JB. Human malaria parasites in continuous culture. *Science* 1976;193:673–675.

42 Centers for Disease Control. Recommendations for prevention of malaria among travelers. *Morbid Mortal Wkly Rep* 1990;39(suppl RR-3):1–10.

43 Wernsdorfer WH, Payne D. The dynamics of drug resistance in *Plasmodium falciparum. Pharmacol Ther* 1991;50:95–121.

44 Subsaeng L, Wernsdorfer WH, Rooney, W, et al. Sensitivity to quinine and mefloquine of *Plasmodium falciparum* in Thailand. *Bull WHO* 1986;64:759–765.

45 Oduola AMJ, Milhous Wk, Salako LA, et al. Reduced *in vitro* susceptibility of West African isolates of *Plasmodium falciparum. Lancet* 1987;2:1304–1305.

46 Pan American Health Organization. Malaria in the Americas. *Epidemiol Bull* 1992;13:1–5.

47 Harinasuta T. Chloroquine resistance in Thailand. *UNESCO 1st Regional Symp on Sci Knowledge of Trop Parasites* 1962;1:143–153.

48 Ringwald P, Le Bras J, Doury JC, et al. Chimiosensibilite du paludisme a *Plasmodium falciparum* en France en 1988. *Bull Epidemiol Hebdom* 1989;23:93–95.

49 Payne D. The history and development of WHO standard *in vivo* and *in vitro* test systems for sensitivity of *Plasmodium falciparum* and other human plasmodia to antimalarial drugs. Thesis dissertation, London School of Hygiene and Tropical Medicine. 1989.

50 Hurwitz ES, Johnson D, Campbell CC, et al. Resistance of *Plasmodium falciparum* to sulfa-doxine-pyremethamine (Fansidar) in a refugee camp in Thailand. *Lancet* 1981;1:1068–1070.

51 Giboda M, Vanista J, Dastych P, et al. The first report of *Plasmodium falciparum* resistant to chloroquine plus sulfadoxine-pyrimethamine. *Trans R Soc Trop Med Hyg* 1988; 82:383.

52 World Health Organization. Advances in malaria chemotherapy. *WHO Tech Rep Ser No 735, 1984.*

53 Giboda M. Biological advantage of *Plasmodium falciparum* isolates resistant to quinine. *Trans R Soc Trop Med Hyg* 1987;81:709.

54 Giboda M, Denis MB. Response of Kampuchean strains of *Plasmodium falciparum* to antimalarials: *in vivo* assessment of quinine and quinine plus tetracycline; multiple drug resistance *in vitro. J Trop Med Hyg* 1988;91: 205–211.

55 Bastien P. Quinine resistant falciparum malaria in Vanuatu? Case report. *Southeast Asian J Trop Med Public Health* 1987;18:101–102.

56 Isaacs RD, Ellis Pegler RB. *Plasmodium falciparum* RI resistance to quinine and sulfadoxine-pyrimethamine in the Solomon Islands. *Med J Aust* 1987;146:449–450.

57 Centers for Disease Control. Change of dosing regimen for malaria prophylaxis with mefloquine. *Morbid Mortal Wkly Rep* 1991; 40:72–73.

58 Schwartz IK. Prevention of malaria. *Infect Dis Clin North Am* 1992;6:313–331.

59 Hoffman SL. Diagnosis, treatment, and prevention of malaria. *Med Clin North Am* 1992;76: 1327–1355.

60 Winstanley PA. Treatment and prevention of falciparum malaria in Africa. *J R Coll Phys Lond* 1992;26:445–449.

61 Amin NM. Prophylaxis for malaria: helping world travelers come home healthy. *Postgrad Med* 1992;92:161–168.

62 Miller KD, Greenberg AE, Campbell CC, et al. Treatment of severe malaria in the United States with a continuous infusion of quinidine gluconate and exchange transfusion. *N Engl J Med* 1989;321:65–70.

63 White NJ, Warrell DA, Chanthavanich P, et al. Severe hypoglycemia and hyperinsulinemia in falciparum malaria. *N Engl J Med* 1983;809:61–66.

64 Warrell DA, Looareensuwan S, Warrell MJ, et al. Dexamethasone proves deleterious in cerebral malaria: a double-blind trial in 100 patients. *N Engl J Med* 1982;206:313–318.

Automated antimicrobial susceptibility testing: what the infectious diseases subspecialist needs to know

MARY JANE FERRARO

INTRODUCTION

The antimicrobial susceptibility test procedures currently used in clinical microbiology laboratories have evolved from classic methods, such as macrobroth and agar dilution, which are highly accurate but cumbersome when testing large numbers of antimicrobial agents. For a number of years, the Subcommittee on Antimicrobial Susceptibility Testing of the National Committee for Clinical Laboratory Standards (NCCLS) has provided laboratories with alternative, well-standardized methods to ensure accurate assessment of bacterial susceptibility. In addition to the classic reference agar dilution and macrobroth dilution methods, the NCCLS standards include guidelines for the performance of disk diffusion (1) and broth microdilution (2) susceptibility tests. These methods allow simultaneous testing of a large battery of antimicrobial agents, provide highly accurate results, and are used by the majority of microbiology laboratories in the United States (3).

The disk diffusion method, first described and standardized by Bauer and colleagues in 1966 (4) and subsequently modified by the NCCLS, is the oldest of these methods. Nevertheless, it is widely used, most likely owing to its accuracy, applicability to a wide variety of bacteria, and flexibility to test a large number of specimens and to easily change the battery of antimicrobial agents. Broth microdilution procedures, employing either commercially or in-house prepared antimicrobial-containing microdilution plates, were used with increased frequency by clinical laboratories from the late 1970s until the late 1980s (3). During that decade, different levels of mechanization or automation for microdilution susceptibility testing also evolved. For some microdilution systems, mechanized panel inoculation, incubation of test panels within an instrument, and automated serial or final interpretation of growth end points became possible. Despite this process, conventional microdilution systems and disk diffusion methods require 16 to 24 hours of incubation before test results are available.

The most profound change to occur in antimicrobial susceptibility testing during the 1980s has been development and increased use of rapid automated susceptibility tests.

Progress in the development of microprocessors, robotics, and microcomputers have allowed manufacturers to develop instruments designed to produce antimicrobial susceptibility results in as little as 3.5 to 4 hours. A variety of nontraditional strategies are employed in rapid susceptibility test systems to provide accurate results in a relatively short time frame. The concentration of bacteria in the test inoculum is usually adjusted upward from the 1 to 5×10^5 CFU/mL used in standard procedures. The actual concentration of the antimicrobial agent in the test well is often manipulated to provide comparable results to standard minimum inhibitory concentration (MIC) tests employing longer incubation periods. MICs are algorithmically derived from growth rate comparisons or the use of fluorogenic compounds for microbial growth detection. The instrument's computer software can allow editing and adjustment of results for some specific drug/microorganism combinations. In some instances, adjustments to the growth medium are made to promote a more rapid growth of certain microorganisms.

Currently, none of the NCCLS Subcommittees or other professional groups oversees the quality control, use, or modification of these rapid susceptibility methods. Following the enactment of the Safe Medical Devices Act of 1990, the rapid susceptibility instruments and their drug panels now require premarket approval (PMA) by the Food and Drug Administration (FDA) for clearance to be marketed in the United States. This PMA has become more difficult to obtain in the 1990s because of new, more stringent FDA controls (5). Extensive studies at 3 separate sites that provide data on the ability of the rapid system to accurately determine susceptibility test results as compared with a reference method (either broth or agar MIC or disk diffusion) are required for PMA. The organisms (500 strains/site) selected for the study must include American Type Culture Collection (ATCC) quality control organisms, a Centers for Disease Control (CDC) challenge set (75–100 organisms) with known mechanisms of resistance, and fresh clinical isolates (300 strains/site) or stock organisms (100 strains/site) that are representative of each antimicrobial agent's spectrum of activity. For penicillins and cephalosporins, at least 10 resistant isolates of *Enterobacter* spp., *Citrobacter freundii*, *Serratia marcescens*, and *Pseudomonas aeuriginosa* must be included. For other antimicrobial agents, at least 20 to 25 organisms representative of each known mode of resistance for that antimicrobial must be tested. It is expected that very major errors (false-susceptible) will be 1.5% or less; major errors (false-resistant), $\leq 3\%$ or less; essential agreement ($\pm$ one $\log_2$ dilution), 90% or more; and growth failures, $\leq 10\%$ or less. For any micro-organisms, antimicrobial agents, or combinations thereof, not meeting these specifications, the labeling (package insert) of the device should include this contraindication and recommend the use of an alternative method for testing. When less than 20 strains representing each known mechanism of resistance for that antimicrobial agent were tested, a statement must be included in the labeling saying that the ability to detect resistance to an agent among these species is unknown because resistant strains were not available at the time of comparative testing.

It has been estimated that nearly one quarter of clinical laboratories in the United States use on a daily basis a rapid, automated susceptibility system for testing certain bacterial groups (6) (Table 5.1). For many physicians, who are the ultimate users of the susceptibility results produced by these systems, the methods involved are somewhat of an enigma and often engender questions with regard to the reliability of reported

Table 5.1   Testing methods used by College of
American Pathologists survey participants,
Bacteriology Survey D-A 1991 [6]

Method	*Percent of total*
Microdilution	46
Disk diffusion	32
Automated rapid	20
Agar/broth dilution	2

results. This chapter focuses on antimicrobial susceptibility methods that produce rapid, automated test results using nontraditional methods.

RAPID AUTOMATED SUSCEPTIBILITY SYSTEMS

The first rapid, automated susceptibility system, the TAAS system, was developed in the early 1970s by Technicon Instruments Corp. (Tarryton, NY), but it was never marketed (7). In this system, bacterial growth after 3 hours in the presence of one concentration of an antibiotic was compared with growth after 3 hours in a control broth with no antibiotic. An index was calculated by comparing the growth in the presence of antimicrobial agent with growth in the control broth. From this index, judgments were made as to whether the bacterium was susceptible or resistant to the given antimicrobial agent.

Subsequent instruments, such as the Autobac System developed and marketed by Pfizer Diagnostics in the early 1970s (later called Autobac Series II; Organon-Teknika, Durham, NC) and the Abbott MS-2 system (later called the Advantage Microbiology Center; Abbott Laboratories Diagnostic Division, Irving, TX), were based on growth detection principles used in TAAS (8). Although these systems enjoy the distinction of being the first rapid automated susceptibility test systems sold and used, they are no longer manufactured and are currently virtually extinct in clinical microbiology laboratories. Systems such as the Vitek System (formerly called the AutoMicrobic System [AMS]; bioMerieux Vitek, Hazelwood, MO) (8,9) and the WalkAway (formerly called the autoSCAN-W/A; Baxter Diagnostics, Inc., Microscan Division, West Sacramento, CA) are now the most widely used rapid susceptibility testing systems in the United States. Both the Vitek and WalkAway systems were initially approved by the FDA for testing most common bacteria and antimicrobial agents prior to the more stringent 1991 PMA requirements. However, all new antimicrobial agents or organisms to be marketed for testing with these systems must undergo the extensive FDA review described previously. Other systems such as the ATB-plus (bioMerieux, France), the Cobas Bact (Roche Diagnostics, Switzerland), and the Sensititre Fluorogenic System (Radiometer America, Inc., West Lake, OH) are used to varying extents throughout the world, but are not approved by the FDA for use in the United States (Table 5.2). Because the companies that market these latter 3 instruments do not intend to seek

Table 5.2 Automated and semi-automated rapid susceptibility systems

System	Manufacturer	Availability
ATB	bioMerieux	Worldwide, *except USA*
WalkAway	Baxter-Microscan	Worldwide
Cobas Bact	Roche Diagnostic	Worldwide, *except USA*
Sensititre	Radiometer America	Worldwide, *except USA*
Vitek	bioMerieux Vitek	Worldwide

FDA PMA approval, the Vitek and WalkAway systems will be used to illustrate 2 different approaches to rapid susceptibility testing.

The Vitek system

The Vitek System (Figure 5.1) was developed by McDonnell-Douglas Corp. in the 1960s under contract from the National Aeronautics and Space Administration. Designed originally to detect and identify common urinary tract pathogens directly from primary urine specimens of astronauts aboard a space craft, it was subsequently introduced as a clinical microbiology laboratory instrument in the mid-1970s. Highly automated and relatively compact, the Vitek system remains, after more than 2 decades, a tribute to its superb engineering. Although slower to develop, the microbiologic capabilities of the system are now commensurate with the hardware. Susceptibility and identification results can be obtained in as early as 4 hours. In addition to a large variety of drug-containing susceptibility test cards for testing gram-negative bacilli or gram-positive cocci, there are biochemical cards for rapid identification of gram-negative bacilli, gram-positive bacteria, and yeasts.

Susceptibility test card The hallmark of the Vitek system is a small, thin, plastic reagent card (Figure 5.2) containing 30 small wells or microcuvettes. The card is closed except for capillaries, through which the bacterial test suspension passes for rehydration and inoculation. Each card has a numeric matrix area, where an instrument-readable sample identification number is written directly onto the card.

Vitek cards are available with a variety of predefined configurations of antimicrobial agents specified by the manufacturer or can be designed by the user with a customized battery of drugs. The wells of the card contain an enriched medium to support growth as well as specific concentrations of each antimicrobial agent. One of the 30 wells is a growth control well, which is used to monitor growth during incubation. The generation of a MIC value for the majority of antimicrobial agents requires testing of 3 concentrations of drug (a few are 1,2, or 5), thus allowing the testing of 9 to 11 agents per card. For laboratories wishing to test a larger number of antimicrobial agents, Vitek offers a combination of 2 cards at a lower unit price, which, when tested together, allow merging of results into 1 report. A 45-well card that will allow testing of 15 to 17 agents will be introduced in late 1933. All susceptibility cards must be stored at 4°C and generally have a shelf-life of 12 months following production.

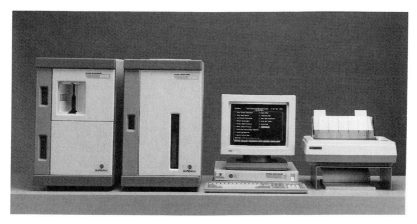

Figure 5.1   Vitek System; 120 test card capacity.

Hardware and software   The Vitek System includes integrated modular hardware consisting of (1) a filling-sealer unit that provides the vacuum for inoculation of up to 10 cards simultaneously and seals them after filling; (2) a reader-incubator module that incorporates a robotic system to move the cards on an hourly basis from a carousel to a position in the instrument where the optical density or biochemical reaction color change for each well is measured by a photometer; (3) a computer control module that receives floppy disk updates of test software; (4) a video display terminal; and (5) a multicopy printer. A variety of Vitek Systems with capacities of 30, 60, 120, or 240 cards are available, all of which can be linked with the main laboratory computer through a standard RS-232 interface. An information management system for storing and retrieving test data for laboratory, pharmacy, and infection control purposes, providing conditional antibiotic reporting capability, as well as printing chartable patient reports is also available.

Inoculum preparation   Perhaps the single most important step to ensure accurate testing with this as well as other rapid automated systems is the standardization of the test inoculum. A densitometer, rather than visual adjustment of turbidity, should be employed for this purpose.

Inocula for the Vitek susceptibility cards are prepared by suspending 3 to 4 fresh colonies in 0.45% to 0.5% saline. The suspension is then adjusted to the equivalent of a number 1.0 McFarland barium sulfate turbidity standard for gram-negative and an 0.5 McFarland standard for gram-positive bacteria. A further dilution of this suspension, resulting in approximately 10^7 CFU/mL, is made. The inoculum is automatically transferred to the test card via a small, straw-like transfer tube during the vacuum cycle of the filling module. The resulting inoculum in each antibiotic test well (25 μL) is approximately 2×10^5 CFU/well.

Growth detection and MIC calculation   Growth in the Vitek card wells is determined by turbidimetry. The Vitek reader measures the optical density or the amount of

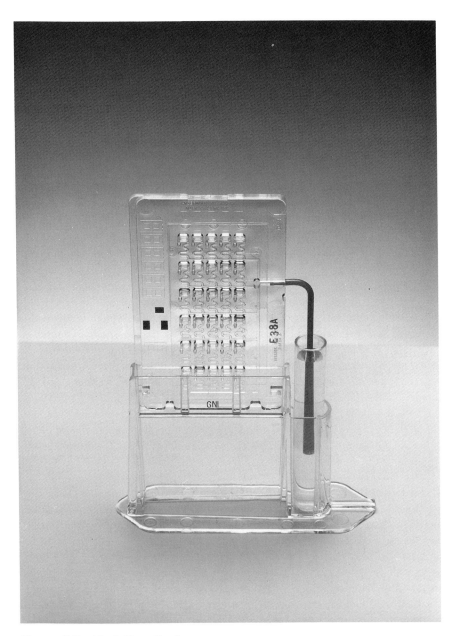

Figure 5.2 Vitek Test Card.

light that passes through each well at each hour, beginning with hour 0, to a maximum of 15 hours. The 0-hour reading usually establishes a baseline value; as growth causes this light to decrease, the differences in hourly readings are expressed as percentages of the maximum reading. When a predetermined minimum threshold percent has been reached in the positive control (PC) well and a minimum number of hours has passed, slope calculations for all wells are made. The hourly percents constitute a growth curve, which is made linear by converting them into $\log_2$ values. The slope of this linear line is then optimized to choose the log phase of the growth curve by magnitude and "least-squared error" comparisons of different sections of the line. Once the well slopes are determined, each drug well is normalized (divided by) the slope of the PC well. This normalizing step allows each well slope to be expressed as a fraction of the PC slope and serves to offset minor card-to-card differences in base broth composition or inoculum size. The slope of any given well can range from 0, indicating no growth, to 1.0, indicating growth equal to the PC well. Finally, a composite slope is determined for each antibiotic by adding the individual normalized slopes of each well containing that drug. If the PC well does not reach the predetermined threshold by hour 15, the card is reported as "insufficient growth."

Linear regression is utilized to calculate the best fit line for relation of the standard MIC to the composite slope. The best fit line is mathematically defined by a coefficient that is stored in the software. When a bacterium of unknown MIC is tested, its growth characteristics in the presence of the drug (composite slope) can be related to the MIC by the stored best fit line coefficients or linear regression analysis, thus resulting in an algorithm-derived MIC.

The user may elect to have susceptibility test results reported as discrete MIC, doubling dilution MIC, or qualitative (i.e., susceptible, intermediate, or resistant) formats.

The WalkAway System

The WalkAway System (Figure 5.3) for rapid susceptibility testing was developed in the late 1980s. This system differs from the Vitek system in that it uses fluorogenic-substrate hydrolysis to detect bacterial growth. The instrument consists of a large computer-controlled panel processor that incubates standard-sized microdilution trays and interprets rapid biochemical or susceptibility results with a fluorogenic reader. Although not discussed herein, the WalkAway System can also read conventional microdilution panels photometrically following overnight incubation. Fluorogenic panels are available that provide susceptibility results for gram-negative bacilli and gram-positive cocci in 3.5 to 15 hours, as well as identification of gram-negative bacilli and gram-positive bacteria as early as 2 hours after incubation.

Susceptibility test panel   The WalkAway System offers a choice of panels containing dilutions of antimicrobial agents and the fluorogenic substrates for MIC susceptibility testing or special "combo" panels, which provide breakpoint susceptibility and organism identification in the same tray (Figure 5.4). Depending on whether one uses an MIC or breakpoint susceptibility test panel, anywhere from 17 to 27 antimicrobials

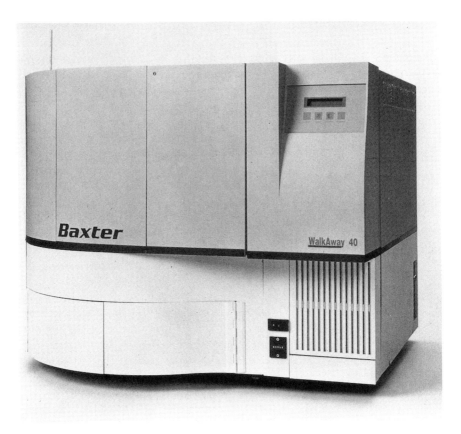

Figure 5.3 WalkAway System; 40 test panel capacity.

may be tested. An instrument-readable bar code label for patient or specimen identification can be printed by the data management system and attached to the side of the test panel. The panels require considerable space for storage at 4°C but have a shelf-life of up to 6 months following manufacture.

Hardware and software   The WalkAway System, available with either 40 or 96 test panel capacity, consists of (1) a large, self-contained incubator-reader unit that incorporates 2 microprocessor chips, an ultrasonic humidifier, a large carousel that rotates the panel holding towers, a bar code scanner, a spectrophotometer, a fluorometric reader, a robotic mechanism or stepper motors to perform discrete, computer-controlled steps, such as to add reagents from the reagent-dispensing subsystem and to access and position trays for reading of growth endpoints under the photometer or fluorometer; (2) a personal computer; (3) video display terminal; and (4) a printer.

The system has a data management system capable of producing chartable patient reports, epidemiologic reports, and antibiograms. In addition, a pharmacy-link program, which allows the pharmacy to interact with the WalkAway system, can be added.

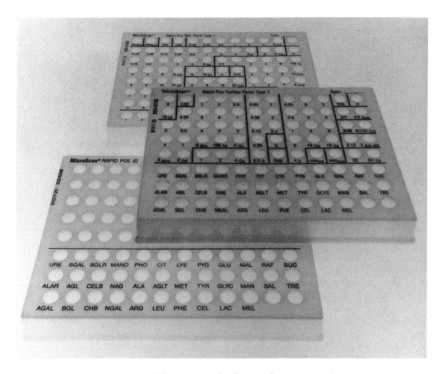

Figure 5.4   WalkAway MIC or "combo" panels.

As with the Vitek System, the WalkAway can be linked with other laboratory computer systems through a one-way or two-way interface.

Inoculum preparation   An inoculum is prepared by suspending 4 to 5 fresh colonies into 0.4% saline with Pluronic (BASF Wyandotte, Wyandotte, MI) to achieve a density equivalent to a 0.5 McFarland standard; an aliquot of this suspension is then inoculated into 25 mL cation-supplemented Mueller-Hinton broth, resulting in a final concentration of approximately $6 \times 10^5 = CFU/mL$ (gram-negative organisms) or $1.8 \times 10^6 \, CFU/mL$ (gram-positive organisms). The inoculum is poured into a disposable seed trough and transferred to the test panel using the RENOK rehydrator/inoculator, a manual pipettor that simultaneously rehydrates and inoculates each panel well with approximately 0.115 mL for a final concentration of approximately $6 \times 10^4 \, CFU/well$ (gram-negative organisms) or $10^5 \, CFU/well$ (gram-positive organisms).

Growth determination   A unique feature of the WalkAway system is the incorporation of amidomethylcoumarin or methylumbelliferyl fluorogenic substrates in the growth medium. Detection of bacterial growth is based on hydrolysis of these fluorogenic substrates (with subsequent release of the fluorophore) by specific bacterial enzymes produced during bacterial growth. As fluorophores are released, fluorescence increases. The fluorometric detection system uses a quartz-halogen incadescent bulb passing through an excitation filter so that ultraviolet light (370 nm) is focused through fiber-optic cables into each of the 96-panel wells. Any free fluorophore present in the wells will emit light at 450 nm, which passes through an emission filter and focuses onto a detector. The lower wavelength excitation light is blocked by the emission filter. In theory, detection of resulting fluorescence is more sensitive than photometric technology, thus allowing more rapid assessment of bacterial growth. However, fluorometric detection of growth is indirect. If for some reason the test bacteria fail to produce sufficient or specific enzymes, fluorophores will not be cleaved and fluorescence will not be detected, despite growth in the presence of an antimicrobial agent. The MIC is recorded as the first well showing inhibition of growth starting at the lowest concentration. Growth is detected as an increase in fluorescence; inhibition of growth is detected as no increase in fluorescence as compared with the growth well. The exact algorithms stored in the WalkAway software and used to assess degree of bacterial growth and antimicrobial susceptibility are proprietary and have not been published.

POTENTIAL ADVANTAGES OF AUTOMATED SUSCEPTIBILITY INSTRUMENTS

Undoubtedly the marked increase in the number of laboratories using rapid automated susceptibility test systems is due to a number of perceived advantages over more standardized traditional methods. It has yet to be definitively demonstrated that rapid susceptibility test results have a major positive impact on patient care. Doern and colleagues (10) found that among 173 patients with bacteremia who were receiving antibiotics, a change in therapy was indicated by the results of a nonautomated, rapid, direct blood culture susceptibility test for 48 of these patients. In 32 of these 48 patients, the indicated change was made approximately 24 hours sooner than if conventional, nonrapid susceptibility tests had been used. Matsen and associates (11), in a questionnaire submitted to physicians caring for 300 patients with culture-proven infections, reported that when a one-day-sooner susceptibility result was received, there was a change in therapy for 20% of patients who were on antimicrobial therapy, by substitution of a more appropriate antibiotic, removal of an unnecessary antibiotic, or change to a less toxic antibiotic. For this same group of patients, 9% had their hospital stay shortened by 1 or more days as determined by the physicians' subjective evaluations. Trenholme and colleagues (12), in a study of 226 patients with bacteremia, found that rapid automated susceptibility results were significantly likely to result in the initiation of appropriate antimicrobial therapy, a change to more effective therapy, or a change to less expensive therapy. Furthermore, better controlled studies must be conducted if the clinical benefits of routine same-day susceptibility testing can be clearly defined. Regardless, rapid generation of any test results in the laboratory can only have clinical impact when linked to a reporting system that also permits rapid transmission of these test results to physicians, preferably not too late in the working day.

   Less controversial is the perception that rapid automated susceptibility test instruments afford laboratories greater opportunities for both intralaboratory and interlaboratory standardization of methods. Because procedures for inoculum preparation, exact length of test incubation in the instrument, and instrument assessment of growth determination are all highly standardized or instrument-controlled, certain subjective components of the more manual test methods are removed.

Perhaps the greatest advantage for high-volume laboratories is that the technologist time required to manually read and interpret routine susceptibility tests is diminished when using an automated system. Because these systems are also capable of performing a simultaneous identification of the organism (13) from the same initial inoculum, the redundancy of separate identification and susceptibility test procedures is removed. The major labor-saving capability of automated instruments, however, results from the potential to establish a link between the microcomputer that controls the function of the instrument and the laboratory computer. This interface eliminates the technologist time required to sort, distribute, and enter results printed on separate report sheets when the instrument is not used with an on-line interface. This approach also allows for a decrease in transcription errors. As with manual entry, verification of susceptibility data by a technologist or supervisory personnel is advisable before automated transfer of data to the patient file.

One of the most exciting, although yet to be fully exploited, advantages of automated susceptibility test systems is the potential use of artificial intelligence to create an expert system (14) for automated review and verification of the data generated. Appropriately programmed software could contain error detection rules akin to those used by knowledgeable microbiologists to detect impossible phenotypes (e.g., penicillin-resistant Group A, C, or G *Streptococcus*) and to correct technical errors that may have occurred in the testing and could otherwise result in interpretation or reporting problems, or both. Similarly, rules could be designed to recognize a rare or unlikely resistance marker (e.g., an imipenem-resistant strain of an *Enterobacteriaceae*) or a rare antibiogram phenotype (e.g., amikacin resistance with gentamicin susceptibility). The recognition by computer programs of potential errors or unusual phenotypes would then result in the printing of a comment on the data terminal or laboratory report. This comment would be reviewed by a technologist or a supervisor, thereby allowing verification of the test results or investigation of the possibility of an unusual resistance mechanism before transmitting data to a patient report. A few laboratories, including our own, have had their own in-house–designed software to perform this function for many years. Incorporation of expert systems into automated instruments would make possible a sophisticated review of laboratory results, even for small laboratories without microbiologists with a high level of expertise in antibiotic resistance.

POTENTIAL DISADVANTAGES OF RAPID, AUTOMATED SUSCEPTIBILITY TESTING SYSTEMS

The movement from traditional methods to rapid automated systems has not come without some disadvantages for clinical laboratories. Laboratories using these systems must purchase antibiotic test panels or cards that are specified by the manufacturer, unless their volume warrants purchase of a more expensive custom panel. To be cost-effective, most laboratories do not want to test more than one test panel or card per organism. Therefore, the number of antimicrobial agents that can be easily tested is also restricted. Flexibility to change their test battery (e.g., when one antimicrobial agent is replaced by another on the hospital formulary) or to quickly begin testing a newly FDA-approved agent is limited.

Another major disadvantage is that these test systems are not applicable for testing all groups of bacteria isolated from clinical specimens. For example, testing of most fastidious bacteria or anaerobes is not yet possible using a rapid automated system. Other organisms, such as *Pseudomonas aeruginosa, Xanthomonas maltophilia,* and some coagulase-negative staphyloccoci, often do not grow well enough in these systems to be tested (15). Therefore, laboratories must have a number of different susceptibility test methods available.

For the most part, a wide range of doubling dilutions or drug concentrations for a given antimicrobial agent are not tested in these rapid systems. MIC values, when produced, are only reliable within the concentrations tested; MICs higher than or lower than the test concentrations can only be expressed as semiquantitative results. The most prudent users of rapid susceptibility systems often only report results using the NCCLS categories (i.e., susceptible, intermediate, and resistant).

Quality control of these test systems is currently dependent on the use of ATCC organisms specified by the manufacturer. As stated previously, the NCCLS has not yet written any standards for laboratories to follow regarding test procedures or quality control for rapid susceptibility test systems. Some of the quality control organisms suggested by manufacturers do not produce on-scale quality control values (i.e., the MIC of the quality control organism may be less than or higher than the concentrations tested by the instrument). Therefore, subtle changes in the precision of the instrument or test panels may not be adequately detected.

When purchased, these systems require a substantial capital investment by the laboratory. The disposables used with the rapid systems may be more expensive than the components needed for manual test methods. In addition to space and electrical requirements, fees for service contracts add to operational costs. The laboratory must also incur the costs to maintain supplies for alternative, emergency test procedures to be used during potential instrument failure.

Package inserts often include frequent disclaimers or limitations for organisms that can be tested on the panel when data for FDA submission showed discrepant MIC values when compared with an overnight reference method. If the antimicrobial agent is critical to patient care, an alternative procedure must be used to assess resistance or the antimicrobial agent cannot be reported. Finally, not all resistance mechanisms in clinically important bacteria are easily detected with rapid susceptibility test methods.

POTENTIAL PROBLEMS IN THE DETECTION OF RESISTANCE WHEN USING RAPID SUSCEPTIBILITY TEST METHODS

A number of problems with detection of resistance have been reported by users of rapid susceptibility test systems. In some cases, false-susceptibility or false-resistance results are sporadic and not easily explained. In many instances, careful review with the technologists of the importance of inoculum preparation from fresh colonies and appropriate inoculum standardization using a nephelometer will correct spurious results. Major problems with the detection of resistance or susceptibility for a given system should have been identified in data submitted to the FDA, at least for known mechanisms of resistance at the time of initial FDA approval. Many of the earlier testing errors with rapid susceptibility methods have been corrected by continual improvement of both growth media and software. Nevertheless, some problems remain. The most troublesome involve detection of some of the newly emerging mechanisms of resistance, which either were not recognized or did not exist at the time of the initial testing of drug/micro-organism combinations for FDA approval. Therefore, it is important that laboratories using these systems re-establish their reliability as bacteria continue to become resistant.

Detection of β-lactamase resistance

The rapid susceptibility test systems often have problems with the detection of intrinsic ampicillin resistance, particularly for certain strains of *Citrobacter, Enterobacter, Morganella,* and *Serratia*. In cases when the organism identification is known, the software of the test system will suppress reporting of this drug. When the identification is unknown, however, false susceptibility of these organisms could be reported if not detected and deleted by technologist review. If a laboratory's cumulative susceptibility statistics reveal more than 5% of unique strains of these genera are testing susceptible to ampicillin, it is most likely due to an error in the testing procedure.

Detection of Type-1 β-lactamases

Certain genera or species, such as *Citrobacter* (primarily *C. freundii*), all species of *Enterobacter*, all species of *Serratia*, indole-positive *Proteus, Providencia,* and *Pseudomonas*, possess type-I, inducible β-lactamases. These enzymes are chromosomal in origin and are induced either by a reversible mechanism when the organism is exposed to an enzyme inducer (e.g., certain cephalosporins) or by a nonreversible mechanism that involves spontaneous mutation resulting in what has been termed *stably derepressed mutants*.

Detection of this mechanism of resistance has been a problem with automated systems, because the inducible type may be missed because it requires a longer period for induction and expression than allowed by the short incubation of rapid methods. Detection of the spontaneous mutants is difficult because the frequency of mutation is approximately 1 in 10^6 to 1 in 10^7 wild-type cells. Both the lower inoculum concentration per well and the short incubation periods can contribute to this detection problem. Detection of these stably depressed mutants can also be a problem with conventional methods. It has been shown, however, that when this selection occurs clinically, the subsequent patient isolates currently in the stably derepressed state are detected by rapid methods in subsequent specimens without any problem (16).

Detection of extended spectrum β-lactamases

Extended spectrum β-lactamases (ESBL) are enzymes that confer resistance to ceftazidime, cefotaxime, and other broad-spectrum cephalosporins and monobactams. These plasmid-mediated enzymes have been shown to be derivatives of the more common SHV-1, TEM-1, and TEM-2 β-lactamases. In some instances, strains with ESBLs will test highly resistant to one antimicrobial agent (e.g., ceftazidime), but display an intermediate or susceptible phenotype for other third-generation cephalosporins. In the latter instance, the actual MICs of agents like cefotaxime may be considerably higher than for strains without ESBLs, and the apparent "susceptibility" of these organisms is due to the fact that current breakpoints are set too high to detect this type of resistance. In either case, treatment failures may result when an ESBL is not detected. This phenomenon has been particularly common in *Klebsiella spp.* and as yet remains a problem for detection in the clinical laboratory, both with rapid as well as conventional methods. The inclusion of indicator drugs such as ceftazidime (not normally tested against members of the family *Enterobacteriaceae*) or aztreonam in the test battery or of companion wells with a low concentration of a third-generation cephalosporin/β-lactamase inhibitor (e.g., clavulanate) may help point out the existence of strains with these enzymes (17).

Detection of aminoglycoside resistance

Initially, errors in the detection of aminoglycoside resistance or susceptibility for *Pseudomonas aeruginosa* were reported sporadically. Companies have become more conscious of the importance of adjustments of the cation content in the growth medium to control these errors, and it is no longer a major problem.

False resistance to aztreonam

False resistance to aztreonam can occur with the rapid systems, especially for *Proteus* and *Morganella spp.* This phenomenon results because the optics in the growth detecting systems actually see the elongation of the cells, which occurs just prior to lysis, as growth. The problem has been partially addressed by software rules, which require a more prolonged incubation for isolates known to be these genera.

False resistance to imipenem

Recently, false resistance to imipenem, especially for *P. aeruginosa* as well as other species, has been reported. Although yet to be elucidated, it is thought that this sporadic false resistance may be due to instability of the antimicrobial agent in the test system. It is recommended that normally susceptible isolates found to be resistant to imipenem be rechecked by an alternative method.

Detection of oxacillin-resistant staphylococci

Although detection of oxacillin-resistant staphylococci was an early problem with rapid automated susceptibility test systems, the inclusion of increased NaCl content in the growth medium has largely corrected this problem. The software of rapid systems also contains rules to look for resistance to multiple antimicrobial agents as a signal for possible oxacillin resistance. However, rapid systems as well as conventional disk or microdilution systems still do not detect all heterorresistant strains because the frequency of methicillin-resistant organisms among some heteroresistant strains (either *S. aureus* or coagulase-negative staphylococci) can be as low as 1 in 10^6 to 1 in 10^8 resistant cells per population (18). Therefore, the inoculum concentration in either conventional or rapid susceptibility test systems may not detect these strains. If heterogenous strains are prevalent in one's hospital, or for isolates recovered from serious infections, it is recommended that laboratories use the NCCLS procedure of a spot screen on Mueller-Hinton agar containing $6\mu g/mL$ oxacillin and 4% NaCl (2) to rule out oxacillin-resistant staphylococci.

Detection of low- or moderate-level vancomycin resistant

The recent emergence of vancomycin resistance in *Enterococcus* spp. has posed a problem for users of rapid susceptibility test systems (19). For the most part, strains with MICs of 8 to 128 $\mu g/mL$ are the most difficult for the systems to detect. Because some vancomycin-resistant strains exhibit inducible resistance, failure to detect them may be due to the short incubation period of rapid methods. This problem is currently being addressed by instrument manufacturers and may be corrected by changes in instrument algorithms or optical reading devices.

Detection of high-level aminoglycoside resistance

A number of problems with the detection of high-level gentamicin or high-level streptomycin resistance for *Enterococcus spp.* have also been reported using rapid susceptibility test instruments (20). These problems have been the result of a combination of factors, such as inappropriate concentration of aminoglycosides in the test medium, the growth medium employed (20), or failure of the optical reading devices to see subtle amounts of growth. As with vancomycin resistance, this problem is currently being addressed by the manufacturers of the test systems and should be correctable.

CONCLUSIONS

Overall, the advent of automated susceptibility systems for clinical microbiology laboratories has been beneficial. Many excellent laboratories use these systems successfully and report accurate results. The most important element to ensure this accuracy, however, is an appropriate understanding of the limitations of the methods and diligent supervisory review of test results as they are generated. Whenever possible, the facilitation of this review by computer software provides an extra measure of safety where there are known problems. As the volume of susceptibility testing increases in the face of pressures to control costs, it may be necessary for more clinical microbiology laboratories to implement further automated testing. Currently, however, an instrument capable of testing a variety of bacteria and detecting all of the known resistance mechanisms is far from reality. As bacteria continue to challenge us with new types of resistance, the manufacturers of rapid, automated susceptibility systems will have to assure microbiologists of both rapid and accurate detection of all mechanisms of resistance. The next generation of instruments may employ DNA probes to determine the presence of genes that are responsible for resistance rather than growth-based detection.

REFERENCES

1 **National Committee for Clinical Laboratory Standards.** *Approved Standard M2-A4: Performance Standards for Antimicrobial Disk Susceptibility Tests.* Villanova: National Committee for Clinical Laboratory Standards, 1990.

2 **National Committee for Clinical Laboratory Standards.** *Approved Standard M7-A2: Methods for Dilution Antimicrobial Susceptibility Tests for Bacteria that Grow Aerobically.* Villanova: National Committee for Clinical Laboratory Standards, 1990.

3 **Jones RN, Edson DC.** Antimicrobial susceptibility testing trends and accuracy in the United States. *Arch Pathol Lab Med* 1991;115:429–436.

4 **Bauer AW, Kirby WMM, Sherris JC, Turck M.** Antibiotic susceptibility by a standardized single disk method. *Am J Clin Pathol* 1966;45:493–496.

5 **Food and Drug Administration.** *Federal Guidelines. Review Criteria for Assessment of Antimicrobial Susceptibility Devices.* Washington, DC: Food and Drug Administration. 1991.

6 **Microbiology Resource Committee.** *Bacteriology CAP Survey Set D-A* Northfield, Il. College of American Pathologists, 1991:14.

7 **Isenberg HD, Reichler A, Wiseman D.** Prototype of a fully automated device for determination of bacterial antibiotic susceptibility in the clinical laboratory. *Appl Microbiol* 1971;22:980–986.

8 **Thornsberry C.** Automated procedures for antimicrobial susceptibility tests. In: Lennette EH, Balows A, Hausler WJ Jr, Shadomy HJ, eds. *Manual of Clinical Microbiology, 4th ed.* Washington, DC: American Society for Microbiology, 1985:1015–1018.

9 **Jorgensen JH.** Antibacterial susceptibility tests: automated or instrument-based methods. In: Balows A, Hausler WJ Jr, Herrmann KL, Isenberg HD, Shadomy HJ, eds. *Manual of Clinical Microbiology, 5th ed.* Washington, DC: American Society for Microbiology, 1991:1166–1172.

10 **Doern GV, Scott DR, Rashad AL.** Clinical impact of rapid antimicrobial susceptibility testing of blood culture isolates. *Antimicrob Agents Chemother* 1982;21:1023.

11 **Matsen JM, Krall BJ, Saxon BA.** The influence of first day susceptibility testing results on antimicrobial therapy and length of patient hospital stay. *Proceedings of the Second International Symposium on Rapid Methods and Automation in Microbiology, Cambridge, England.* Oxford, England: Learned Information (Europe) Ltd, 1976.

12 **Trenholme GM, Kaplan RL, Karakusis PH, et al.** Clinical impact of rapid identification and susceptibility testing of bacterial blood culture isolates. *J Clin Microbiol* 1989;27:1342–1345.

13 **Stager CE, Davis JR.** Automated systems for identification of microorganisms. *Clin Microbiol Rev* 1992;5:302–327.

14 **Courvalin P.** Interpretive reading of antimicrobial susceptibility tests. *Am Soc Microbiol News* 1992;58:368–375.

15 **Visser MR, Bogaards L, Rozenberg-Arska M, Verhoef J.** Comparison of the autoSCAN-W/A and Vitek Automicrobic Systems for identification and susceptibility testing of bacteria. *Eur J Clin Microbiol Infect Dis* 1992;11:979–984.

16 **Washington JA II, Knapp CC, Sanders CC.** Accuracy of microdilution and the Automicrobial System in detection of β-lactam resistance in gram-negative bacterial mutants with depressed β-lactamase. *Rev Infect Dis* 1988;10:824–829.

17 **Ferraro MJ, Jacoby GA, Katsanis G, Solliday JT, Spargo J, Gayral JP.** Improving the reliability of extended-spectrum β-lactamase detection by the Vitek System. Abstracts from the 32nd

Interscience Conference on Antimicrobial Agents and Chemotherapy, Anaheim, California, 1992.

18 **Tomasz A, Nachman S, Leaf H.** Stable classes of phenotypic expression in methicillin-resistant clinical isolates of staphylococci. *Antimicrob Agents Chemother* 1991;35:124–129.

19 **Tenover FC, Tokars J, Swenson J, Paul S, Spitalny K, Jarvis W.** Ability of clinical laboratories to detect antimicrobial-resistant enterococci. *J Clin Microbiol* 1993;31: 1695–1699.

20 **Weissmann D, Spargo J, Wennersten C, Ferraro MJ.** Detection of enterococcal high-level aminoglycoside resistance with MicroScan freeze-dried panels containing newly modified medium and Vitek gram-positive susceptibility cards. *J Clin Microbiol* 1991;29:1232–1235.

Hepatitis C virus and chronic liver disease

STANLEY M. LEMON
EDWIN A. BROWN

VIROLOGY

Historical perspective

Recognition of a third form of viral hepatitis rapidly followed the development of sensitive serologic tests for detection of hepatitis A and B infections in the mid 1970s as it became apparent that the vast majority of cases of viral hepatitis developing after blood transfusion were neither hepatitis A nor hepatitis B (1). In the absence of a better name, this form of hepatitis became known as "non-A, non-B hepatitis" (NANB). Studies in chimpanzees confirmed the transmissible nature of NANB hepatitis (2,3) and demonstrated that NANB infections could persist in humans over many years. Multiple clinical studies suggested that NANB infections could lead to chronic active hepatitis and other serious forms of chronic liver disease (4–8). By 1980, it was apparent that a considerable proportion of cases of community-acquired hepatitis, with no prior history of transfusion, were also due to an NANB agent (9,10). The responsible virus was shown a decade later to be identical to that causing post-transfusion NANB hepatitis. Finally, by the mid 1980s, several investigators had recognized an association between post-transfusion NANB hepatitis and subsequent development of hepato-cellular carcinoma (11,12).

Despite advances in characterizing the clinical manifestations of NANB hepatitis, little progress was made in the search for a specific serologic marker for this infection. Many reports of such markers appeared in the literature, but none were able to withstand the rigors of testing a coded panel of sera developed at the National Institutes of Health. Finally, in the late 1980s, Michael Houghton's laboratory at Chiron Corporation, working closely with Dan Bradley of the Centers for Disease Control, succeeded in identifying the first virus-specific antigen associated with NANB infection (13). These investigators adopted a sophisticated molecular strategy for identification of an NANB antigen, using high-titered, pedigreed infectious chimpanzee plasma as source material. Their success after many failures represents one of the great triumphs of modern molecular biology. As evidence continued to accrue linking this new viral antigen with most cases of post-transfusion NANB hepatitis (14–16), the newly discovered agent became widely accepted as "hepatitis C virus" (HCV). Early "first-generation" enzyme-linked immunosorbent assays (ELISA) for HCV antibodies provided a great deal of new information about the natural history of HCV infection, but have since been replaced by more sensitive and specific second-generation ELISA assays (17,18).

Shortly after the recognition of post-transfusion NANB hepatitis, a very different form of enterically transmitted NANB hepatitis was described in northern India (19,20). Enterically transmitted NANB hepatitis was distinct epidemiologically from post-transfusion NANB hepatitis observed in well-developed countries and more closely resembled hepatitis A virus with respect to its apparent mode of transmission and the lack of an association with chronic hepatitis. The virus responsible for enterically transmitted NANB hepatitis was subsequently identified by Balayan and coworkers (21) in the feces in an infected human volunteer. This virus, now known as hepatitis E virus (HEV), has recently been molecularly cloned and shown to be completely distinct from HCV (22).

HCV genome structure and organization

HCV is an enveloped, positive-stranded RNA virus with a genome length of approximately 9.4 kb (13,23–26). The general organization of the genome is similar to that of the flaviviruses (i.e., viruses that include dengue and yellow fever virus), but even more so to the pestiviruses (which include bovine viral diarrhea virus and hog cholera virus, veterinary pathogens of substantial importance) (27,28). The HCV genome contains a single, large open-reading frame that follows a relatively lengthy 5′ nontranslated region of approximately 342 bases (Figure 6.1). Recent evidence suggests that this 5′ nontranslated region has an important role in controlling virus translation (29,30) and may be analogous in this respect to the 5′ nontranslated region of the picornaviruses. Although still controversial, it now seems likely that viral translation is initiated in a 5′ m7G cap-independent fashion, as in the picornaviruses, which include hepatitis A virus. If true, this aspect of HCV replication would be distinctly different from replication of flaviviruses. Flavivirus RNAs have a 5′ cap and a much shorter 5′ noncoding region.

The open-reading frame of HCV encodes a large polyprotein, which undergoes post-translational cleavage mediated by both cellular and virus-specified proteases (31,32). The structural proteins are located within the amino third of the polyprotein, and include a 21-kd core (nucleocapsid) protein (C) and 2 envelope glycoproteins (E1 and E2 [or NS1]) (see Figure 6.1). These proteins are cleaved from each other via the action of signal peptidase in the endoplasmic reticulum, and E1 and E2 subsequently become heavily glycosylated. E1 and E2 are thought to represent surface proteins present in the lipid envelope of the HCV particle, whereas C appears to be an internal protein resembling the core protein of hepatitis B. The remainder of the polyprotein contains a number of nonstructural viral proteins involved in the replication of the virus, including viral proteases, a putative helicase, and an RNA polymerase. Different strains of HCV demonstrate a remarkable degree of genetic diversity. At least 5 genotypes of HCV have been identified thus far (33). Genetic variation is most pronounced in

Hepatitis C Virus Genome

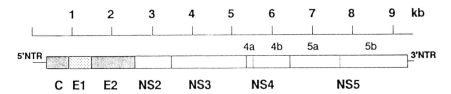

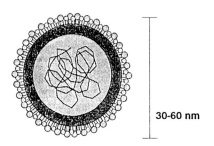

30-60 nm

Figure 6.1 Genetic and physical organization of hepatitis C virus. The single-stranded RNA genome is approximately 9.4 kb in length, and positive sense. It encodes a single large polyprotein that contains at the amino end a series of 3 structural proteins (C, E1, and E2), which are cleaved by signal peptidase, followed by 4 to 6 nonstructural proteins, which include NS3 (putatively a protease/helicase) and NS5 (the viral RNA polymerase). NTR = nontranslated region.

a "hypervariable" region of E2 (possibly reflecting substantial antigenic variation), and is least evident in the 5′ nontranslated region, which is highly conserved among different strains (34,35).

There is no well-established system for in vitro propagation of HCV. However, limited replication of the virus has been reported in primary hepatocyte explants obtained from chimpanzees (36), as well as cultured human T-cell lines (37). This currently remains an intensive area of investigation.

EPIDEMIOLOGY

Percutaneous transmission

Hepatitis C virus was first recognized in the context of percutaneous transmission. Multiple studies suggest that HCV accounts for approximately 90% of post-transfusion hepatitis cases after exclusion of hepatitis B surface antigen (HBsAg)–positive units by current methods of donor screening (16,17,38). Studies carried out in the 1970s suggested that NANB hepatitis developed in as many as 7% of transfusion recipients and that up to 1% of blood units might contain the responsible virus (4). Introduction of donor screening for elevations of serum alanine aminotransferase (ALT) and anti-bodies to hepatitis B core protein (both surrogate markers of NANB) reduced the risk of transfusion-acquired NANB prior to the advent of specific donor screening for hepatitis C by approximately 40% to 50%. Specific donor screening for anti-HCV has probably reduced the transmission of hepatitis C by 80% to 90% (16,39). HCV has also been transmitted with administration of other blood products, particularly early preparations of clotting factor concentrates. The majority of multitransfused hemophiliac patients who received factor concentrates prior to the advent of heat treatment for virus inactivation became infected with HCV (40,41). Single-unit transfusions of cryoprecipitate or plasma carried lower but still substantial risks of HCV infection. Notably, human immune globulin has been free of any apparent risk of HCV transmission.

The high risk of hepatitis C infection associated with transfusion is due to the fact that HCV commonly establishes persistent infection with continuous or intermittent viremia. The magnitude of this viremia has been difficult to quantitate, but estimates range from 10^2 to 10^8 virus particles per ml plasma, based on chimpanzee challenge studies as well as direct detection of HCV RNA in serum by polymerase chain reaction (PCR)–based techniques (42,43). Viremia may be greater during flares in the level of activity of chronic liver disease, but this correlation is imperfect.

In recent years, the advent of screening tests for detection of HCV infection in blood donors and the use of heat treatment and solvent/detergent virus inactivation procedures in the production of clotting factor concentrates have substantially lessened but not completely eliminated the risk of post-transfusion HCV infection. A low frequency of HCV infection (0.3% of recipients) continues to accompany blood transfusion due to the presence of infectious donors who are not detected by currently available antibody screening tests (16,17).

Concordant with the blood-borne nature of HCV, health care workers with frequent exposure to blood are also at risk for acquiring infection, although there are no comprehensive seroprevalence studies of these groups. Dentists, particularly oral surgeons, have been shown to be substantially more likely to have antibodies to HCV than the general population (44). In addition, intravenous drug users frequently have serologic evidence of HCV infection. In one study carried out in patients attending an inner-city emergency room, 83% of intravenous drug users had antibodies to HCV (45). In contrast, only 6% were HBsAg-positive.

Nonpercutaneous transmission

NANB hepatitis is often acquired in the absence of apparent parenteral exposures. Recent data from the Centers of Disease Control indicate that approximately 41% of patients with community-acquired acute hepatitis C do not report recognizable parenteral exposures (46). However, the precise means by which virus is transmitted nonpercutaneously remain obscure. No more than 6% of these patients report possible sexual or household exposures. The risk of transmission associated with sexual activity has been investigated carefully in a number of studies, none of which provide convincing evidence for very efficient sexual transmission of hepatitis C (47–50). HCV infection was found with somewhat higher frequency in prostitutes in Taiwan (3.5% vs 0.95% for blood donors) (51), but it is difficult to exclude confounding risk factors such as parenteral drug abuse. Some studies have suggested that spouses of HCV-infected persons are at significantly higher risks for having antibodies to HCV than other members of households (47,52). Transmission was inefficient; only 18% to 21% of spouses tested positive for antibodies. However, sequence comparisons in one study suggested that spousal couples were infected with the same virus strain (47). Evidence for transmission appears to be greatest among older couples with many years of marriage (52). In contrast to these studies, which were carried out in Asia, Everhart and associates (48) found no antibodies in 42 monogamous heterosexual partners of patients with chronic hepatitis C infection. Nonsexual, household contacts appear to be at very low risk for infection (≤2%) (48,52).

Substantial data also argue strongly against efficient perinatal transmission of HCV, although it appears clear from a number of reports that the virus is occasionally transmitted from infected mothers to their children during birth or shortly thereafter (53–56). However, these studies may be complicated by the fact that the antibody response to viral proteins in infected neonates may be weak or nonexistent.

CLINICAL MANIFESTATIONS

Acute infection

Acute hepatitis C is clinically indistinguishable from acute hepatitis A or hepatitis B in individual patients. However, several general features of hepatitis C set it apart from other forms of hepatitis. The incubation period for acute hepatitis C averages approximately 6 weeks, based on studies of transfusion recipients (17) and is thus intermediate between types A and B hepatitis. Symptoms of the infection are usually gradual in their onset and often milder than symptoms of either hepatitis A or B. Similarly, biochemical measures of hepatocellular dysfunction, including elevations of serum ALT activities and bilirubin levels, are generally less pronounced in patients with hepatitis C. Prospective studies of transfusion recipients show that more than 75% of acute hepatitis C infections are anicteric, and 50% or more would be missed without careful screening of aminotransferase abnormalities (17). It is not surprising that sporadic cases of acute hepatitis C presenting without antecedent history of blood transfusion tend to be more severe (approximately 75% of cases are jaundiced) (46). This finding undoubtedly reflects a reporting artifact, because it is likely that most acute HCV infections in the general population are not recognized clinically. Although 20% to 30% of cases of fulminant hepatitis lack markers of acute hepatitis A or hepatitis B, the frequency with which HCV causes fulminant hepatitis is controversial. One study from Japan suggested that HCV infection was present in one-third of patients with fulminant hepatitis (57), whereas a second study carried out in the United States failed to document HCV infection in patients with fulminant hepatitis (58). Extrahepatic manifestations of acute hepatitis C infection have not been recognized.

The development of assays for viral RNA and antibodies to viral proteins has thus far provided only a partial picture of the virologic events occurring during acute hepatitis C infection. In chimpanzees, viral RNA can be found in serum within 1 to 2 weeks of inoculation (59–61). Viremia appears to be maximal at the onset of hepatitis. It is reduced in magnitude later in the course of the infection but is usually not eliminated. Current estimates suggest that at least 50%, and perhaps as many as 70% to 80%, of infected individuals fail to clear the virus during the acute phase of the illness (17,46,59,61). Antibodies to the core protein, C, and several nonstructural proteins, including NS3 and NS4, usually develop and are maintained in these individuals. In contrast, individuals who clear the infection during the acute phase often have a more limited antibody response. First-generation ELISA assays that utilize an NS4 antigen (c100-3 antigen) are often only transiently positive in patients who appear to clear the infection (59). However, a more long-lived antibody response to C and NS3 antigens included in second-generation ELISA assays usually develops in these patients (62). Seroconversion is often detected several weeks earlier in second-generation tests, but antibodies develop relatively late in the course of the infection. Even in second-generation ELISA tests, detectable antibodies develop in only approximately 75% of patients within 6 weeks of the onset of symptoms (46). Transient immunoglobulin M (IgM) responses to the core protein have been described following acute infection (63) and may eventually prove useful as a diagnostic marker.

Thus far, no good tests have been described for antibodies that react with the envelope glycoproteins of HCV. The antigens displayed by these glycoproteins are likely to be highly conformational, perhaps dependent on proper glycosylation, and not readily mimicked by synthetic peptides or proteins derived from recombinant complementary DNA (cDNA).

Chronic HCV infection

Persistent infection occurs in the majority of infected individuals. The typical picture is that of a relapsing-remitting infection with recurrent bouts of hepatitis marked by periodic fluctuations in serum aminotransferase activities. During quiescent periods, serum ALT levels may be normal or near normal. Thus, the absence of ALT abnormalities does not preclude chronic HCV infection (40). In fact, clinical studies evaluating the utility of ALT as a surrogate marker for NANB infections in blood donors suggest that more than half of all viremic patients have normal ALT levels (64). Serum ALT activities are also very poor indicators of the severity of chronic liver disease associated with HCV infection, because ALT and aspartate aminotransferase (AST) levels are often normal or near normal even in patients with advanced liver disease (65). Measurement of serum albumin concentrations or prothrombin time, or both, are much better measures of the severity of liver disease, but these values become abnormal only late in the course of the disease.

Recent studies suggest that most patients (95%) with chronic HCV infection have levels of antibodies to HCV antigens that are detectable by currently available second-generation ELISA assays (18,66). In addition, viral RNA is usually detectable in serum or plasma by sensitive PCR-based assays (66). However, reports describing such PCR assays vary with the criteria for patient selection, the oligonucleotide primers and methodologies utilized, and probably the quality of the serum samples tested. Viremia is often constant but may be detected only intermittently in some patients who are studied over extended periods (59).

Type II or III essential cryoglobulinemia appears to be frequently associated with chronic HCV infection (67,68). These patients are generally viremic, with circulating RNA detectable by PCR assays. However, a large portion of these patients appear to lack antibodies detectable in even second-generation assays (68). Membranoproliferative glomerulonephritis has been shown recently to be associated with HCV-related cryoglobulinemia (67,69). Chronic HCV infection may also be a common cause of sporadic (type 1) porphyria cutanea tarda (70).

Late hepatic sequelae of HCV infection

Many studies have confirmed the presence of chronic liver disease, including chronic hepatitis and cirrhosis, in individuals with HCV infection (46,71,72). In addition, multiple studies from Japan and elsewhere document an association between chronic HCV infection and subsequent development of primary hepatocellular carcinoma (73–75). However, there is currently considerable controversy surrounding the natural history of chronic hepatitis C infection. It is clear that this is a serious infection; however, it is equally clear that the late sequelae of end-stage liver cirrhosis or hepatocellular carcinoma usually take many years to develop. The impact of HCV strain differences, genetic factors, dietary exposures, or even other coinfecting viruses on the natural history of the disease remain largely undefined. Although the literature provides a general sense that the disease may be more severe in Japan than in the United States, there are no comprehensive comparative studies.

Clinical studies carried out in the late 1970s documented the development of chronic persistent hepatitis as well as chronic active hepatitis in many patients with post-transfusion NANB hepatitis (5,7,8). Although the initial impression was that this form of chronic viral hepatitis was relatively benign, a greater appreciation of the potential severity of chronic NANB hepatitis was derived from studies evaluating such patients over a number of years. With the advent of specific serologic tests for HCV infection, numerous studies have documented a high prevalence of HCV infection among patients with chronic active hepatitis and cryptogenic liver cirrhosis. Surprisingly, a very high prevalence of HCV infection was found in patients with chronic liver disease and had been considered clinically to be related to alcohol use (76–78). These observations have led to the concept that chronic HCV infection and alcohol abuse may work synergistically in the pathogenesis of chronic liver disease (79). Early studies also suggested a high prevalence of antibodies to HCV among patients with autoimmune forms of chronic hepatitis, but this association is suspect on the grounds that patients with autoimmune disease might have false-positive serologic test results, particularly with first-generation assays for anti-HCV antibodies (80,81).

Liver biopsy and histopathologic examination provide the only certain means of evaluating the extent of liver disease in patients with chronic HCV infection. This invasive procedure is probably warranted in patients with serologic evidence of HCV infection who demonstrate elevated levels of serum aminotransferases over periods of 6 to 12 months. It is also helpful in selecting patients who may be good candidates for therapy with reombinant interferon-α (see below). However, the prognosis for patients showing histologic evidence of chronic active hepatitis, or even early cirrhosis, is far from clear. Such patients may follow relatively benign courses extending over a decade or longer, without obvious clinical evidence of hepatic decompensation.

Seeff and co-workers recently described the long term follow-up of patients who developed posttransfusion NANB hepatitis during the mid 1970s (82). These patients were participants in several prospective studies of transfusion-transmitted virus infections that were carried out at that time. Although the individual studies had long since been terminated, Seeff and co-workers documented clinical outcomes in previously enrolled patients after an average follow-up of 18 years through a rigorous examination of Social Security records, and a variety of other national and local data bases. Using a case-control approach, 586 patients who developed chemical evidence of NANB hepatitis following transfusion were matched with 984 transfused control patients who did not develop NANB hepatitis. Death certificates were obtained for 97% of the deceased patients. Surprisingly, these authors found no difference between the overall long term mortalities (51%) of patients who did and did not develop posttransfusion NANB hepatitis. Only a slight increase in death due to liver disease was noted in patients with NANB hepatitis (3.3% vs 1.5%). Taken at face value, these data suggest that NANB hepatitis, presumably hepatitis C, is a relatively benign infection.

Serologic evaluation of this cohort has been completed recently, and provides a somewhat different view of the risks associated with chronic HCV infection. A large proportion of the HCV-infected patients identified in this study have been shown to have elevated ALT levels, and liver biopsies have demonstrated serious chronic liver disease in many of those studied thus far. Thus it is likely that continued observation will document substantial morbidity and perhaps mortality due to HCV in this cohort. An additional problem is that individuals with a history of alcohol abuse were excluded from several of the individual prospective studies that form the core of this large clinical follow-up study (82). As mentioned, alcohol abuse appears to be a very important co-factor in the development of HCV-related chronic liver disease (76–79).

Hurwitz and colleagues (83), at the Centers for Disease Control, recently estimated the contribution of HCV to deaths related to severe chronic liver disease in the United States. Chronic liver disease represented the 9th leading cause of death and years of potential life lost in the United States between 1979 and 1988. The most important factor in these deaths was assumed to be alcohol abuse in the past. However, based on reports of the prevalence of HCV infection in patients with chronic liver disease, Hurwitz and colleagues estimated that approximately 41% of deaths in which chronic liver disease was listed as the underlying cause may have had chronic HCV infection as an important factor, or co-factor, in the pathogenesis in their disease (83). Approximately 12% of these patients may be coinfected with hepatitis B virus. Extrapolating this analysis to population-wide rates for death due to chronic liver disease as reported to the National Center for Health Statistics, the authors suggested that chronic HCV infection may be linked to the deaths of approximately 13,000 Americans from chronic liver disease each year. The existence of a chronic viral infection of the liver did not seem to be appreciated by attending physicians in most of these patients.

Resolution of the somewhat discordant views of the natural history of HCV infection provided by the study of Seeff and associates (82) and studies of selected patient cohorts that suggest a much greater association between chronic HCV infection and severe forms of liver disease, currently remains a central issue in the field. It is likely that these different views of the clinical impact of HCV infection reflect the fact that chronic HCV infection usually leads to severe liver disease only after a period of many years, perhaps even decades. A better understanding of the natural history of chronic hepatitis C infection is urgently needed so that a more informed assessment may be made of the relative risks and benefits of therapies, such as interferon-alpha.

Although there is a definite association between chronic HCV infection and primary hepatocellular carcinoma (73–75,84), substantial questions remain concerning the frequency with which this association occurs, as well as the specific mechanisms of carcinogenesis involved. Worldwide, chronic HBV infection is perhaps the leading factor in the development of primary liver cancer. Nonetheless, in Japan, approximately 60% to 70% of patients with hepatocellular carcinoma who lack detectable serum HBsAg have serologic evidence of chronic HCV infection, compared with only 10% of patients with other forms of cancer (73). Similar results were obtained in a study carried out in Italy: HCV infection was found in 71% of patients with liver cancer, and HBsAg in only 15% (75). Both studies utilized first-generation ELISA assays for HCV antibodies, but a second-generation assay confirmed an even greater prevalence of HCV infection in hepatitis B–negative patients with hepatocellular carcinoma. Strong evidence also exists for an association between HCV infection and primary liver cancer in the United States (85). Several studies have shown serologic evidence of chronic HCV infection in approximately 50% of American patients with hepatocellular carcinoma who do not have primary biliary cirrhosis, autoimmune hepatitis, hemochromatosis or alpha-antitrypsin deficiency (85,86).

Nonetheless, Seeff and colleagues (82) found that patients with post-transfusion NANB hepatitis did not have a measurable risk for development of liver cancer over a period of follow-up averaging 18 years. Again, these apparently contradictory observations can be reconciled by the hypothesis that hepatocellular carcinoma develops only after many years of chronic HCV infection. This finding is consistent with early case reports, which noted intervals of 17 and 19 years between acute post-transfusion NANB hepatitis and the subsequent development of liver cancer (11,12).

What are the mechanisms by which chronic HCV infection could lead to hepatocellular carcinoma? HCV is a positive-stranded RNA virus with a replication cycle likely to be confined to the cytoplasm of infected cells. There is no suggestion that the HCV genome might encode a transforming protein, nor is there any likelihood that HCV genetic information would become integrated into cellular chromosomes. However, a possible mechanism of carcinogenesis is provided by the work of Chisari and colleagues (87), who have studied the development of hepatocellular carcinoma in transgenic mice that express high levels of cytoplasmic HBsAg. This work suggests that chronic hepatocellular injury and inflammation of the liver may be key factors common to both hepatitis B– and hepatitis C–related hepatocarcinogenesis. According to this model, cellular inflammatory infiltrates, which are present in the liver in both chronic hepatitis B and chronic hepatitis C, are associated with premature hepatocellular death (possibly by apoptosis), leading to regeneration of hepatocytes and thus an overall increase in the rate of proliferation and turnover of the hepatocyte population. At the same time, inflammatory cells, particularly monocytes and macrophages, which are present in the liver, generate free hydroxyl radicals, which are capable of damaging cellular DNA and may be the proximate cause of malignant transformation. Significantly, although the inflammatory response may be triggered by antigen-specific T cells responding to the presence of viral antigens, much of the intrahepatic inflammatory response may be nonspecific and cytokine-mediated (particularly interferon-γ). This hypothetical mechanism of viral hepatocarcinogenesis is consistent with the observation that primary liver cancer commonly develops within a background of chronic hepatic inflammation and cirrhosis in both hepatitis B and hepatitis C infections (84). If correct, this mechanism has important implications for the management of patients with chronic hepatitis C, because it would support the use of antiviral agents and therapeutic approaches that lessen the extent of chronic inflammatory changes in the liver. This mechanism would also account for the association between alcohol abuse and progression of HCV infection to primary liver cancer (79).

IMMUNE RESPONSE TO HCV INFECTION

Serologic tests for the measurement of antibody responses to HCV proteins differ from those for other types of viral hepatitis because they are based entirely on the use of recombinant proteins or synthetic peptides as antigen. This difference is due to the absence of an in vitro system for propagation of HCV (unlike hepatitis A virus) and insufficient quantities of viral antigen present in infected tissues or serum to form the basis for a serologic test (unlike all other types of viral hepatitis). However, antibodies reactive with several structural and nonstructural protein antigens of HCV that have been expressed from recombinant cDNA or synthesized as oligopeptides generally develop in infected individuals. First-generation ELISA assays measured antibodies directed predominantly against NS4 (c100-3 antigen) (14), whereas current second-generation ELISA assays detect antibodies reactive with the core protein (c22-3 antigen) and the nonstructural protein NS3 (c33-C or c200 antigens) as well (18,88). As indicated, even antibodies detected in second-generation tests develop relatively late in the course of infection and do not include antibodies reactive with the surface of the virion (E1 and presumably E2 glycoproteins). Thus, antibodies measured by currently available assays would not be expected to include antibodies with viral neutralizing activity.

Neutralizing antibodies to HCV have never been clearly identified. However, at least one early clinical study suggested that administration of immune globulin to patients receiving multiple transfusions could protect against subsequent development of NANB hepatitis as well as chronic liver disease (7). Another study, carried out among American soldiers stationed in Korea, suggested that administration of immune globulin conferred protection against nonparenterally transmitted NANB hepatitis of undetermined type (89). Although it is difficult to discount these observations, further evidence for the presence of protective antibodies in immune globulin is required before their existence can be generally accepted.

Several groups of investigators have addressed the issue of immunity by serial challenge of HCV-infected chimpanzees with various viral inocula (90,91). These studies indicate that reinfection (i.e., reappearance of hepatocellular pathology or HCV viremia, or both) is common following rechallenge of previously infected animals. Nonetheless, manifestations of HCV infection were generally significantly reduced in secondary compared with primary infections. These data collectively suggest that immunity does develop following primary HCV infection, but that it is incomplete. Reinfection could be demonstrated with homologous as well as heterologous virus rechallenges, indicating that poor immunity is not related simply to antigenic variation among different strains of HCV. Such data have important implications for vaccine development efforts. However, it is important to view these observations from the perspective of chronic HBV infections. HBsAg-positive carriers can become super-infected with hepatitis delta virus (which shares a common envelope antigen with hepatitis B virus) and possibly different strains of hepatitis B virus. Nonetheless, solid immunity against hepatitis B does develop in those individuals who successfully clear the infection. Currently, it is not known whether a more complete form of immunity against HCV might develop in the small proportion of individuals who completely clear the infection, or whether such immunity could be conferred by immunization with properly presented envelope glycoproteins of HCV.

The role of cell-mediate immunity in chronic HCV infection is being vigorously explored by several research groups (92,93). The presence of CD8+ cytotoxic T lymphocytes in the liver has been clearly demonstrated, and several T-cell epitopes have been defined. The relative contributions of this T-cell response to immunity and to disease pathogenesis, however, remain uncertain. Although interest in the development of T-cell vaccines for HCV has been driven by the lack of evidence for virus-neutralizing antibodies, the rechallenge studies described (91,94) do not paint a very rosy picture for this approach to vaccine development.

PATHOLOGY

The typical histologic features of chronic hepatitis C include a mild lymphocytic inflammatory pattern with prominent lymphoid aggregates or lymphoid follicles within portal tracts (71,72). Macrovesicular fatty changes and damage to bile ducts are found in many biopsies, as are acidophilic changes in hepatocytes and acidophil bodies. In a series of 54 biopsies from 45 chronically infected patients with antibodies to HCV detected in second-generation assays, Scheuer and colleagues (71) arrived at an overall histologic diagnosis of acute hepatitis in 1 (2%) patient; mild or moderate chronic persistent, chronic lobular or chronic active hepatitis in 29 (54%) biopsy specimens; and severe chronic active hepatitis or cirrhosis, or both, in 5 (9%) biopsy specimens. The 19 (35%) remaining biopsy specimens showed well-established cirrhosis. These findings are similar to those of Bach and associates (72), who found cirrhosis in 58% of patients with chronic hepatitis C. Patients who have undergone liver biopsy are likely to represent a highly selective subset of all patients with chronic hepatitis C, but these findings provide strong evidence for an association between persistent HCV infection and serious chronic liver disease.

One view of the frequency with which HCV infection progresses to chronic liver disease comes from a recent study that prospectively followed patients presenting with acute NANB hepatitis (46). Chronic hepatitis developed in 60 of 97 (62%) HCV-infected patients followed for 9 to 48 months. Liver biopsies were done in 30 patients: only 1 patient was found to have cirrhosis, 10 had chronic active hepatitis, and 19 patients were thought to have chronic persistent or lobular hepatitis. Nonetheless, serial biopsies in small numbers of patients (46,71) and long-term clinical follow-up of patients who have undergone liver biopsy previously suggest that the liver disease progresses at no more than a very slow rate.

Much less information is available concerning the histologic picture in acute hepatitis C infection. Histopathologic examination of serial liver samples from experimentally infected chimpanzees demonstrated rare foci of liver cell necrosis within 1 week of inoculation, when significant elevations of ALT first became apparent (95). Intralobular necrosis with hepatocellular degeneration and mild lymphocytic infiltrates were most prominent 1 week later.

Viral RNA is readily demonstrated in liver tissue by PCR-based techniques (96). A modified nonisotopic in situ hybridization approach using a synthetic oligonucleotide probe demonstrated the presence of cytoplasmic viral RNA in the majority of hepatocytes within 48 hours of inoculation of experimentally infected chimpanzees (95). The number of RNA-positive cells declined sharply over a period of several weeks, but then fluctuated substantially in subsequent follow-up. The presence of viral RNA within the cytoplasm of hepatocytes did not correlate well with detection of viral RNA in serum or the extent of inflammatory changes in the liver, but did correlate roughly with serum ALT elevations in 2 chimpanzees. HCV antigens (C, E1, or NS3) have been identified in the cytoplasm of hepatocytes in about approximately one fourth of liver biopsy specimens from patients with chronic hepatitis C (65). Generally, only small numbers of widely scattered hepatocytes were found to contain these antigens. Biopsy specimens containing antigen-positive cells were more likely to have higher scores for intralobular inflammation and fibrosis. Examination of liver biopsy specimens for the presence of viral RNA or viral antigens, or both, may ultimately prove useful in following patients who receive antiviral therapy, but more information is needed concerning the clinical correlates of these laboratory observations.

DIAGNOSTIC METHODS

Serodiagnosis of HCV infections

The various antigens present in first- and second-generation ELISA assays have been described. First-generation assays utilized a recombinant fusion protein representing part of the NS4 nonstructural protein fused to the human enzyme superoxide dismutase (c100-3 antigen) (14). These first-generation assays were quite sensitive; they detected the presence of anti-HCV in approximately 80% to 90% of blood donors suspected of transmitting HCV infection (16). However, false-positive test results were relatively common, particularly in patients with autoimmune diseases, in older stored serum samples, and in sera collected in the tropics. Improvements in both sensitivity and specificity were attained by the addition of peptide antigens representative of additional antigenic domains within the core and NS3 proteins. These second-generation ELISA assays are considerably more sensitive, particularly for the early diagnosis of primary HCV infection, because seroconversion occurs earlier to the C and NS4 antigens than to c100-3 (62). Second-generation ELISA tests were positive in 98% of patients with chronic NANB hepatitis in one study, whereas the first-generation ELISA was positive in only 89% (66). Second-generation tests are also less likely to give false-positive results.

ELISA assays were developed primarily as screening tests to exclude HCV infection in blood donations, and the utility of the ELISA as a clinical diagnostic tool has been limited in several respects. Perhaps the greatest limitation has been the absence of a readily available confirmatory test. The most widely used confirmatory test for detection of antibodies to HCV has been the recombinant immunoblot assay (RIBA). The RIBA test employs a plastic strip coated with individual bands of each of the antigens included in the ELISA. The c100-3 superoxide dismutase-fusion protein and related 5-1-1 antigens are present in individual bands, whereas a third band contains superoxide dismutase alone as a control (97). Additional peptide antigens are included in individual bands in the second-generation RIBA (66). The RIBA assay generally allows determination of the specific antigens to which antibodies are reacting in the ELISA assay and has been particularly helpful in excluding sera that give false-positive ELISA results due to reactivity of antibodies with superoxide dismutase. The sensitivity of the second-generation RIBA approximates that of the second-generation ELISA tests. However, the RIBA assay is not a true confirmatory test in the sense that the Western blot is for serologic diagnosis of human immunodeficiency virus infection, because it contains only antigens that are present in the ELISA assay. A true confirmatory test should use additional antigens not present in the primary screening ELISA.

Detection of HCV RNA

An alternative approach to confirmation of HCV infection is provided by PCR-based methods for detection of viral RNA in serum or plasma (59,98,99). The virus appears to be much less stable than antibody, making it essential that blood specimens be processed promptly and that serum or plasma specimens be stored under appropriate conditions prior to testing by PCR. Reports on this subject are somewhat conflicting, but there are suggestions that extended refrigeration at 4°C, or multiple freeze-thaw cycles may substantially limit the sensitivity of PCR-based detection of viral RNA.

PCR-based tests begin by the extraction of RNA from a small volume of serum or plasma under highly denaturing conditions that are likely to inactivate circulating RNases. Complementary DNA is synthesized from the RNA using reverse transcriptase (RT) and a specific oligonucleotide primer. This first-strand cDNA product is then used as template for amplification of a double-stranded DNA via conventional PCR, using pairs of HCV-specific primers, which are complementary to opposing strands of the viral RNA. These primers are usually positioned several hundred bases distant from each other within the linear map of the HCV genome and usually represent sequences located in the conserved 5′ nontranslated region (100). Following an initial round of PCR, typically involving 30 to 35 amplification cycles, a small fraction of the amplification product is removed and subjected to a second round of PCR using a second set of oligonucleotide primers that are nested within and do not overlap with the primers used for the first PCR round. This nested PCR approach offers the advantages of extreme sensitivity, as well as high specificity. The major difficulties with the procedure are that it is time-consuming, laborious, expensive, and generally limited to research laboratories. In addition, PCR "carry-over" or other sources of contamination leading to false-positive results remain major concerns for laboratories engaged in RT-PCR detection of HCV. To a great extent, the risk of false-positive RT-PCR results due to contamination may be prevented by careful attention to proper techniques. Nonetheless, each positive result must be reproducible and ideally shown to be dependent on inclusion of the RT step.

RT-PCR has proven very useful in confirming the diagnosis of hepatitis C infection in a large number of clinical studies and has provided a great deal of information concerning the natural history of this infection. Most patients with chronic hepatitis and persistent anti-HCV antibodies have circulating RNA detectable by RT-PCR (59,66,101). However, some patients become persistently RT-PCR–negative following acute HCV infection, and many patients show evidence of fluctuating levels of viremia with intermittently negative RT-PCR results. Thus, a negative RT-PCR result should be viewed with caution and certainly does not exclude the presence of virus infection in the liver or even low-level viremia. Another problem is that nested PCR is inherently nonquantitative and incapable of providing an estimate of titer of virus present without additional modifications. However, when dilutions of serum are tested by RT-PCR, estimates of the titer of RNA correlate well with the infectious titer determined by chimpanzee inoculation (43). A new branched-chain DNA hybridization assay. In detection of HCV DNA may be more quantitative, although not as sensitive, as RT-PCR.

As discussed, there has been some success in direct detection of viral antigens or nucleic acids in infected liver tissue (65,95,96). However, these methods are not sufficiently well developed, nor are clinical correlations sufficiently well established to warrant their routine use in diagnosis or management of HCV infections.

Approach to clinical diagnosis

There are several key principles relating to the serologic diagnosis of HCV infections. First, when confronted with a patient with acute NANB hepatitis, it is important to keep in mind that antibodies that are detectable by second-generation ELISA assays may not appear for a number of weeks after the onset of symptoms (46). This delay severely limits the ability to diagnose acute primary HCV infection. Documentation of primary, acute hepatitis C will generally require testing of follow-up serologies 6 and 12 weeks after the onset of clinical symptoms. The diagnosis should not be excluded unless the patient has normal ALT levels and remains seronegative at 6 months. If available, RT-PCR detection of circulating RNA may be the best means for diagnosis of early infection.

Second, in the context of chronic hepatitis, the presence of anti-HCV should be construed as indicative of persistent infection with the virus. In particular, anti-c100-3 positivity (determined by RIBA) should be considered a marker of persistent virus infection. However, in the absence of better tests, all antibody-positive patients should be considered to be potentially viremic, whether clinical evidence of hepatocellular disease is present. Clinicians should also remember that antibodies detected in anti-HCV ELISAs are reactive with nonstructural proteins expressed during viral replication or with the core protein, which is an internal component of the virus particle. These antibodies are not likely to provide immunity against hepatitis C. As discussed, the presence and extent of immunity following natural infection with HCV remains very poorly defined.

TREATMENT

A number of clinical studies document the efficacy of recombinant interferon-α in the treatment of chronic hepatitis C (102–105). In general, these studies indicate that administration of interferon-α at doses approximating 3 million units three times weekly for periods of 6 months or longer will result in significant reductions in aminotransferase abnormalities in approximately 40–70% of patients. Improvements in the extent of inflammation within the liver have been documented in follow-up biopsy specimens. In addition, substantial reductions in the level of HCV viremia have been found in patients who experience a clinical response, suggesting that the effects of interferon may be due in part to a direct antiviral action (42,43,106,107). However, approximately half of all patients who initially respond to interferon-α relapse in the first few months following cessation of therapy. The overall response rate after 12 months is therefore 40% or lower, but long-term remissions (3–6 yrs) without return of detectable circulating HCV RNA have recently been documented (106).

The Food and Drug Administration's approval of recombinant interferon-α for treatment of chronic hepatitis C has resulted in this therapy becoming widely available to many patients and their physicians. However, there are many unanswered questions concerning the use of interferon-α in this setting (108,109). Interferon therapy is not without side effects, although they generally have not limited the extent of therapy. In addition, the costs of treatment and monitoring can be considerable. The conflicting results of clinical studies assessing natural history make long-term prognosis very unclear for patients with chronic hepatitis C; thus, it is difficult to compare the costs with the benefits of interferon therapy. The most dramatic and serious consequences of chronic HCV infection develop after many years of infection. Whether interferon therapy might reduce the risk of these late sequelae is uncertain and is likely to remain so for many years. Moreover, the lack of firm selection criteria makes it particularly difficult to judge the potential value of interferon in individual patients. It is more likely that interferon therapy would benefit patients with persistently elevated or fluctuating ALT abnormalities and inflammatory infiltrates on liver biopsy specimen than patients who have normal ALT levels and more advanced stages of liver fibrosis or cirrhosis. In addition, interferon therapy may be most advantageous for younger patients with many years of potential life before them. However, even these distinctions are uncertain, because the potential impact of interferon therapy on subsequent development of hepatocellular carcinoma, if any, is unknown. There is some suggestion that interferon responsiveness may vary among different strains of HCV and that determining the genotype of infecting HCV strains by analysis of the sequence of PCR amplifiers may help identify patients who are most likely to benefit from a course of interferon therapy (107). However, most strains of HCV in the United States fall into a single genotype; thus, this approach is unlikely to prove very helpful in the future. The decision to attempt interferon therapy is one that must be reached after careful consultation between the patient and an expert hepatologist. Historically, infectious disease specialists usually have had little input into this decision, but this separation is likely to change in the future.

There has also been interest in the potential offered by ribavirin for treatment of chronic hepatitis C (110,111). In part, this interest stems from the broad antiviral spectrum of ribavirin against a number of positive-stranded RNA viruses. One uncontrolled study demonstrated an apparent reduction in serum alanine aminotransferase activities during a 3-month treatment course. However, within 6 weeks of the end of the treatment, aminotransferase activities had returned to levels that were not significantly different from those before treatment. A second uncontrolled trial demonstrated an antiviral effect; levels of circulating HCV RNA were reduced 10-fold with therapy (111). Although these results are encouraging, no significant improvement was noted in histologic scores. Whether ribavirin provides a useful alternative to interferon-α will require the results of controlled studies that are now in progress. Theoretically, combination therapy with ribavirin and interferon could offer significant advantages, because the antiviral mechanisms of the 2 therapies are probably unrelated and the toxicities are unlikely to be synergistic.

COUNSELING AND FOLLOW-UP OF HCV-INFECTED PATIENTS

Given our current level of understanding, practicing physicians are faced with a number of dilemmas concerning HCV. A common situation confronting infectious disease physicians is management of patients found to be anti-HCV–positive after donating a unit of blood. The issues include (1) whether the test result truly reflects HCV infection; (2) whether the infection is associated with active liver disease and, if so, what to do about it; and (3) whether a patient represents an infectious risk to their personal contacts. Substantial gaps in our understanding of hepatitis C limit physicians' ability to address each of these issues.

Positive serologies for anti-HCV should be confirmed by repeat testing. If possible, positive results should be confirmed by RIBA analysis. However, this test is not commonly carried out by blood banks, and in fact is not currently licensed for clinical use within the United States. Infection may also be confirmed by PCR analysis, as discussed, but this is also not generally available to practicing physicians. In the absence of either RIBA or PCR confirmation, individuals who are found to be repeatedly positive for anti-HCV should be considered to be infected with the virus, regardless of the presence or absence of liver disease.

The extent of ongoing hepatic inflammation should be assessed by multiple determinations of serum ALT activities. Serum ALT levels should be monitored at several points over a period of 6 to 12 months, because aminotransferase abnormalities may be present only intermittently in chronic hepatitis C. In addition, serum concentrations of bilirubin and albumin and the prothrombin time should be measured to determine whether there are any serious deficiencies in liver conjugating and synthetic functions. Those patients who are found to have persistent or recurrent ALT elevations should undergo liver biopsy if therapy with interferon is under consideration.

No simple answer can be provided concerning the potential long-term value of interferon-α therapy for patients who are found to have an active histologic lesion, as discussed. This is a decision that must be reached after careful discussion of the potential benefits and risks with patients. Only compliant and reliable patients should be seriously considered for interferon therapy, and patients should be carefully followed during and after treatment. The optimal duration of interferon therapy is not clear, but is probably in the range of 6 to 12 months. Ideally, patients should be treated at centers that are able to monitor levels of HCV viremia by RT-PCR. Given the multiple associations between severe chronic liver disease, liver cancer, alcohol abuse, and persistent HCV infection (76–79), physicians should strenuously counsel HCV-infected patients to avoid alcohol. If followed, it is possible that such advice may be more useful than any therapeutic course of interferon.

With regard to the potential infectiousness of anti-HCV–positive patients, the most important consideration is that such patients should not donate blood or serve as organ donors. Administration of immune serum globulin may provide some level of protection against parenteral exposure to HCV (7), but this effect is far from certain (112). In addition, any protective benefit of immune globulin may be eliminated by changes in donor selection, which exclude HCV antibody–positive donor units from the plasma pools used for manufacture of immune globulin.

A substantial proportion of hepatitis C infections are acquired in the community in the absence of a recognized percutaneous exposure, but specific risk factors for such infection remain poorly defined. As discussed, the risk of household contacts acquiring infection appears to be much lower than with chronic hepatitis B. The risk of transmission to sexual contacts appears to be substantially greater, but is still relatively low (48,52). We believe that the data currently do not support universally recommending the use of condoms for individuals engaged in stable monogamous sexual relationships, although others may argue differently. Individuals in unstable sexual relationships or who have multiple sex partners should routinely use condoms as much for protection against human immunodeficiency virus infection as for prevention of hepatitis C transmission. No firm guidance can be provided concerning the testing of long-term sexual partners or spouses for anti-HCV antibodies, but this would seem to be a reasonable practice given our current state of knowledge.

FUTURE DIRECTIONS

Intensive efforts are now underway to characterize better the immune response to HCV and to develop a vaccine capable of preventing this infection. This will not be an easy task. Many of the problems that confound the development of vaccines for human immunodeficiency virus also impede the development of a hepatitis C vaccine. Among others, these problems include the genetic and antigenic heterogeneity of virus isolates, the lack of clearly definable protective immunity following natural infection, and difficulties in producing effective synthetic immunogens. Although it is too early to assume a pessimistic view concerning the likelihood for development of an effective vaccine, it will certainly be many years before such a vaccine becomes available. In the interim, physicians should look forward to an increasing understanding of the epidemiology and modes of transmission of this virus during the next few years, coupled with better approaches for the diagnosis and treatment of patients who are chronically infected. Development of a simple procedure for detection of viral antigen in blood would be particularly useful. The virus presents several potential targets for development of new antivirals (e.g., the protease, NS3), and advances in this area are likely.

Physicians and their patients should keep in mind that our current, meager knowledge of the natural history of hepatitis C can be credited, to a very large extent, to the explosion in understanding and exploitation of molecular biology that has occurred during the past decade. It is very likely that continuing advances in this rapidly expanding field will impact favorably on the ability of physicians to recognize, treat, and possibly prevent this infection in the future.

REFERENCES

1 Feinstone SM, Kapikian AZ, Purcell RH, Alter HJ, Holland PV. Transfusion-associated hepatitis not due to viral hepatitis type A or B. N Engl J Med 1975; 292:767–770.

2 Alter HJ, Holland PV, Purcell RH, Popper H. Transmissible agent in non-A, non-B hepatitis. Lancet 1978;1:459–463.

3 Tabor E, Gerety RJ, Drucker JA, et al. Transmission of non-A, non-B hepatitis from man to chimpanzee. Lancet 1978;1:463–466.

4 Aach RD, Kahn RA. Post-transfusion hepatitis: current perspectives. Ann Intern Med 1980;92:539–546.

5 Berman M, Alter HJ, Ishak KG, Purcell RH, Jones EA. The chronic sequelae of non-A, non-B hepatitis. Ann Intern Med 1979;91:1–6.

6 Kim HC, Saidi P, Ackley AM, Bringelsen KA, Gocke DJ. Prevalence of type B and non-A, non-B hepatitis in hemophilia: relationship to chronic liver disease. Gastroenterology 1980;79:1159–1164.

7 Knodell RG, Conrad ME, Ishak KG. Development of chronic liver disease after acute non-A, non-B post-transfusion hepatitis: role of [gamma]-globulin prophylaxis in its prevention. Gastroenterology 1977;72:902–909.

8 Rakela J, Redeker AG. Chronic liver disease after acute non-A, non-B viral hepatitis. Gastroenterology 1979;77:1200–1202.

9 Villarejos VM, Vison KA, Eduarte ACA, Provost PJ, Hilleman MR. Evidence for viral hepatitis other than type A or type B among persons in Costa Rica. N Engl J Med 1975;293:1350–1352.

10 Alter MJ, Gerety RJ, Smallwood LA, et al. Sporadic non-A, non-B hepatitis: frequency and epidemiology in an urban U.S. population. J Infect Dis 1982;145:886–893.

11 Kiyosawa K, Akahane Y, Nagata A, Furata S. Hepatocellular carcinoma after non-A, non-B hepatitis. Am J Gastroenterol 1984;79:777–781.

12 Resnick RH, Stone K, Antonucci D. Primary hepatocellular carcinoma following non-A,

non-B posttransfusion hepatitis. *Dig Dis Sci* 1983;28:908–911.

13   Choo Q-L, Kuo G, Weiner AJ, Overby LR, Bradley DW, Houghton M. Isolation of a cDNA clone derived from a blood-borne non-A, non-B viral hepatitis genome. *Science* 1989;244:359–362.

14   Kuo G, Choo Q-L, Alter HJ, et al. An assay for circulating antibodies to a major etiologic virus of human non-A, non-B hepatitis. *Science* 1989;244:362–364.

15   Weiner AJ, Kuo G, Bradley DW, et al. Detection of hepatitis C viral sequences in non-A, non-B hepatitis. *Lancet* 1990;335:1–3.

16   Alter HJ, Purcell RH, Shih JW, et al. Detection of antibody to hepatitis C virus in prospectively followed transfusion recipients with acute and chronic non-A, non-B hepatitis. *N Engl J Med* 1989;321:1494–1500.

17   Aach RD, Stevens CE, Hollinger FB, et al. Hepatitis C virus infection in post-transfusion hepatitis—an analysis with first- and second-generation assays. *N Engl J Med* 1991;325:1325–1329.

18   Chien DY, Choo Q-L, Tabrizi A, et al. Diagnosis of hepatitis C virus (HCV) infection using an immunodominant chimeric polyprotein to capture circulating antibodies: reevaluation of the role of HCV in liver disease. *Proc Natl Acad Sci USA* 1992;89:10011–10015.

19   Khuroo MS. Study of an epidemic of non-A, non-B hepatitis: possibility of another human hepatitis virus distinct from post-transfusion non-A, non-B type. *Am J Med* 1980;68:818–824.

20   Wong DC, Purcell RH, Sreenivasan MA, Prasad SR, Pavri KM. Epidemic and endemic hepatitis A in India: evidence for a non-A, non-B hepatitis virus etiology. *Lancet* 1980;2:876–879.

21   Balayan MS, Andzhaparidze AG, Savinskaya SS, et al. Evidence for a virus in non-A, non-B hepatitis transmitted via the fecal-oral route. *Intervirology* 1983;20:23–31.

22   Reyes GR, Purdy MA, Kim JP, et al. Isolation of a cDNA from the virus responsible for enterically transmitted non-A, non-B hepatitis. *Science* 1990;247:1335–1339.

23   Ogata N, Alter HJ, Miller RH, Purcell RH. Nucleotide sequence and mutation rate of the H strain of hepatitis C virus. *Proc Natl Acad Sci USA* 1991;88:3392–3396.

24   Okamoto H, Kurai K, Okada S-I, et al. Full-length sequence of a hepatitis C virus genome having poor homology to reported isolates: comparative study of four distinct genotypes. *Virology* 1992;188:331–341.

25   Houghton M, Weiner A, Han J, Kuo G, Choo Q-L. Molecular biology of the hepatitis C viruses: implications for diagnosis, development and control of viral disease. *Hepatology* 1991;14:381–388.

26   Kato N, Hijikata M, Ootsuyama Y, et al. Molecular cloning of the human hepatitis C virus genome from Japanese patients with non-A, non-B hepatitis. *Proc Natl Acad Sci USA* 1990;87:9524–9528.

27   Choo Q-L, Richman KH, Han JH, et al. Genetic organization and diversity of the hepatitis C virus. *Proc Natl Acad Sci USA* 1991;88:2451–2455.

28   Miller RH, Purcell RH. Hepatitis C virus shares amino acid sequence similarity with pestiviruses and flaviviruses as well as members of two plant virus supergroups. *Proc Natl Acad Sci USA* 1990;87:2057–2061.

29   Tsukiyama-Kohara K, Iizuka N, Kohara M, Nomoto A. Internal ribosome entry site within hepatitis C virus RNA. *J Virol* 1992;66:1476–1483.

30   Yoo BJ, Spaete RR, Geballe AP, Selby M, Houghton M, Han JH. 5′ end-dependent translation initiation of hepatitis C viral RNA and the presence of putative positive and negative translational control elements within the 5′ untranslated region. *Virology* 1992;191:889–899.

31   Hijikata M, Kato N, Ootsuyama Y, Nakagawa M, Shimotohno K. Gene mapping of the putative structural region of the hepatitis C virus genome by *in vitro* processing analysis. *Proc Natl Acad Sci USA* 1991;88:5547–5551.

32   Grakoui A, Wychowski C, Lin C, Feinstone SM, Rice CM. Expression and identification of hepatitis C virus polyprotein cleavage products. *J Virol* 1993;67:1385–1395.

33   Cha T-A, Beall E, Irvine B, et al. At least five related, but distinct, hepatitis C viral genotypes exist. *Proc Natl Acad Sci USA* 1992;89:7144–7148.

34   Hijikata M, Kato N, Ootsuyama Y, Nakagawa M, Ohkoshi S, Shimotohno K. Hypervariable regions in the putative glycoprotein of hepatitis C virus. *Biochem Biophys Res Commun* 1991;175:220–228.

35   Han JH, Shyamala V, Richman KH, et al. Characterization of the terminal regions of hepatitis C viral RNA: identification of conserved sequences in the 5′ untranslated region and poly(A) tails at the 3′ end. *Proc Natl Acad Sci USA* 1991;88:1711–1715.

36   Jacob JR, Burk KH, Eichberg JW, Dreesman GR, Lanford RE. Expression of infectious viral particles by primary chimpanzee hepatocytes

isolated during the acute phase of non-A, non-B hepatitis. *J Infect Dis* 1990;161:1121–1127.

37 Shimizu YK, Iwamoto A, Hijikata M, Purcell RH, Yoshikura H. Evidence for *in vitro* replication of hepatitis C virus genome in a human T-cell line. *Proc Natl Acad Sci USA* 1992;89:5477–5481.

38 Esteban JI, Gonzalez A, Hernandez JM, et al. Evaluation of antibodies to hepatitis C virus in a study of transfusion-associated hepatitis. *N Engl J Med* 1990;323:1107–1112.

39 Barrera JM, Bruguera M, Ercilla MG, et al. Incidence of non-A, non-B hepatitis after screening blood donors for antibodies to hepatitis C virus and surrogate markers. *Ann Intern Med* 1991;115:596–600.

40 Rumi MG, Colombo M, Gringeri A, Mannucci PM. High prevalence of antibody to hepatitis C virus in multitransfused hemophiliacs with normal transaminase levels. *Ann Intern Med* 1990;112:379–380.

41 Tedder RS, Briggs M, Ring C, et al. Hepatitis C antibody profile and viraemia prevalence in adults with severe haemophilia. *Br J Haematol* 1991;79:512–515.

42 Brillanti S, Garson JA, Tuke PW, et al. Effect of alpha-interferon therapy on hepatitis C viraemia in community-acquired chronic non-A, non-B hepatitis: a quantitative polymerase chain reaction study. *J Med Virol* 1991;34:136–141.

43 Shindo M, Di Bisceglie AM, Cheung L, et al. Decrease in serum hepatitis C viral RNA during alpha-interferon therapy for chronic hepatitis C. *Ann Intern Med* 1991;115:700–704.

44 Klein RS, Freeman K, Taylor PE, Stevens CE. Occupational risk for hepatitis C virus infection among New York City dentists. *Lancet* 1991;338:1539–1542.

45 Kelen GD, Green GB, Purcell RH, et al. Hepatitis B and hepatitis C in emergency department patients. *N Engl J Med* 1992;326:1399–1404.

46 Alter MJ, Margolis HS, Krawczynski K, et al. The natural history of community-acquired hepatitis C in the United States. *N Engl J Med* 1992;327:1899–1905.

47 Akahane Y, Aikawa T, Tsuda F, Okamoto H, Mishiro S. Transmission of HCV between spouses. *Lancet* 1992;339:1059–1060.

48 Everhart JE, Di Bisceglie AM, Murray LM, et al. Risk for non-A, non-B (type C) hepatitis through sexual or household contacts with chronic carriers. *Ann Intern Med* 1990;112:544–545.

49 Pachucki CT, Lentino JR, Schaaff D, et al. Low prevalence of sexual transmission of hepatitis C virus in sex partners of seropositive intravenous drug users. *J Infect Dis* 1991;164:820–821.

50 Brettler DB, Mannucci PM, Gringeri A, et al. The low risk of hepatitis C virus transmission among sexual partners of hepatitis C-infected hemophilic males: an international, multi-center study. *Blood* 1992;80:540–543.

51 Chen D-S, Kuo GC, Sung J-L, et al. Hepatitis C infection in an area hyperendemic for hepatitis B and chronic liver disease: the Taiwan experience. *J Infect Dis* 1990;162:817–822.

52 Kao J-H, Chen P-J, Yang P-M, et al. Intrafamilial transmission of hepatitis C virus: the important role of infections between spouses. *J Infect Dis* 1992;166:900–903.

53 Thaler MM, Park C-K, Landers DV, et al. Vertical transmission of hepatitis C virus. *Lancet* 1991;338:17–18.

54 Novati R, Thiers V, D'Arminio Monforte A, et al. Mother-to-child transmission of hepatitis C virus detected by nested polymerase chain reaction. *J Infect Dis* 1992;165:720–723.

55 Wejstl R, Widell A, Mnsson A-S, Hermodsson S, Norkrans G. Mother-to-infant transmission of hepatitis C virus. *Ann Intern Med* 1992;117:887–890.

56 Reinus JF, Leikin EL, Alter HJ, et al. Failure to detect vertical transmission of hepatitis C virus. *Ann Intern Med* 1992;117:881–886.

57 Yanagi M, Kaneko S, Unoura M, et al. Hepatitis C virus in fulminant hepatic failure. *N Engl J Med* 1991;324:1895–1896.

58 Wright TL, Hsu H, Donegan E, et al. Hepatitis C virus not found in fulminant non-A, non-B hepatitis. *Ann Intern Med* 1991;115:111–112.

59 Farci P, Alter HJ, Wong D, et al. A long-term study of hepatitis C virus replication in non-A, non-B hepatitis. *N Engl J Med* 1991;325:98–104.

60 Shindo M, Di Bisceglie AM, Biswas R, Mihalik K, Feinstone SM. Hepatitis C virus replication during acute infection in the chimpanzee. *J Infect Dis* 1992;166:424–427.

61 Abe K, Inchauspe G, Shikata T, Prince AM. Three different patterns of hepatitis C virus infection in chimpanzees. *Hepatology* 1992;15:690–695.

62 Farci P, London WT, Wong DC, et al. The natural history of infection with hepatitis C virus (HCV) in chimpanzees: comparison of serologic responses measured with first- and second-generation assays and relationship to HCV viremia. *J Infect Dis* 1992;165:1006–1011.

63 Chen P-J, Wang J-T, Hwang L-H, et al. Transient immunoglobulin M antibody response to hepatitis C virus capsid antigen in

posttransfusion hepatitis C: putative serological marker for acute viral infection. *Proc Natl Acad Sci USA* 1992;89:5971–5975.

64   Aach RD, Szmuness W, Mosley JW, et al. Serum alanine aminotransferase of donors in relation to the risk of non-A, non-B hepatitis in recipients: the Transfusion-Transmitted Viruses Study. *N Engl J Med* 1981;304:989–994.

65   Hiramatsu N, Hayashi N, Haruna Y, et al. Immunohistochemical detection of hepatitis C virus-infected hepatocytes in chronic liver disease with monoclonal antibodies to core, envelope and NS3 regions of the hepatitis C virus genome. *Hepatology* 1992;16:306–311.

66   Nakatsuji Y, Matsumoto A, Tanaka E, Ogata H, Kiyosawa K. Detection of chronic hepatitis C virus infection by four diagnostic systems: first-generation and second-generation enzyme-linked immunosorbent assay, second-generation recombinant immunoblot assay and nested polymerase chain reaction analysis. *Hepatology* 1992;16:300–305.

67   Misiani R, Bellavita P, Fenili D, et al. Hepatitis C virus infection in patients with essential mixed cryoglobulinemia. *Ann Intern Med* 1992;117:573–577.

68   Agnello V, Chung RT, Kaplan LM. A role for hepatitis C virus infection in type II cryoglobulinemia. *N Engl J Med* 1992;327:1490–1495.

69   Johnson RJ, Gretch DR, Yamabe H, et al. Membranoproliferative glomerulonephritis associated with hepatitis C virus infection. *N Engl J Med* 1993;328:465–470.

70   Fargion S, Piperno A, Cappellini MD, et al. Hepatitis C virus and porphyria cutanea tarda: evidence of a strong association. *Hepatology* 1992;16:1322–1326.

71   Scheuer PJ, Ashrafzadeh P, Sherlock S, Brown D, Dusheiko GM. The pathology of hepatitis C. *Hepatology* 1992;15:567–571.

72   Bach N, Thung SN, Schaffner F. The histological features of chronic hepatitis C and autoimmune chronic hepatitis: a comparative analysis. *Hepatology* 1992;15:572–577.

73   Saito I, Miyamura T, Ohbayashi A, et al. Hepatitis C virus infection is associated with the development of hepatocellular carcinoma. *Proc Natl Acad Sci USA* 1991;87:6547–6549.

74   Jeng J-E, Tsai J-F. Hepatitis C virus antibody in hepatocellular carcinoma in Taiwan. *J Med Virol* 1991;34:74–77.

75   Simonetti RG, Camm C, Fiorello F, et al. Hepatitis C virus infection as a risk factor for hepatocellular carcinoma in patients with cirrhosis. A case-control study. *Ann Intern Med* 1992;116:97–102.

76   Mendenhall CL, Seeff L, Diehl AM, et al. Antibodies to hepatitis B virus and hepatitis C virus in alcoholic hepatitis and cirrhosis: their prevalence and clinical relevance. *Hepatology* 1991;14:581–589.

77   Nishiguchi S, Kuroki T, Yabusako T, et al. Detection of hepatitis C virus antibodies and hepatitis C virus RNA in patients with alcoholic liver disease. *Hepatology* 1991;14:985–989.

78   Laurent-Puig P, Dussaix E, Lecoz Y, Martes P, Buffet C. Prevalence of anti-hepatitis C virus antibodies among patients with alcoholic liver disease, supplemented by 4-RIBA. *Dig Dis Sci* 1992;37:156–157.

79   Takase S, Tsutsumi M, Kawahara H, Takada N, Takada A. The alcohol-altered liver membrane antibody and hepatitis C virus infection in the progression of alcoholic liver disease. *Hepatology* 1993;17:9–13.

80   Nishiguchi S, Kuroki T, Ueda T, et al. Detection of hepatitis C virus antibody in the absence of viral RNA in patients with autoimmune hepatitis. *Ann Intern Med* 1992;116:21–25.

81   Davis GL. Hepatitis C virus antibody in patients with chronic autoimmune hepatitis: pitfalls in diagnosis and implications for treatment. *Mayo Clin Proc* 1991;66:647–650.

82   Seeff LB, Buskell-Bales Z, Wright EC, et al. Long-term mortality after transfusion-associated non-A, non-B hepatitis. *N Engl J Med* 1992;327:1906–1911.

83   Hurwitz ES, Holman RC, Neal JJ, Strine TW, Margolis HS. Chronic liver disease deaths associated with viral hepatitis in the United States, 1979–1988. Abstracts of the 1992 ICAAC. 1992.

84   Okuda K. Hepatocellular carcinoma: recent progress. *Hepatology* 1992;15:948–963.

85   Tabor E, Kobayashi K. Hepatitis C virus, a causative infectious agent of non-A, non-B hepatitis: prevalence and structure—summary of a conference on hepatitis C virus as a cause of hepatocellular carcinoma. *JNCI* 1992;84:86–90.

86   Hasan F, Jeffers LJ, de Medina M, et al. Hepatitis C-associated hepatocellular carcinoma. *Hepatology* 1990;12:589–598.

87   Chisari FV, Filippi P, Buras J, et al. Structural and pathological effects of synthesis of hepatitis B virus large envelope polypeptide in transgenic mice. *Proc Natl Acad Sci USA* 1987;84:6909–6913.

88   Alter HJ. New kit on the block: evaluation of second-generation assays for detection of antibody to the hepatitis C virus. *Hepatology* 1992;15:350–353.

89 Conrad ME, Lemon SM. Prevention of endemic icteric viral hepatitis by administration of immune serum globulin. *J Infect Dis* 1987;156:56–63.

90 Farci P, Alter HJ, Govindarajan S, et al. Lack of protective immunity against reinfection with hepatitis C virus. *Science* 1992;258:135–140.

91 Prince AM, Brotman B, Huima T, Pascual D, Jaffery M, Inchausp G. Immunity in hepatitis C infection. *J Infect Dis* 1992;165:438–443.

92 Koziel MJ, Dudley D, Wong JT, et al. Intrahepatic cytotoxic T lymphocytes specific for hepatitis C virus in persons with chronic hepatitis. *J Immunol* 1992;149:3339–3344.

93 Shirai M, Akatsuka T, Pendleton CD, et al. Induction of cytotoxic T cells to a cross-reactive epitope in the hepatitis C virus nonstructural RNA polymerase-like protein. *J Virol* 1992;66:4098–4106.

94 Nassal M. Conserved cysteines of the hepatitis B virus core protein are not required for assembly of replication-competent core particles nor for their envelopment. *Virology* 1992;190:499–505.

95 Negro F, Pacchioni D, Shimizu Y, et al. Detection of intrahepatic replication of hepatitis C virus RNA by *in situ* hybridization and comparison with histopathology. *Proc Natl Acad Sci USA* 1992;89:2247–2251.

96 Hosoda K, Omata M, Yokosuka O, Kato N, Ohto M. Non-A, non-B chronic hepatitis is chronic hepatitis C: a sensitive assay for detection of hepatitis C virus RNA in the liver. *Hepatology* 1992;15:777–781.

97 van der Poel CL, Cuypers HTM, Reesink HW, et al. Confirmation of hepatitis C virus infection by new four-antigen recombinant immunoblot assay. *Lancet* 1991;337:317–319.

98 Garson JA, Tedder RS, Briggs M, et al. Detection of hepatitis C viral sequences in blood donations by "nested" polymerase chain reaction and prediction of infectivity. *Lancet* 1990;335:1419–1422.

99 Cristiano K, Di Bisceglie AM, Hoofnagle JH, Feinstone SM. Hepatitis C viral RNA in serum of patients with chronic non-A, non-B hepatitis: detection by the polymerase chain reaction using multiple primer sets. *Hepatology* 1991;14:51–55.

100 Okamoto H, Okada S, Sugiyama Y, et al. The 5′-terminal sequence of the hepatitis C virus genome. *Jpn J Exp Med* 1990;60:167–177.

101 Widell A, Mansson A-S, Sundstrom G, Hansson BG, Nordenfelt E. Hepatitis C virus RNA in blood donor sera detected by the polymerase chain reaction: comparison with supplementary hepatitis C antibody assays. *J Med Virol* 1991;35:253–258.

102 Di Bisceglie AM, Martin P, Kassianides C, et al. Recombinant interferon alfa therapy for chronic hepatitis C: a randomized, double-blind, placebo-controlled trial. *N Engl J Med* 1989;321:1506–1510.

103 Sez-Royuela F, Porres JC, Moreno A, et al. High doses of recombinant alpha-interferon or gamma-interferon for chronic hepatitis C: a randomized, controlled trial. *Hepatology* 1991;13:327–331.

104 Makris M, Preston FE, Triger DR, Underwood JCE, Westlake L, Adelman MI. A randomized controlled trial of recombinant interferon-alpha in chronic hepatitis C in hemophiliacs. *Blood* 1991;78:1672–1677.

105 Viladomiu L, Genesc J, Esteban JI, et al. Interferon-alpha in acute posttransfusion hepatitis C: a randomized, controlled trial. *Hepatology* 1992;15:767–769.

106 Shindo M, Di Bisceglie AM, Hoofnagle JH. Long-term follow-up of patients with chronic hepatitis C treated with alpha-interferon. *Hepatology* 1992;15:1013–1016.

107 Yoshioka K, Kakumu S, Wakita T, et al. Detection of hepatitis C virus by polymerase chain reaction and response to interferon-alpha therapy: relationship to genotypes of hepatitis C virus. *Hepatology* 1992;16:293–299.

108 Di Bisceglie AM, Hoofnagle JH. Therapy of chronic hepatitis C with alpha-interferon: the answer? Or more questions. *Hepatology* 1991;13:601–603.

109 Rakela J, Douglas DD. Therapy of acute hepatitis C with interferon: how good is it really. *Hepatology* 1992;16:497–498.

110 Reichard O, Andersson J, Schvarcz R, Weiland O. Ribavirin treatment for chronic hepatitis C. *Lancet* 1991;337:1058–1061.

111 Di Bisceglie AM, Shindo M, Fong T-L, et al. A pilot study of ribavirin therapy for chronic hepatitis C. *Hepatology* 1992;16:649–654.

112 Immunization Practices Advisory Committee. Protection against viral hepatitis. *MMWR* 1990;39:23.

Nodular lymphangitis: clinical features, differential diagnosis and management

HOWARD M. HELLER
MORTON N. SWARTZ

INTRODUCTION

A variety of clinical syndromes can occur when pathogenic micro-organisms are introduced into humans by cutaneous inoculation. Some organisms, such as *Staphylococcus aureus* and *Streptococcus* species, commonly cause local cellulitis, often with regional erythematous lymphangitic streaking and adenopathy. Some organisms, such as *Treponema pallidum* and *Francisella tularensis*, may cause chancriform or ulcerative lesions at the site of inoculation and accompanying regional adenopathy. Other infections, such as cat scratch disease, are typically associated with regional adenopathy but with minimal or no obvious cutaneous lesions. Another pattern of infection sometimes seen after cutaneous inoculation of micro-organisms is nodular lymphangitis (i.e., superficial cutaneous nodular lesions that progress as the infection ascends the dermal and subcutaneous lymphatic channels). The first organism to be clearly associated with a nodular lymphangitic process was *Sporothrix schenckii*, and sporotrichosis remains the protypical infection causing this entity. Other infections that were subsequently associated with similar nodular lesions occurring in a lymphangitic pattern have been described as "sporotrichoid."

Nodular lymphangitis can occur in any area where inoculation occurs, but the hands and the upper extremities are by far the most common sites of infection. *S. schenckii* and *Mycobacterium marinum* are the most frequently encountered organisms in cases of nodular lymphangitis, although infections with other organisms, including *Nocardia spp.*, *Leishmania*, *M. kansasii*, *M. chelonae*, *M. avium-intracellulare*, *M. tuberculosis*, *Cryptococcus neoformans*, *Histoplasma capsulatum*, *Coccidioides immitis*, *Blastomyces dermatitis*, dematiaceous fungi (chromomycoses), *Staphylococcus aureus*, *F. tularensis*, and cowpox virus, have also been reported.

The typical presentation of sporotrichoid lymphangitis involves development of superficial nodular lesions of a distal extremity. These advance indolently, ascending along the route of the lymphatic channel. The individual nodules vary in size from 2 to 15 mm or more and may or may not exhibit overlying erythema. The larger lesions are more likely to be erythematous than the smaller ones; erythematous lesions usually involve the superficial skin to which they are adherent. Smaller lesions without overlying erythema may be freely movable in the subcutaneous tissues and not bound to the overlying superficial skin layers. A history of injury at the site of the early (primary inoculation) lesions can usually be elicited. A careful study of the circumstances surrounding the injury along with the characteristic appearance of nodular lymphangitis is often adequate for arriving at a clinical diagnosis.

Very rarely, other processes may superficially resemble nodular lymphangitis in appearance. For example, we have seen several nodular subcutaneous lesions in an upper extremity, arranged in what might have been a lymphangitic distribution, that were in fact the subcutaneous lesions of cysticercosis. Also, we have seen several subcutaneous nodular lesions in an upper extremity that represented fortuitously positioned metastatic nodular neoplastic lesions from a primary malignancy located elsewhere in the body. In both the foregoing instances, the nodules were nonerythematous, freely movable, and any intervening lymphatic channels were not palpable or thickened. In another patient with mycobacterial tenosynovitis, linearly arranged violaceous nodules along several fingers and the wrist mimicked nodular lymphangitis; but pain on movement of the fingers, limitation of motion, and absence of a primary cutaneous lesion are distinguishing features.

The histopathologic picture typically seen with most of the causes of nodular lymphangitis involves some degree of granuloma formation, as might be expected in an indolent, often chronic, infectious process. Varying degrees of neutrophilic reaction are seen in the different infections. The specific pathologic and clinical characteristics of each infection are described.

COMMON PATHOGENS

Sporothrix schenckii (sporotrichosis)

Microbiology   *S. schenckii* is a dimorphic fungus that grows as a mold in nature and at room temperature but as a yeast at body temperature or when incubated at 37°C. It grows well on Sabouraud agar and other simple media, usually within 1 week. In tissue, the yeast appear oval or cigar-shaped and are 4 to 6 μm wide.

Epidemiology   *S. schenckii* is generally found in soil and botanical material. Infection in humans most commonly occurs when the fungus is inoculated cutaneously; it is therefore frequently associated with contact with thorned material, such as rose bushes or sphagnum moss. Outbreaks of cutaneous sporotrichosis have been reported in plant nursery workers, miners, and other handlers of botanical material. The largest reported outbreak (84 people) in the United States occurred in 1988 and was related to contact with sphagnum moss that had come from a single source in Wisconsin (1). Pulmonary infection can occur after inhalation of spores, and ocular infection can occur as a result of conjunctival inoculation.

Cats are particularly susceptible to infection with *S. schenckii* and shed large numbers of organisms from ulcerated lesions and even in feces. Several reports of transmission from cats to humans have been reported (2).

Sporotrichosis is found in a wide geographic distribution, although it appears to be more common in certain areas, such as the Missouri and Mississippi River valleys and Oklahoma (3) in the United States, and in Mexico and Central America.

Clinical features

Localized (fixed cutaneous) and lymphocutaneous disease   Fixed cutaneous disease with *S. schenckii* occurs as a result of direct cutaneous inoculation of fungal spores. After a variable incubation period of 1 to 12 weeks, a nontender, red-purple papule develops at the site of inoculation. The papule enlarges, may drain serosanguinous fluid, and then may ulcerate or become plaque-like, or both. If untreated, the infection usually progresses proximally along a lymphangitic channel, producing erythematous, sometimes tender and warm nodular lesions (Figure 7.1). Significant adenopathy or systemic signs of infection are usually not present (4).

Fixed cutaneous infections occur much less commonly than nodular lymphocutaneous disease. The lymphangitic progression of the infection is dependent on several characteristics of host and pathogen, including site of infection, immune status of the host, prior exposure and sensitization of the host to *S. schenckii*, and thermosensitivity

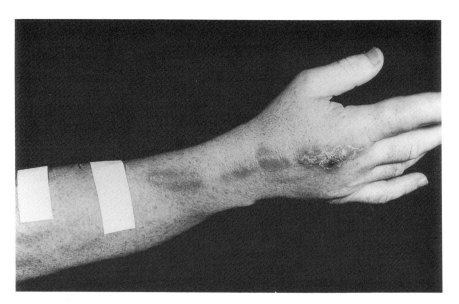

Figure 7.1   Nodular lymphangitis due to *Sporothrix schenckii* (Courtesy of Richard Johnson, MD). **(a)** The lesions are linearly arranged and the inflamed lymphatics are erythematous and thickened. The earlier, more distal lesion shows ulceration. **(b)** The linear array of descrete, erythematous nodular lesions is evident, and some thickening of the involved lymphatics between individual nodules is palpable.

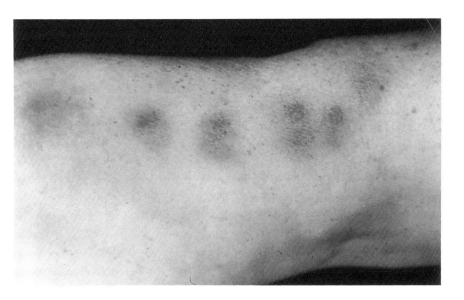

of the infecting organisms. Isolates from fixed cutaneous lesions tend to grow poorly at 37°C, in contrast to isolates from lymphocutaneous infections (5).

Extracutaneous and disseminated sporotrichosis   Monoarticular arthritis and polytenosynovitis due to *S. schenckii* result from hematogenous dissemination. There is usually no prior history of distal localized or lymphocutaneous disease. Pulmonary sporotrichosis may result from inhalation of spores and typically is associated with thin-walled pulmonary cavities. Ocular infection can occur after direct mucosal inoculation or less frequently as a result of hematogenous dissemination. Chronic meningitis due to *S. schenckii* has been reported and it presumably occurs after subclinical hematogenous dissemination (3).

Disseminated sporotrichosis has been reported in alcoholics, patients receiving immunosuppressive medications, and patients with human immunodeficiency virus infection (6). It usually presents with disseminated nodular cutaneous lesions and frequently with monoarticular arthritis.

Diagnosis   The diagnosis of sporotrichosis is made by demonstrating the organism in biopsy specimen or by isolating it in culture from drainage or from tissue. Serologic tests and tests of cutaneous hypersensitivity are not helpful clinically in diagnosis and management of cutaneous disease but may be helpful in cases of deeply invasive or systemic infection.

Pathology   Histopathologic examination of the nodular lesions usually reveals granuloma formation with giant and epithelioid cells. A prominent neutrophilic infiltration may also be present. Yeast cells are frequently not seen, and only rarely are hyphae seen. "Asteroid bodies" composed of fungal spores surrounded by eosinophilic material in a radiate pattern are often seen in the center of granulomas and are almost pathogno-monic for sporotrichosis (7). The eosinophilic material is an example of the Splendore-Hoeppli reaction and consists of a precipitate of fungal antigen, host antibody, and possibly other plasma proteins (8). Similar phenomena are seen with other infections, including mycetoma, nasofacial zygomycosis, dermatophytosis, and schistosomiasis. Such structures should be distinguished from the "asteroid bodies" or "asteroid inclu-sion bodies" described particularly in sarcoidosis (but also in other types of granulomas) (9). In sarcoidosis, these inclusion bodies have usually been found within giant cells of either the foreign-body type or the Langhans' type.

Treatment   Spontaneous resolution of fixed cutaneous lesions may occur, but nodu-lar lymphangitic lesions require treatment. Local application of heat with the use of a heating pad at 39°C to 42°C for several hours per day is sometimes adequate to achieve cure of fixed cutaneous or lymphocutaneous disease. Saturated solution of potassium iodide (SSKI) in doses of up to 1.8 gm/day is also effective, but gastrointestinal toxicity and potential thyroid toxicity limit its utility. SSKI is administered at a dose of 5 drops orally 3 times daily after meals and increased by 3 to 5 drops daily up to 120 drops daily or the maximum tolerated dose. Dilution of the SSKI in unsweetened grapefruit juice may help mask the unpleasant taste of the medication. Itraconazole (100–200 mg/day) (10,11) or ketoconazole (200–400 mg/day) (12) have also been demonstrated to be effective against sporotrichosis and are easier to administer and generally better toler-ated than potassium iodide. Itraconazole is now licensed for clinical use and may supplant SSKI as the preferred initial therapy for lymphonodular cutaneous sporotricho-sis. Amphotericin B is usually effective treatment for S. *schenckii* infections, but its use is generally confined to cases of disseminated disease. The duration of therapy required varies depending on the severity of disease, but 1.5 to 3 months is adequate for most cases in immunocompetent hosts. In general, treatment is continued until the lesions have been healed for 4 weeks.

Mycobacterium marinum

Microbiology   *Mycobacterium marinum* is a photochromogenic bacterium that grows optimally at 32°C on Lowenstein-Jensen or Middlebrook culture media. It forms colonies within 10 to 21 days, and after exposure to light, the cream-colored colonies turn yellow-orange. It is acid-fast on Kinyoun or Ziehl-Neelsen stain.

Epidemiology   M. *marinum* is a ubiquitous aquatic micro-organism that has been isolated from freshwater and marine environments and from fish and animals that inhabit them, as well as from swimming pools and aquariums. The organism was first identified in 1926, but the first association with human disease was in 1951, when it was isolated from skin lesions in swimmers using a contaminated swimming pool. It occurs in all parts of the world; however, most cases reported in the literature have been from North America and Europe. Aquarium-acquired infections are more likely to occur from saltwater aquariums than freshwater ones (13).

Clinical features   After an average incubation period of 2 weeks (range, 1–8 weeks), a reddish blue papule appears and then slowly enlarges to form a nodule. Surrounding satellite lesions may appear and often coalesce. The lesions are tender in fewer than half of patients, and ulceration with purulent drainage may occur (14–17). The infection progresses to nodular lymphangitis in approximately 25% of patients. Regional adenopathy is rare. In fishermen, aquarium owners, and other fish handlers ("fish-handler's disease" or "fish-tank granuloma"), lesions occur most commonly on the fingers and the hands. In others, such as those who acquire infection while swimming in seawater or in swimming pools ("swimming pool granuloma"), the lesions tend to occur at elbows, knees, toes, and other bony prominences that are sites more prone to trauma. Its preferential growth at 32°C accounts for its propensity to cause disease in superficial and therefore cooler areas of the body. Infection may spread to deeper tissues, causing tenosynovitis, particularly when the hand is involved (18).

Dissemination occurs extremely rarely, even in immunocompromised hosts, probably as a result of its poor growth at 37°C. The disease in immunocompromised patients may be more aggressive but appears to respond readily to appropriate therapy (19–21).

Diagnosis   Acid-fast bacilli cannot be demonstrated in tissue reliably in patients with *M. marinum* infection. Definitive diagnosis is made by isolating the organism from drainage or from tissue specimens obtained on biopsy. The organism is often difficult to grow in the laboratory. The microbiology laboratory staff must be alerted to the possibility of *M. marinum* so that appropriate cultures can be prepared and incubated at 30°C to 32°C.

Cutaneous tests for evidence of cell-mediated immunity are not very sensitive. Approximately 50% of patients will react to standard mycobacterial purified protein derivative. Use of specific *M. marinum*–derived antigen increases sensitivity to approximately 75%. *M. marinum* skin testing is positive in up to 25% of people with extensive seawater exposure (22).

Because organisms often are not seen on biopsy, and because the ability to isolate the organism is variable, definite diagnosis may not be possible in some patients. Therefore, the exposure history to acquarium water or to fish or other acquatic animals can provide important epidemiologic clues that may help clinicians arrive at the correct diagnosis.

Pathology   The pathologic changes seen in lesions vary from acute suppurative infiltrates to well-formed granulomas. Granulomas are more likely to be seen in chronic lesions that have progressed over several weeks to months. Bacteria can be visualized in only approximately 10% of patients (23).

Treatment   Spontaneous cure of minor localized infections may occur. Local application of heat can be beneficial as adjunctive therapy, along with antibiotics. Susceptibility to antimicrobial agents is variable (24,25). Oral minocycline (100 mg twice daily) or cotrimoxazole (320 mg trimethoprim, 1600 mg sulfamethoxazole twice daily) have been used successfully. Rifampin (15 mg/kg day orally; usually 600 mg once daily in an adult) in combination with ethambutol (25 mg/kg day) is usually effective, and this combination might be preferred, particularly in individuals who have not shown some clinical improvement after a few weeks of treatment with cotrimoxazole or minocycline. The newer macrolides—clarithromycin and azithromycin—and fluoroquinolones, such as ciprofloxacin, are effective *in vitro*, but clinical evidence of efficacy is lacking. Adequate treatment requires 1 to 4 months of antimicrobial administration. In patients with synovial involvement, surgical debridement may be needed to achieve cure (22,26). Surgical excision can be used to treat localized lesions, but instances of lymphangitic spread following trauma to localized lesions have been reported (18,21).

UNCOMMON PATHOGENS

Leishmania species

Leishmaniasis is a protozoal disease caused by any of several species of *Leishmania*. Infection can result in localized cutaneous disease, mucocutaneous disease, or visceral disease, (also known as kala azar). The manifestations of the disease depend on the interaction between the host and the particular species of *Leishmania* involved. Infection with *Leishmania tropica*, also called Old World leishmaniasis, occurs in tropical and subtropical areas of Africa, the Middle East, and Asia. In Central and South America, the disease is caused by the *L. brasiliensis* and the *L. mexicana* complexes and is known as New World or American leishmaniasis. Both types of cutaneous leishmaniasis are transmitted by sandflies, and the primary reservoirs of the parasite are rodents.

Cutaneous infection typically starts as a small papule at the site of the sandfly bite, usually following an incubation period of 2 to 8 weeks. The incubation period of Old World leishmaniasis can be several months or, rarely, even years. Inoculation occurs on any area of the body that may be exposed and susceptible to sandfly bites. The papule gradually enlarges, and then crusts and ulcerates. The ulcer is shallow, with raised borders and granulation tissue at its base. Papular nodules are often seen proximal to or surrounding an ulcerated lesion. The nodules are firm, nontender, mobile, and may appear to have follicular plugging. In American leishmaniasis, lymphangitic spread with the formation of nodules is common (27–29), whereas it is rarely seen with Old World leishmaniasis (30,31). The nodular lesions are typically 0.5 to 2 cm in diameter and may be scaly, crusted, or ulcerated. Regional adenopathy is usually absent.

Diagnosis is made by biopsy of a lesion and direct visualization of the *Leishmania* amastigotes within histocytes in the tissue or by visualizing the organism in a Giemsa-stained scraping taken from the base of an ulcer. The organism can be grown in tissue culture or in hamsters. The Montenegro leishmanin skin test is positive in 58% to 100% of patients with cutaneous disease.

Localized disease can be successfully treated sometimes with cryotherapy or with local application of heat (40°C to 41°C at skin surface for intervals of 2–3 hr for a total of 25–30 hr) (32). Extensive disease requires systemic therapy, and the most effective agents are the pentavalent antimonials, such as stibogluconate sodium (Pentostam) or meglumine antimoniate (Glucantime), 20 mg/kg daily intravenously or intramuscularly for an adult for 20 to 28 days. Alternative therapies include amphotericin B (0.25–1 mg/kg daily or every other day, up to a cumulative dose of 1.5–2 gm) or pentamidine isethionate (2–4 mg/kg intramuscularly or intravenously daily for 15 days) (33). Oral ketoconazole (400–600 mg/day for 28 days) may also be effective (34).

Nocardia

Nocardia species are ubiquitous soil organisms that can be pathogenic in humans, especially in immunocompromised hosts. They can enter the body either by inhalation or by direct cutaneous inoculation and can disseminate hematogenously. As with S. schenckii, cutaneous infection most commonly occurs by direct inoculation after contact with botanical materials, especially ones that are likely to puncture the skin, or after a cat scratch. The distal extremities are the most commonly involved areas. Both N. asteroides and N. brasiliensis cause cutaneous infection, although the latter is more common (35).

The most common manifestation of cutaneous infection with N. asteroides or N. brasiliensis is localized chronic granuloma formation, but several cases of nodular lymphangitis have also been reported (35–41). The nodular lesions develop 2 to 4 weeks after inoculation and are typically warm, erythematous, and tender. They may be firm or fluctuant. Purulent drainage is often present at the site of the initial inoculation, and pus may be expressed from the nodular lesions if they are fluctuant. Pathognomonic sulfur granules are often evident in the pus. Regional adenopathy is frequently present.

Diagnosis can be made by biopsy of the nodular lesion for histologic examination or culture, or both. Gram positive, thin, beaded, branching rods can frequently be identified in tissue and can usually be isolated from culture. *Nocardia* usually stain with a modified Ziehl-Neelsen stain in which the decolorization is done with 1.0% sulfuric acid instead of acid alcohol. *Nocardia* grow well on most media. However, because it may take several days for colonies to be visible on solid media, it is important to alert the microbiology laboratory staff that *Nocardia* is suspected so the culture plates can be processed appropriately and examined for at least several days for colonies that resemble those of *Nocardia*. Histopathologic examination of nodular lesions usually reveals neutrophilic infiltration with some epithelioid and giant cells.

Nocardia infection generally responds readily to antimicrobial therapy with sulfadiazine (6 gm/day orally or intravenously) or cotrimoxazole (480 mg trimethoprim, 2.4 gm sulfamethoxazole 4 times daily orally or intravenously); these are the drugs usually employed in therapy. Minocycline may be an alternative. Imipenem is effective, and the third-generation cephalosporins may also be effective (42–45). Susceptibility to β-lactam drugs is variable so they should only be used after *in vitro* susceptibility is demonstrated. Surgical drainage may be needed if subcutaneous abscess formation is extensive (35–39).

Other Mycobacteria

Although *M. marinum* is by far the most common mycobacterium to cause nodular lymphangitis, the other mycobacteria can also be associated with a similar process.

Despite the environmental ubiquity of the nontuberculous "atypical" mycobacteria, *M. marinum* causes cutaneous infection more commonly, probably as a result of its preferential growth at temperatures below 37°C. Because the other atypical mycobacteria grow optimally at 37°C or higher, the relatively cooler temperature of the skin may be less conducive to the development of infection.

Both *M. chelonae* (45–48) and *M. kansasii* (49,50) have been associated with nodular lymphangitic infection. As with other environmental pathogens, infection usually begins after percutaneous inoculation of the organism following trauma. Immunocompromised patients, especially those receiving corticosteroids, appear to be at higher risk for development of infection. The lesions develop insidiously and often resolve spontaneously. Dissemination can occur in immunocompromised patients.

The histologic picture is usually a mixture of epithelioid granuloma formation with neutrophilic infiltration. Acid-fast bacilli can frequently be seen on Kinyoun or Ziehl-Neelsen stain. A single instance of *M. avium-intracellulare* causing nodular lymphangitis in a cardiac transplant patient has been reported. In this patient, the reactive histiocytes were spindle cells; only a few Langhans' giant cells were seen on histopathologic examination (51).

Localized cutaneous infection usually resolves spontaneously or with localized care. In immunocompromised patients who might be at greater risk of dissemination, treatment with systemic antibiotics may be more essential, and the choice of agents should be guided by *in vitro* susceptibility testing. *M. kansasii* is typically susceptible to the antituberculous antimicrobial agents isoniazid, rifampin, and ethambutol. *M. chelonae* is usually resistant to the antituberculous agents, and cefoxitin and amikacin are usually the preferred treatment. Fluoroquinolones, doxycycline, and the newer macrolides, clarithromycin and azithromycin, may be active against strains of *M. chelonae*.

Rarely, cutaneous *M. tuberculosis* infection can present with gumma formation in a lymphangitic pattern (52). Initially, the lesions may be fluctuant, but they then ulcerate and crust. Unlike skin infection with atypical mycobacteria, cutaneous tuberculosis occurs as a result of hematogenous dissemination from a primary pulmonary lesion to a focus on the skin, with subsequent local lymphangitic spread.

RARE PATHOGENS

Fungi

Although *S. schenckii* is much more likely to cause nodular lymphangitis than fixed localized cutaneous disease, other dimorphic fungi have the opposite propensity. *Blastomyces dermatiditis*, *Cryptococcus neoformans*, *Histoplasma capsulatum*, and *Coccidioides immitis* generally cause localized lesions in the area of inoculation, and subsequent lymphangitic spread occurs only rarely (53–56). Primary cutaneous lesions start as small papules, which then develop into ulcerative or chancriform lesions. Tender regional adenopathy may be present, but systemic signs of infection are generally absent. The inflammatory response consists of histiocytes with plasma cells and lymphocytes. Reported cases have always involved infections of the hands acquired secondary to trauma.

Chromomycosis or chromoblastomycosis are the collective terms used to describe infections with the dematiaceous or "black" fungi. The dematiaceous fungi cause cutaneous infections more frequently than the dimorphic fungi but are just as unlikely to spread with the development of nodular lymphangitis. Lesions start as small, scaly, pink papules on the foot or leg. These papules enlarge to form purplish nodules and verrucous plaques, which usually are pruritic. Satellite lesions form and frequently coalesce. Only rarely do the satellite lesions appear to follow a lymphangitic pattern (57). Lymph nodes are rarely involved.

The most common infection involving *Pseudoallescheria boydii* is mycetoma. The infection usually begins as an idolent, nontender, logically invasive nodule or subcutaneous swelling. It then gradually spreads to involve the subcutaneous tissues and ligaments, forming fistulous tracts and abscesses. Deep tissues are usually not involved. A single case of nodular lymphangitic spread has been reported (58).

Staphylococcus aureus (botryomycosis, bacterial pseudomycosis)

Botryomycosis produced by *Staphylococcus aureus* has been reported as a cause of nodular lymphangitic infection only rarely. Botryomycosis is a chronic suppurative disease in which grains resembling actinomycotic granules are seen within a suppurative focus. The granules, consisting of clusters of swollen bacterial cells surrounded by eosinophilic material, are seen histopathologically (59,60). The cutaneous nodules may be scaly, ulcerated, or crusted.

Botryomycosis was originally described as a chronic pulmonary disease of horses. The clusters of large cocci (*botryos*, from the Greek meaning "bunch of grapes") seen histopathologically were mistakenly thought to be fungal. Because the true etiology of the infection has been established, the term *bacterial pseudomycosis* is perhaps more accurate.

In humans, botryomycosis most frequently involves the skin and the soft tissues. Visceral involvement rarely occurs. Trauma or the presence of a foreign body frequently precedes the development of botryomycosis. In most reported cases, patients have had no obvious immunodeficiency.

In hematoxylin and eosin–stained tissues, the botryomycotic granules may appear similar to actinomycotic granules. However, when stained with modified gram stains, such as Brown-Hopps stain, the swollen cocci of *Staphylococcus* can easily be distinguished from the filaments of *Actinomyces*. The source of the amorphous eosinophilic material has not been clearly established, but it is believed to result from an unusual balance between the organism, (perhaps with decreased virulence), local tissue factors, and possibly high levels of antistaphylococcal antibodies (60).

Francisella tularensis (Tularemia)

The most common clinical form of tularemia is the ulceroglandular pattern, consisting of a cutaneous ulcer and regional lymphadenopathy. Nodular lymphangitis has been reported earlier this century to occur in 7.5% (61) to 23% (62) of patients with tularemia but was not observed in any of 88 cases observed more recently (1949–1979)

(63). *F. tularensis* is a small, gram-negative pleomorphic coccobacillus that requires cysteine for growth (glucose-cysteine blood agar). Attempts to isolate the organism from blood, skin ulcers, or suppurative lymph nodes should be made only by an experienced bacteriologist in a facility with an appropriate safety hood in view of the danger of laboratory-acquired infection. The principal sources of infection are contact with animals (particularly rabbits, voles, and squirrels, but also domestic animals such as cats) and bites by ticks or deer flies. The disease occurs in the United States (except Hawaii), Canada, Europe (particularly Scandinavia) exclusive of the United Kingdom, and Japan.

After an incubation period of 3 to 6 days, the illness begins with constitutional symptoms (fever, malaise, headache) and early bacteremia. A small red papule develops at the site of inoculation (usually on the hand or the arm), enlarges, and ulcerates. Enlarged regional lymph nodes are evident, but visible erythematous lymphangitis streaks are not a feature unless secondary bacterial infection (streptococcal or staphylococcal) has supervened. Untreated, the illness would run a febrile course of 2 to 4 weeks; during this period, the nodular lymphangitis might develop. These nodules are initially movable and firm, become fixed to overlying skin, and would ultimately suppurate in more than half of patients (61).

The rarity of tularemia currently as a cause of nodular lymphangitis (63) most likely stems from acute febrile presentation, early clinical diagnosis, and institution of antimicrobial therapy with streptomycin or gentamicin (the drugs of choice) or tetracycline or chloramphenicol (alternatives), in contrast to before the antibiotic era.

Cowpox virus

A single case of cowpox infection presenting with nodular lymphangitis spread on the face has been reported (64).

CONCLUSIONS

In evaluating patients with nodular lymphangitis, particular attention to a few key features can help point in the direction of the diagnosis (Table 7.1). Infection occurring in the distal extremities, especially if there is a history or evidence of prior trauma, suggests infection with an environmental pathogen. History of trauma with horticultural material would most likely be associated with *Sporothrix*, *Nocardia*, or atypical mycobacteria. All 3 may be associated with a prior history of cat scratch. A history of contact with cats, even without scratch, may be associated with sporotrichosis or cowpox. A history of contact with dogs may raise a suspicion of blastomycosis because dogs are more susceptible to *B. dermatiditis* and disseminated disease can develop. A history of exposure to an aquatic environment, especially contact with saltwater fish or crustaceans, would be most suggestive of *M. marinum* infection. Concern about *Leishmania* would depend on a geographic exposure risk—travel to the Middle East, Africa, or rural areas of South and Central America.

Table 7.1 Nodular lymphangitis

Organism	Exposure history	Clinical features	Pathology	Diagnosis	Treatment
S. schenckii	Peat moss; soil; flowers, especially thorned; infected cats	Papules with ulceration; serosanguinous drainage	Granulomas, asteroid bodies	Culture on Sabouraud at 32°C	Heat; SSKI; itraconazole
M. marinum	Fish, shellfish, aquariums, swimming pools, seawater	Red-blue papule develops into nodule; satellite nodules, which may coalesce and ulcerate with purulent drainage	Varies: acute suppuration, granulomas; bacilli rarely seen	Culture on Middlebrook or Lowenstein-Jensen at 32°C	Heat; rifampin + ethambutol; minocycline; cotrimoxazole
Leishmania	Travel to Mid-East, Africa, or Central/S. America (especially near forested areas)	Ulceration with surrounding nodules; nontender; no adenopathy; lymphangitic lesions may be scaly/crusted	Amastigotes within histiocytes	Scraping of ulcer, biopsy of lesion, leishmanin skin test	Cryotherapy; heat; pentavalent antimonials; amphotericin B; pentamidine; ketoconazole
Nocardia spp.	Soil, botanicals, cat scratch	Tender, purulent drainage with sulfur granules	Epithelioid and giant cells; neutrophils	Culture on most media	Cotrimoxazole, sulfadiazine; imipenem; third-generation cephalosporin

Table 7.1 *continued*

Organism	Exposure history	Clinical features	Pathology	Diagnosis	Treatment
1. *M. chelonae*	Soil, water, cat scratch	Warm, tender, often with purulence	Epithelioid granulomas; neutrophils	Culture on Middle-brook or Lowenstein-Jensen media	1. Cefoxitin; amikacin; ?macrolide
2. *M. kansasii*					2. Isoniazid; rifampin; ethambutol
3. *M. avium-intracellulare*					3. Macrolide; ethambutol; rifampin
M. tuberculosis	Tuberculosis	Fluctuant; then ulcerative and crusting	Gummas	Culture on Middle-brook or Lowenstein-Jensen media	Isoniazid; rifampin; pyrazinamide; ethambutol
C. neoformans, B. dermatiditis, C. immitis, H. capsulatum, Chromomycosis	Soil, infected animals	Chancriform ulcer	Histiocytes; plasma cells; lymphocytes	Culture on Sabouraud media	Azoles (itraconazole, fluconazole); amphotericin B
P. boydii	Soil, decayed vegetation	Nontender, subcutaneous abscesses with ulceration and crusting	Neutrophils	Culture on Sabouraud media	Debridement; ? azoles (itraconazole, ketoconazole)
S. aureus	No unusual exposure	Scaly; ulcerated; crusted lesions	Botryomycotic granules	Culture on routine media	Antistaphylococcal β-lactam; vancomycin

| F. tularensis | Ticks, deer flies, wild rabbits, voles, squirrels, cats | Fever, bacteremia, 1-degree nodule with ulceration; erythematous lymphangitic nodules, often with suppuration; prominent regional lymphadenopathy | Granulomatous reaction with epithelioid cells, multinucleated giant cells; neutrophils early; focal areas of necrosis | Four-fold rise in agglutination titer or titer of ≥ 1:160 in acute phase; isolation of F. tularensis from ulcer or blood in lab with safety hood | Streptomycin or gentamicin |
| Cowpox | Cattle; cats | Ulcer with regional adenopathy | | Electron microscopy, serology | Supportive |

SSKI = saturated solution of potassium iodide.

The appearance of the lesions may also afford some clues (65). A prominent purulent component of the infection would be most likely to occur with *Nocardia* infection or possibly the atypical mycobacteria. The presence of an ulcer distal to the nodular lymphangitis would be most commonly seen with the dimorphic fungi or *Leishmania*.

Because infection with *M. marinum* and *S. schenckii*, the two most common causes of nodular lymphangitis, may respond to conservative management (i.e., localized application of heat), invasive and expensive diagnostic procedures may not be mandatory in mild, uncomplicated cases, especially if the history is strongly suggestive of exposure to those organisms. If the infection is severe, (i.e., if there is evidence of progression or of bone or synovial involvement), if there are signs of dissemination, or if the patient is immunocompromised, precise and rapid diagnosis is more essential. Usually diagnosis can be accomplished by punch biopsy of a nodule or a primary lesion for histopathologic examination and culture. Small mobile nodules, without attachment to overlying skin, may roll and escape from sampling by the skin punch. In this circumstance, a regular wedge biopsy should be performed. It is important to alert the microbiology laboratory staff to the organisms that are being sought. Some may require special incubation techniques (i.e., for *M. marinum*, *S. schenckii*), special laboratory precautions (i.e., for *C. immitis*), or prolonged observation of the cultures (i.e., for *Nocardia*). In nonimmunocompromised patients, if the etiology of the nodular lymphangitis is promptly ascertained, the infection can almost always be cured with conservative or antibiotic therapy. Rarely will surgical intervention with debridement of deeper tissues be required.

Patients with nodular lymphangitis often go undiagnosed for many weeks, months, or even years (15). It is not uncommon for patients to undergo prolonged treatment with inappropriate antibiotics before the correct diagnosis is made, and then often only after referral to a dermatologist or an infectious disease specialist. By recognizing the distinct pattern of nodular lymphangitis and focusing on the broad but limited differential diagnosis, accurate diagnosis can usually be made promptly and appropriate therapy can be instituted.

REFERENCES

1 Dixon DM, Salkin IF, Duncan RA, et al. Isolation and characterization of *Sporothrix schenckii* from clinical and environmental sources associated with the largest U.S. epidemic of sporotrichosis. *J Clin Microbiol* 1989;29:1106–1113.

2 Caravalho J, Caldwell JB, Radford BL, Feldman AR. Feline-transmitted sporotrichosis in the southwestern United States. *West J Med* 1991;154:462–465.

3 Scott EN, Kaufman L, Brown AC, Muchmore HG. Serologic studies in the diagnosis and management of meningitis due to *Sporothrix schenckii*. *N Engl J Med* 1987;317:935–940.

4 Winn WE. Sporotrichosis. *Infect Dis Clin North Am* 1988;2:89–911.

5 Kwon-Chung KJ. Comparison of isolates of *Sporothrix schenckii* obtained from fixed cutaneous lesions with isolates from other types of lesions. *J Infect Dis* 1979;139:424–431.

6 Heller HM, Fuhrer J. Disseminated sporotrichosis in patients with AIDS: case report and review of the literature. *AIDS* 1991;5:1243–1246.

7 Lurie HI. Histopathology of sporotrichosis. *Arch Pathol* 1963;75:421–437.

8 Lurie HI, Still WJS. The "capsule" of *Sporotrichum schenckii* and the evolution of the

asteroid body: a light and electron microscopic study. Sabouraudia 1969;7:64–70.

9 Freiman DG. Sarcoidosis. *N Engl J Med* 1948;239:664–671.

10 Restrepo A, Robledo J, Gomez I, et al. Itraconazole therapy in lymphangitic and cutaneous sporotrichosis. *Arch Dermatol* 1986;122: 413–417.

11 Baker JH, Goodpasture HC, Kuhns HR, Rinaldi MG. Fungemia caused by an amphotericin B-resistant isolate of *Sporothrix schenckii*, successful treatment with itraconazole. *Arch Pathol Lab Med* 1989;113:1279–1281.

12 Calhoun DL, Waskin H, White MP. Treatment of systemic sporotrichosis with ketoconazole. *Rev Infect Dis* 1991;13:47–51.

13 Huminer D, Pitlik SD, Block C, Kaufman L, et al. Aquarium-borne *Mycobacterium marinum* skin infection. *Arch Dermatol* 1986;122: 698–703.

14 Glickman FS. Sporotrichoid mycobacterial infections; case report and review. *J Am Acad Dermatol* 1983;8:703–707.

15 Raz I, Katz M, Aram H, Haas H. Sporotrichoid *Mycobacterium marinum* infection: report of a ten-year case. *Int J Dermatol* 1984;23:554–555.

16 Kern W, Vanek E, Jungbluth H. Fish breeder granuloma: infection caused by *Mycobacterium marinum* and other atypical mycobacteria in the human. Analysis of 8 cases and review of the literature. *Med Klin* 1989;84:578–583.

17 Dickey RF. Sporotrichoid mycobacteriosis caused by *M. marinum* (balnei). *Arch Dermatol* 1968;98:385–391.

18 Aaronson CM, Park CH. Sporotrichoid infection due to *Mycobacterium marinum*: lesion exacerbated by corticosteroid infiltration. *South Med J* 1974;67:117–118.

19 Dompmartin A, Lorier E, de Raucourt S, et al. Sporotrichoid form of *M. marinum* infection in a patient treated with cyclosporin following kidney transplantation. *Ann Dermatol Venereol* 1991;118:339–377.

20 Zukervar P, Canillot S, Gayrard L, Perrot H. Sporotrichoid *Mycobacterium marinum* infection in a patient with human immunodeficiency virus. *Ann Dermatol Venereol* 1991; 118:111–113.

21 Murdock DK, Sexton M, Marks JG Jr. Persistent nodule on the toe following trauma: sporotrichoid *Mycobacterium marinum* infection. *Arch Dermatol* 1992;128:848–849;851–852.

22 Clark RB, Spector H, Friedman DM, Oldrath KJ, Young CL, Nelson SC. Osteomyelitis and synovitis produced by *Mycobacterium mari-*

num in a fisherman. *J Clin Microbiol* 1990;28:2570–2572.

23 Travis WD, Travis LB, Roberts GD, Su DW, Weiland LW. The histopathologic spectrum in *Mycobacterium marinum* infection. *Arch Pathol Lab Med* 1985;109:1109–1113.

24 Izumi AK, Hanke W, Higaki M. *Mycobacterium marinum* infections treated with tetracycline. *Arch Dermatol* 1977;113:1067–1077.

25 Ljungberg B, Christensson B, Grubb R. Failure of doxycycline in aquarium-associated *Mycobacterium marinum* infections. *Scand J Infect Dis* 1987;19:539–543.

26 Chow SP, Stroebel MB, Lau JHK, Collins RJ. *Mycobacterium marinum* infection of the hand involving deep structures. *J Hand Surg* 1983;8:568–573.

27 Kerdel-Vegas F. American leishmaniasis. *Int J Dermatol* 1982;21:291–303.

28 Spier S, Medenica M, McMillan S, et al. Sporotrichoid leishmanisis. *Arch Dermatol* 1977;113:1104–1105.

29 Parks A, Camisa C. Sporotrichoid leishmaniasis: report of a case in an American graduate student. *J Am Acad Dermatol* 1987; 17:855–856.

30 Kubba R, el-Hassan AM, al-Gindan Y, et al. Dissemination in cutaneous leishmaniasis; I. Subcutaneous nodules. *Int J Dermatol* 1987; 26:300–304.

31 Kibbi A-G, Karam PG, Kurban AK. Sporotricoid leishmaniasis in patients from Saudi Arabia: clinical and histological features. *J Am Acad Dermatol* 1987;17:759–764.

32 Neva FA. Diagnosis and treatment of cutaneous leishmaniasis. In: Remington JS, Swartz MN, eds. *Current Clinical Topics in Infectious Diseases, vol. 3.* New York: McGraw-Hill, 1982.

33 Abramowitz M. Drugs for parasitic infections. *Med Lett* 1992;34:17–26.

34 Saenz RE, Paz H, Berman JD. Efficacy of oral ketoconazole against *Leishmania braziliensis panamensis* cutaneous leishmaniasis. *Am J Med* 1990;89:147–155.

35 Kalb RE, Kaplan MH, Grossman ME. Cutaneous nocardiosis: case reports and review. *J Am Acad Dermatol* 1985;13:125–133.

36 Moore M, Conrad AH. Sporotrichoid nocardiosis caused by *Nocardia brasiliensis*. *Arch Dermatol* 1967;95:390–393.

37 Zecler E, Gilboa Y, Elkina L, Atlan G, Sompolinsky D. Lymphocutaneous nocardiosis due to *Nocardia brasiliensis*. *Arch Dermatol* 1977;113:642–643.

38 **Sachs MK.** Lymphocutaneous *Nocardia brasiliensis* infection acquired from a cat scratch: a case report and review. *Clin Infect Dis* 1992;15:710–711.

39 **el Baze P, Leroux G, Carles D, Lacour JP, Ortonne JP.** Nocardiose cutanee primitive sporotrichoide a *Nocardia asteroides*. *Ann Dermatol Venereol* 1987;114:17–23.

40 **Neubert U, Schaal KP.** Sporotrichoid infection caused by *Nocardia brasiliensis*. *Hautzart* 1982;33:548–552.

41 **Wlodaver CG, Tolomeo T, Benear JB.** Primary cutaneous nocardiosis mimicking sporotrichosis. *Arch Dermatol* 1988;124:659–660.

42 **Kim J, Minamoto GY, Hoy CD, Grieco MH.** Presumptive cerebral *Nocardia asteroides* infection in AIDS: treatment with ceftriaxone and minocycline. *Am J Med* 1991;90:656–658.

43 **Fried J, Hinthorn D, Ralstin J, Gerjarusak P, Liu C.** Cure of brain abscess caused by *Nocardia asteroides* resistant to multiple antibiotics. *South Med J* 1988;81:412–413.

44 **Kikuchi N, Sharasawa T, Suruga Y, Shono K, Nishino T, Narita M.** A case of bronchopulmonary nocardiosis successfully treated with cefotaxime. *Respir Res* 1987;6:1273–1276.

45 **Greer KE, Gross GP, Martensen SH.** Sporotrichoid cutaneous infection due to *Mycobacterium chelonei*. *Arch Dermatol* 1979;115: 738–739.

46 **Jop-McKay AG, Randell P.** Sporotrichoid cutaneous infection due to *Mycobacterium chelonei* in renal transplant patient. *Aust J Dermatol* 1990;31:105–109.

47 **Bendelac A, Cambazard F, Fougerat J, Forestier JY, Thivolet J.** Infectious cutanees a *Mycobacterium chelonei*; revue general a propos d'un cas. *Ann Dermatol Venereol* 1985;112: 319–324.

48 **Murdoch ME, Leigh IM.** Sporotrichoid spread of cutaneous *Mycobacterium chelonei* infection. *Clin Exp Dermatol* 1989;14:309–312.

49 **Owens DW, McBride ME.** Sporotrichoid cutaneous infection with *Mycobacterium kansasii*. *Arch Dermatol* 1969;100:54–58.

50 **Dore N, Collins JP, Mankiewicz E.** A sporotrichoid-like *Mycobacterium kansasii* infection of the skin treated with minocycline hydrochloride. *Br J Dermatol* 1979;101:75–79.

51 **Wood C, Nickoloff BJ, Todes-Taylor NR.** Pseudotumor resulting from atypical mycobacterial infection: a "histoid" variety of *Mycobacterium avium-intracellulare* complex infection. *Am J Clin Pathol* 1985;83:524–527.

52 **Premalatha S, Rao NR, Somasundaram V, Razack EMA, Muthuswami TC.** Tuberculous gumma in sporotrichoid pattern. *Int J Dermatol* 1987;26:600–601.

53 **Shuttleworth D, Philpot CM, Knight AG.** Cutaneous cryptococcosis: treatment with oral fluconazole. *Br J Dermatol* 1989;120:683–687.

54 **Graham WR, Callaway JL.** Primary inoculation blastomycosis in a veterinarian. *J Am Acad Dermatol* 1982;7:785–786.

55 **Wilson JW, Smith CE, Plunkett OA.** Primary cutaneous coccidioidomycosis; the criteria for diagnosis and a report of a case. *Calif Med* 1953;79:233–239.

56 **Wilson JW.** Cutaneous (chancriform) syndrome in deep mycoses. *Arch Dermatol* 1963;87:121–125.

57 **McGinnis MR.** Chromoblastomycosis and phaeohyphomycosis: new concepts, diagnosis and mycology. *J Am Acad Dermatol* 1983; 8:1–16.

58 **Conti-Diaz A.** Micetomas y procesos premicetomatoses en el Uruguay. *Mycopathologia* 1980;72:59–64.

59 **Tanaka S, Mochizuki T, Watanabe S.** Sporotrichoid pyogenic bacterial infection. *Dermatologica* 1989;178:228–230.

60 **Harman RRM, English MP, Halford M, Saihan EM, Greenham LW.** Botryomycosis: a complication of extensive follicular mucinosis. *Br J Dermatol* 1980;102:215–222.

61 **Foshay L.** Tularemia: a summary of certain aspects of the disease including methods for early diagnosis and the results of serum treatment in 600 patients. *Medicine* 1940;19:1–83.

62 **Kavanaugh CN.** Tularemia: a consideration of one hundred and twenty-three cases, with observation at autopsy in one. *Arch Intern Med* 1935;55:651–683.

63 **Evans ME, Gregory DW, Schaffner W, McGee ZA.** Tularemia: a 30-year experience with 88 cases. *Medicine* 1985;64:251–269.

64 **Motley RJ, Holt PJA.** Cowpox presenting with sporotrichoid spread: a case report. *Br J Dermatol* 1990;122:705–707.

65 **Kostman JR, DiNubile MJ.** Nodular lymphangitis: a distinctive but often unrecognized syndrome. *Ann Intern Med* 1993;118:883–888.

Human herpesvirus 6

WILLIAM S. ROBINSON

INTRODUCTION

Human herpesvirus 6 (HHV-6) was discovered in 1986 (1) during studies to identify viruses in lymphocytes of patients with diseases of the lymphoid system. Cytopathic changes developed in cultures of lymphocytes from some patients with lymphoproliferative disorders, including acquired immunodeficiency syndrome (AIDS). Examination of such cells by electron microscopy revealed particles with the appearance of a herpesvirus within inclusion bodies in the cell cytoplasm and the nucleus. Virus in the culture medium readily infected phytohemagglutinin (PHA)-stimulated peripheral blood lymphocytes (PBL) but not cell lines. Serum from patients with the virus reacted in an immunofluorescent assay with cells containing the virus-like particles. The virus was shown to be serologically distinct from known human herpesviruses, and the virus was first called human B-lymphotropic virus (HBLV) because it was thought to be a virus of B cells (1). It was later recognized to infect primarily T cells, and the name was changed to human herpesvirus 6. This name indicates that HHV-6 is the sixth human herpesvirus to be discovered after herpes simplex virus (HSV) types 1 and 2, varicella-zoster virus (VZV), human cytomegalovirus (CMV), and Epstein-Barr virus (EBV). The cell culture isolation and discovery of HHV-6 was fortuitous, and, like the isolation of other T-cell tropic viruses such as HTLV (2) and human immunodeficiency virus (HIV) (3), HHV-6 isolation in cell culture was made possible by the earlier discovery of the T cell growth factor interleukin 2 (IL-2) (4) and the subsequent development of culture methods to grow T cells (5), including mitogen activation of T cells and stimulation of their growth by IL-2. Since its discovery, there has been significant progress in understanding the molecular structure of HHV-6 and its behavior in vivo, as well as disease associations and other epidemiologic features. HHV-6 shares many properties of other herpes viruses, including an ability to persist in cells of infected hosts for many years without clinically apparent pathologic effects. HHV-6 has been found to infect almost all children by age 2 years in all populations studied around the world. It has been established as the etiologic agent of exanthem subitum and acute febrile illness without rash in young children, but the clinical and biologic significance of its apparent association with numerous other syndromes, including some chronic illnesses, remains to be shown.

VIRUS STRUCTURE

HHV-6 has the typical structure of a herpesvirus, with a virion diameter of approximately 160 to 200 nm and an envelope from 20 to 40 nm in thickness surrounding a nucleocapsid of 90 to 110 nm in diameter (6–8). An internal core with a diameter of approximately 65 nm has an appearance similar to that of herpes simplex virus. Viral nucleocapsids are observed in the nucleus of infected cells, the viral envelope is acquired in membranes of cell cytoplasm, and mature virions are released from the cell surface membrane by exocytosis (7,8).

The viral genome is a double-stranded DNA of approximately 160 to 170 kilobase pairs (kb) (9–13). The DNA has guanine and cytosine content of 43% to 44% (10,13–16), which is significantly lower than that of any other human herpesvirus. No hybridization was observed between HHV-6 DNA and the DNA of any other human herpesviruses (17), except for a fragment of the CMV genome, which has homology with a subgenomic region of HHV-6 (15). The HHV-6 genome contains a 115-kb sequence that is collinear with and homologous to a portion of the CMV genome (11–13), although the CMV genome is 50% longer than that of HHV-6, CMV appears to have greater genetic complexity, and it has many genes with no counterpart in HHV-6. However, the sequence homology in the two genomes indicates that HHV-6 is more closely related to CMV than to other human herpes viruses. HHV-6 DNA also has some homology with the DNA of Marek's disease virus, a herpesvirus of chickens (18). Analysis of virion proteins revealed at least 29 polypeptides ranging in size from 30 to 180 kd (19). Some crossreactive epitopes have been detected between HHV-6 and EBV DNA polymerases (20,21) and between HHV-6 and CMV cell-associated antigens (22) using monoclonal antibodies. Despite these crossreactions between specific epitopes, there is no significant serologic crossreactivity detected between different herpesviruses and HHV-6 when polyvalent virus-specific antisera are used (23,24).

INFECTION OF CELLS IN CULTURE AND IN VIVO

Originally, HHV-6 was thought to infect and replicate only in primary human lymphocytes from peripheral blood (1). The virus was later found to also grow in lymphocytes of chimpanzees (25,26). More recently, human diploid lung fibroblast cell line MRC5 has been found to support primary virus isolation (27). Individual HHV-6 isolates vary in their ability to grow in different cell types; some replicate only primary peripheral blood lymphocytes, whereas others are able to infect T- and B-cell lines and certain other cell lines in culture. Tissue culture–adapted virus more readily grows in cell lines. Tissue culture–adapted HHV-6 strains may grow in continuous cell lines of T- and B-cell origin, MRC5, glioblastoma, neuroblastoma, megakaryocytes, and some other cell lines

(25,27–35). Levels of virus replication are low in many such lines. Certain HHV-6–resistant B-cell lines have become susceptible after infection with EBV (29,30). Different HHV-6 strains may have different cell line preferences. Although HHV-6 was originally thought to infect B cells most readily, it is now clear that CD4+ T cells are the cells most readily infected in tissue culture (36–38), and virus appears to replicate less well in cells of other T-cell subsets. Monoclonal antibodies that bind CD4 do not block the ability of HHV-6 to infect CD4+ cells (39), and HeLa cells expressing CD4 are not infected by HHV-6 (40), indicating that the CD4 molecule is not directly required for cell infection. HHV-6 growth in primary lymphocytes requires stimulation of the cells (e.g., by PHA and then growth in IL-2) (35). HHV-6 infection of cells appears to induce a growth advantage of infected cells compared with uninfected cells for several days, but eventually host cell DNA synthesis is shut off by HHV-6 infection and infected cells eventually die and lyse (1,6,41).

During acute HHV-6 infection in vivo, the major target cell appears to be T cells, and most of the infected T cells are CD4+. Examination of cells from peripheral blood of infected patients has revealed that most HHV-6–infected lymphocytes are CD4+ (36–38). HHV-6 antigens or DNA, or both, have been detected in several cell types and tissues of infected patients, including T cells, monocytes, macrophages, lymph nodes, liver, kidney, salivary glands, bronchial glands, and brain (36–38,42–46), indicating that each of these and perhaps other cells and organs can be infected under some circumstances. HHV-6 has been isolated from saliva of most (e.g., 85%) seropositive individuals in some studies (47–49) and from the urine of 50% of seropositive individuals in one study (40).

HOST RANGE

HHV-6 infects humans, chimpanzees (25,26), and several species of monkeys. Studies of sera of wild monkeys has shown antibodies to HHV-6 in 100% of squirrel monkeys and lower prevalences in other species (50); these results suggest that certain monkeys may be a natural host for HHV-6 or a similar serologically crossreacting virus of monkeys. No infection of lower mammalian or other species has been observed.

EPIDEMIOLOGY

HHV-6 is a ubiquitous virus, and specific antibody is found in sera of human populations throughout the world. Using sensitive and specific serologic tests, antibody to HHV-6 has been found in 90% or more of individuals over the age of 2 years in all populations studied (51–58). Newborns appear to be protected by maternal antibody, and new infections become frequent at about 5 or 6 months of age (53,54,59–61). Many infants have detectable serum antibody to HHV-6 at birth, and the prevalence declines to less than 10% by age 6 months (53) as maternal antibody is lost. From that age, the prevalence of antibody increases rapidly by age and usually exceeds 90% by 2 years (51–58). Antibody prevalence may decrease in older age groups (62). In most adult populations, there appears to be at least a small fraction of individuals that have never been infected with HHV-6 and who remain susceptible to primary infection.

Specific routes of HHV-6 transmission are not established, but whatever the routes, they operate effectively in early childhood. This finding suggests that the virus is frequently present in the household environment of infants. HHV-6 has been detected by in situ hybridization in salivary glands of seropositive individuals (43,44) and has been isolated from saliva of more than 85% of seropositive individuals (47–49), suggesting that maternal saliva may be a common source of virus for infant infections. Seroconversions have been documented in infants who did not receive breast milk (63), indicating that breast feeding is not required for transmission. Whether virus is present in breast milk and can be transmitted by that route has not been tested. The finding of HHV-6 antigens in renal tissue (45) and its isolation from urine of 50% of seropositive individuals (40) suggest that urine could be the source of virus for some household infections. Finally, the persistence of HHV-6 in blood suggests that routes which are common for other blood-borne viruses, such as by parental exposure with needles, use of blood products, and other routes common for blood-born viruses, such as HIV and hepatitis B virus, are potential routes for HHV-6 infection.

INFECTION AND DISEASE

Most primary HHV-6 infections appear to be silent or subclinical, or mild febrile illnesses in infants and small children. Virus may persist in lymphocyte or monocyte/macrophage populations and in salivary glands and kidney, with low level virus replication for years or for the lifetime of infected individuals (45). This characteristic is similar to other human herpesviruses, such as EBV and CMV, which appear to persist in lymphoid and other cells for the life of at least many individuals following primary infection.

Although HHV-6 has been associated with a number of different diseases, an etiologic role of the virus in most of these diseases remains unproven and appears to be unlikely. Good evidence, however, indicates that HHV-6 is the etiologic agent of exanthem subitum (i.e., roseola infantum or sixth disease), which is the most common exanthem of children between the ages of 6 months and 2 years (64). The typical illness features a rapid onset of high fever lasting 3 to 5 days, followed by a decrease in temperature to normal and appearance of an erythematous macular or maculopapular erythematous rash that persists for up to 48 hours. The association of HHV-6 infection with exanthem subitum was first recognized in Japan in 1988 (65) when HHV-6 was isolated from peripheral blood of children with exanthem subitum and all were noted to seroconvert to HHV-6. Viral neutralizing antibody was first detected 3 days after onset of fever, was detected in each of 26 patients by 6 to 8 days after disease onset, and persisted in all patients (66,67). HHV-6 was isolated from peripheral blood lymphocytes (PBLs) in all 26 patients during the period of fever and could no longer be isolated after the fifth day following onset of illness (66). Numerous other studies have confirmed the seroconversion to HHV-6 at the time of exanthem subitum as well as virus isolation during the disease. Seroconversions have also been noted in infants with high fever that resolves without rash (68,69), suggesting that primary HHV-6 infection can be associated with fever without the typical rash of exanthem subitum.

Some evidence indicates that HHV-6 can infect liver, and there are rare reports of acute hepatitis associated with evidence of primary HHV-6 infection. A 3-month-old infant with fulminant hepatitis was shown to have increases in titers of both immunoglobulin G (IgG) and IgM antibody to HHV-6 (46). HHV-6 was isolated in tissue culture from lymphocytes of the patient, and HHV-6 DNA was detected in liver and brain. There was no evidence of infection with other viruses associated with viral hepatitis. Evidence of hepatitis has also been reported in association with exanthem subitum in a young child (70). In addition, adult cases of hepatitis without evidence of infection with other viruses associated with viral hepatitis have been shown to have serologic evidence of primary HHV-6 infection (71–73). Thus, it appears that primary HHV-6 infection in infants can be (rarely) associated with acute hepatitis, and sometimes the disease can be fulminant. Whether primary infection of seronegative adults is ever a cause of acute hepatitis, as the few reported cases of serologic responses in adults suggest, remains to be more thoroughly established.

Several cases of an infectious mononucleosis–like illness with fever, lymphadenopathy, and other features consistent with infectious mononucleosis but without evidence of EBV or CMV infection have been associated with serologic responses consistent with primary HHV-6 infection, including both IgM and IgG antibody titer increases (72,73). That these cases may represent a syndrome caused by primary HHV-6 infection of seronegative older children and adults is a significant possibility that deserves further investigation.

Increased titers of IgG antibody to HHV-6 and sometimes a higher prevalence of antibody than in control subjects have been reported for a number of lymphoproliferative disorders, including leukemia, Hodgkin's and non-Hodgkin's lymphomas (including EBV-negative Burkitts lymphoma), and follicular large-cell and angioimmunoblastic lymphomas; HHV-6 has been isolated from lymphocytes from several such patients (29,74–76). Similar findings have been made in patients with diseases such as sarcoidosis, Sjögren's syndrome, systemic lupus erythematosis, and chronic fatigue syndrome (29,49,76–78). These findings raise the question of whether any of these syndromes may be caused by HHV-6 infection or whether HHV-6, present since earlier primary infection, is in some way activated, leading to increases in specific antibody titers in patients with such disorders. The latter seems more likely, but further investigation is required to more completely exclude an etiologic role for HHV-6 in any of these diseases and to elucidate the basis for the increased antibody titers.

Increases in HHV-6 IgG antibody titers have been reported in organ transplantation patients, including recipients of heart, liver, kidney, and bone marrow transplants (45,46,55,79,80). In many instances, HHV-6 was isolated in cell culture from lymphocytes of such patients several days or weeks after transplantation. These findings are consistent with activation of prior HHV-6 infection in these patients following transplantation and therapeutic immunosuppression, but in some cases susceptible (seronegative) recipients may have been infected by virus in the donor tissue. An unanswered question is whether activation of endogenous HHV-6 following organ transplantation or primary infection from virus in donor tissue causes disease of any kind or contributes to transplant rejection. In this regard, increases in antibody titer to HHV-6 were found in 8 of 21 renal transplant recipients, and rejection of a transplant occurred in all 8 (45). Virus was isolated from lymphocytes of some of these patients, and HHV-6 antigens were detected in renal tissue in some. These cases are consistent with HHV-6 infection of the transplanted kidneys, but whether the virus had a role in graft rejection is not as clear. Whether donor organs or tissue can be the source of HHV-6 for primary infections in HHV-6–seronegative or susceptible organ transplantation recipients is an important question that has not been answered. In this regard, bone marrow transplant recipients have been reported to have HHV-6 antibody titer increases and HHV-6 isolation from lymphocytes coincident with fewer and erythematous macular rash 2 weeks after transplantation (46). The antibody status of these patients before transplantation was not reported; therefore, proof that these cases represented disease associated with primary HHV-6 infection was not established. HHV-6 was detected in macrophages and other cells in the lungs of patients with interstitial pneumonitis following bone marrow transplantation (80). What role HHV-6 had in the pulmonary disease is not clear, and whether the virus represented old or new infection cannot be answered. However, these and the other cases described demand that the issue of the pathogenic role of HHV-6 in transplant recipients be more carefully investigated.

There has been much interest in whether coinfection with HHV-6 can alter the course of infection and disease caused by HIV or other viruses. Evidence has been presented that HHV-6 can increase HIV transcription and gene expression (81,82); the mechanism may be transactivation of the principal transcriptional enhancer of the HIV long terminal repeat (LTR), which is the kB enhancer (i.e., the binding sequence for the cellular transcription factor NFkB) by an HHV-6 gene product (83). Despite this evidence for the ability of HHV-6 to activate HIV transcription and gene expression, most studies of dual viral infection of tissue culture cells suggest that HHV-6 inhibits HIV replication in cell culture (17,84–86). A single study suggested increased HIV replication and earlier cell death of coinfected cells compared with cells infected with HIV alone (82). HHV-6 was said to induce expression of CD4 in CD4− CD8+ lymphocytes (87), which could in theory result in an increase in the number of HIV-susceptible cells. There is no evidence, however, that such a mechanism takes place in vivo and alters HIV infection. Numerous studies of HIV-infected patients have led to conflicting results concerning HHV-6 antibody titers and prevalence of antibody to HHV-6 compared with control subjects (29,49,76,88–90). There is no evidence that the course of HIV infection or occurrence of HIV-associated disease or its severity is altered by HHV-6 infection.

ANTIVIRAL THERAPY

Cell culture studies have shown suppression of HHV-6 replication with concentrations of gangcyclovir, phosphonoacetic acid, and phosphonoformic acid that are achievable in serum of patients receiving therapeutic doses of each respective drug (91–93). HHV-6 is relatively resistant to acyclovir (91,93,94), as is human CMV. The overwhelming majority of primary HHV-6 infections in young children are relatively benign, and antiviral therapy is not indicated. Rare cases of fulminant disease in infants (36,95), if recognized to be associated with primary HHV-6 infection, might be treated with gangcyclovir, although there is no clinical evidence demonstrating effectiveness of such therapy. If HHV-6 is shown in the future to cause disease or transplant rejection in patients following organ transplantation (or disease in other immunosuppressed or other hosts), antiviral therapy might have a useful role, but there is currently no justification for antiviral therapy of any such patients.

PROSPECTS FOR THE FUTURE

Important issues to be addressed in the future include better antigenic characterization of HHV-6 to determine the degree of antigenic variation among HHV-6 isolates, and whether different strains or antigenic types exist. This is important information that can affect the development of serodiagnostic testing. Further studies are needed to determine whether HHV-6 infection imports protective and long-lasting immunity or whether reinfections with disease can occur. It will be important to better understand how long HHV-6 persists in patients following primary infection, in what cell types it may persist, the state of the virus in such cells (e.g., replicating or nonreplicating forms of virus), whether natural infection can cause any form of disease long after primary infection, and whether late activation of virus by immunosuppression or other factors can cause acute disease (or organ transplant rejection). Finally, whether primary infections in older children and adults leads to disease syndromes other than those observed in young children is an important issue to be resolved. The need for developing a vaccine and effective antiviral therapy will depend on answers to some of these questions and on future evidence of the pathogenetic potential of this virus.

REFERENCES

1 Salahuddin SZ, Ablashi DV, Markham PD, et al. Isolation of a new virus, HBLV, in patients with lymphoproliferative disorders. *Science* 1986;234:596–600.

2 Poiesz BJ, Ruscetti FW, Gazdar AF, Bunn PA, Minna JD, Gallo RC. Isolation of type-C retrovirus particles from cultured and fresh lymphocytes of a patient with cutaneous T-cell lymphoma. *Proc Natl Acad Sci USA* 1980; 77:615.

3 Barre-Sinoussi F, Chermann J-C, Rey F, et al. Isolation of T-lymphotropic retrovirus from a patient at risk for acquired immune deficiency syndrome (AIDS). *Science* 1983;220:868.

4 Morgan DA, Ruscetti FW, Gallo RC. Selective *in vitro* growth of T-lymphocytes from normal human bone marrows. *Science* 1976; 193:1007.

5 Ruscetti FW, Morgan DA, Gallo RC. Functional and morphologic characterization of human T-cells continuously grown in vitro. *J Immunol* 1977;119:131.

6 Biberfeld P, Kramarsky B, Salahuddin SZ, Gallo RC. Ultrastructural characterization of a new human B lymphotropic DNA virus (HBLV) isolated from patients with lymphoproliferative disease. *J Natl Cancer Inst* 1987; 79:93–94.

7 Yoshida M, Uno F, Bai ZL, et al. Electron microscopic study of a herpes-type virus isolated from an infant with exanthem subitum. *Microbiol Immunol* 1989;33:147–154.

8 Roffman E, Albert J, Foff J, Frenkel N. Putative site for the acquisition of human herpesvirus 6 virion tegument. *J Virol* 1990; 64:6308–6313.

9 Josephs SF, Ablashi DV, Salahuddin SZ, et al. Molecular studies of HHV-6. *J Virol Methods* 1989;21:179–190.

10 Lindquester GJ, Pellett PE. Properties of the human herpesvirus 6 strain Z29 genome: G+C content, length, and presence of variable-length directly repeated terminal sequence elements. *Virology* 1991;182:102–110.

11 Martin MED, Thompson BJ, Honess RW, et al. The genome of human herpesvirus 6: maps of unit-length and concatemeric genomes for nine restriction endonucleases. *J Gen Virol* 1991;72:157–168.

12 Neipel F, Ellinger K, Fleckenstein B. The unique region of the human herpesvirus 6 genome is essentially collinear with the U_L segment of human cytomegalovirus. *J Gen Virol* 1991;72:2293–2297.

13 Teo IA, Griffin BE, Jones MD. Characterization of the DNA polymerase gene of human herpesvirus 6. *J Virol* 1991;65:4670–4680.

14 Lopez C, Honess R. Human herpesvirus 6. In: Fields NN, Knipe DM, Chanock RM, et al., eds. *Virology*. 2nd ed, vol 2. New York: Raven, 1990: 2062–2205.

15 Efstathiou S, Gompels UA, Craxton MA, Honess RW, Ward K. DNA homology between a novel human herpesvirus (HHV-6) and human cytomegalovirus. *Lancet* 1988;1: 63–64.

16 Lawrence GL, Chee M, Craxton MA, Gompels UA, Honess RW, Barrell BG. Human herpesvirus 6 is closely related to human cytomegalovirus. *J Virol* 1990;64:287–299.

17 Lopez C, Pellett P, Stewart J, et al. Characteristics of human herpesvirus-6. *J Infect Dis* 1988;157:1271–1273.

18 Kishi M, Harada H, Takahashi M, et al. A repeat sequence, GGGTTA, is shared by DNA of human herpesvirus 6 and Marek's diseases virus. *J Virol* 1988;62:4824–4827.

19 Shiraki K, Okuno T, Yamanishi K, Takahashi M. Virion and nonstructural polypeptides of human herpesvirus-6. *Virus Res* 1989;13: 173–178.

20 Williams MV, Ablashi DV, Salahuddin SZ, Glaser R. Demonstration of the human herpesvirus 6-induced DNA polymerase and DNase. *Virology* 1989;173:223–230.

21 Tsai CA, Williams MV, Glasser R. A monoclonal antibody that neutralizes Epstein-Barr virus, human cytomegalovirus, human herpesvirus 6 and bacteriophage T4 DNA polymerases. *Proc Natl Acad Sci USA* 1990; 87:7963–7967.

22 Yamamoto M, Black J, Stewart J, Lopez C,

Pellett P. Identification of a nucleocapsid protein as a specific serological marker of human herpesvirus 6 infection. *J Clin Microbiol* 1990;28:1957–1962.

23 Irving WL, Ratnamohan VM, Hueston LC, Chapman JR, Cunningham AL. Dual antibody rises to cytomegalovirus and human herpesvirus type 6: frequency of occurrence in CMV infections and evidence for genuine reactivity to both viruses. *J Infect Dis* 1990; 161:910–916.

24 Linde A, Fridell E, Dahl H, Anderson J, Biberfeld P, Wahren B. Effect of primary Epstein-Barr virus infection on human herpesvirus-6, cytomegalovirus, and measles virus immunoglobulin G titers. *J Clin Microbiol* 1990;28:211–215.

25 Levy JA, Ferro F, Lennette ET, Oshiro L, Poulin L. Characterization of a new strain of HHV-6 (HHV-6$_{SF}$) recovered from the saliva of an HIV-infected individual. *Virology* 1990; 178:113–121.

26 Lusso P, Markham PD, DeRocco SE, Gallo RC. In vitro susceptibility of T lymphocytes from chimpanzees (Pantroglodytes) to human herpesvirus 6 (HHV-6): a potential animal model to study the interaction between HHV-6 and human immunodeficiency virus type 1 in vitro. *J Virol* 1990;61:2751–2758.

27 Luka J, Okano M, Thiele G. Isolation of human herpesvirus-6 from clinical specimens using human fibroblast cultures. *J Clin Lab Anal* 1990;4:483–486.

28 Ablashi DV, Salahuddin SZ, Josephs SF, et al. HBLV (or HHV-6) in human cell lines. *Nature* 1987;329:207.

29 Ablashi DV, Josephs SF, Buchbinder C, et al. Human B-lymphotropic virus (human herpesvirus-6). *J Virol Methods* 1988;21:29–48.

30 Ablashi DV, Lusso P, Hung C, et al. Utilization of human hematopoietic cell lines for the progagation and characterization of HBLV (human herpesvirus 6). *Int J Cancer* 1988; 42:787–791.

31 Ablashi DV, Lusso P, Hung CL, et al. Utilization of human hematopoietic cell lines for the propagation and characterization of HBLV (human herpesvirus 6). *Dev Biol Stand* 1989;70:139–146.

32 Downing RG, Sweankambo N, Serwadda D, et al. Isolation of human lymphotropic herpesviruses from Uganda. *Lancet* 1987;2:390.

33 Tedder RS, Briggs M, Cameron CH, Honess R, Robertson D, Whittle H. A novel lymphotropic herpesvirus. *Lancet* 1987;2:390–392.

34 Asada H, Yalcin S, Balachandra K, Higashi K, Yamanishi K. Establishment of titration system

for human herpesvirus 6 and evaluation of neutralizing antibody response to the virus. *J Clin Microbiol* 1989;27:2204–2207.

35 Black JB, Sanderlin KC, Goldsmith CS, Gary HE, Lopez C, Pellett PE. Growth properties of human herpesvirus-6 strain Z29. *J Virol Methods* 1989;26:133–145.

36 Lusso P, Salahuddin SZ, Ablashi DV, Gallo RC, Veronese F, Markham PD. Diverse tropism of humn B-lymphotropic virus (human herpesvirus-6). *Lancet* 1987;2:743–744.

37 Lusso P, Markham PD, Tschachler E, et al. In vitro cellular tropism of human B-lymphotropic virus (human herpesvirus-6). *J Exp Med* 1988;167:1659–1670.

38 Takahashi K, Sonoda S, Higashi K, et al. Predominant CD4 T-lymphocyte tropism of human herpesvirus 6-related virus. *J Virol* 1989;63:3161–3163.

39 Lusso P, Gallo R, DeRocco SW, Markham PD. CD4 is not the membrane receptor for HHV-6. *Lancet* 1989;1:730.

40 Pellett PE, Black JB, Yamamoto M. Human herpesvirus 6: the virus and the search for its role as a human pathogen. *Adv Virus Res* 1992;41:1–52.

41 Di Luca D, Katsafanas G, Schirmer EC, Balachandran N, Frenkel N. The replication of viral and cellular DNA in human herpesvirus 6-infected cells. *Virology* 1990;175:199–210.

42 Kikuta H, Itami N, Matsumoto S, Chikaraishi T, Togashi M. Frequent detection of human herpesvirus 6 DNA in perpheral blood mononuclear cells from kidney transplant patients. *J Infect Dis* 1991;163:925.

43 Fox JD, Briggs M, Ward PA, Tedder RS. Human herpesvirus 6 in salivary glands. *Lancet* 1990;336:590–593.

44 Krueger GRF, Wassermann K, deClerck LS, et al. Latent herpesvirus-6 in salivary and bronchial glands. *Lancet* 1990;336:1255–1256.

45 Okuno T, Higashi K, Shiraki K, et al. Human herpesvirus 6 infection in renal transplantation. *Transplantation* 1990;49:519–522.

46 Asano Y, Hoshikawa T, Suga S, Yazaki T, Kondo K, Yamanishi K. Fatal fulminant hepatitis in an infant with human herpesvirus-6 infection. *Lancet* 1990;335:862–863.

47 Pietroboni GR, Harnett GB, Bucens MR, Honess RW. Antibody to human herpesvirus-6 in saliva. *Lancet* 1988;1:1059.

48 Harnett GB, Farr TJ, Pietroboni GR, Bucens MR. Frequent shedding of human herpesvirus 6 in saliva. *J Med Virol* 1990;30:128–130.

49 Levy JA, Ferro F, Greenspan D, Lennette ET.

Frequent isolation of HHV-6 from saliva and high seroprevalence of the virus in the population. *Lancet* 1990;335:1047–1050.

50 Higashi K, Asada H, Kurata T, et al. Presence of antibody to human herpesvirus 6 in monkeys. *J Gen Virol* 1989;70:3171–3176.

51 Saxinger C, Plesky H, Edby N, et al. Antibody reactivity with HBLV (HHV-6) in U.S. populations. *J Virol Methods* 1988;21:199–208.

52 Andre M, Matz B. Antibody responses to human herpesvirus 6 and other herpesviruses. *Lancet* 1988;2:1426.

53 Briggs M, Fox J, Tedder RS. Age prevalence of antibody to human herpesvirus 6. *Lancet* 1988;1:1058–1059.

54 Balachandra K, Ayuthaya PI, Auwanit W, et al. Prevalence of antibody to human herpesvirus 6 in women and children. *Microbiol Immunol* 1989;33:515–518.

55 Chou SW, Scott KM. Rises in antibody to human herpesvirus 6 detected by enzyme immunoassay in transplant recipients with primary cytomegalovirus infection. *J Clin Microbiol* 1990;28:851–854.

56 Yoshikawa T, Suga S, Asano Y, Yazaki T, Ozaki T. Neutralizing antibodies to human herpesvirus-6 in healthy individuals. *Pediatr Infect Dis J* 1990;9:589–590.

57 Yanagi K, Harada S, Ban F, Oya A, Okabe N, Toninai K. High prevalence of antibody to human herpesvirus-6 and decrease in titer with increase in age in Japan. *J Infect Dis* 1990;161:153–154.

58 Dahl H, Linde A, Sundqvist VA, Wahren B. An enzyme-linked immunosorbent assay for antibodies to human herpes virus 6. *J Virol Methods* 1990;29:313–323.

59 Knowles WA, Gardner SD. High prevalence of antibody to human herpesvirus-6 and seroconversion associated with rash in two infants. *Lancet* 1988;2:912–913.

60 Okuno T, Takahashi K, Balachandra K, et al. Seroepidemiology of human herpesvirus 6 infection in normal children and adults. *J Clin Microbiol* 1989;27:651–653.

61 Yoshikawa T, Suga S, Asano Y, Yazaki T, Kodama H, Ozaki T. Distribution of antibodies to a causative agent of exanthem subitum (human herpesvirus-6) in healthy individuals. *Pediatrics* 1989;84:675–677.

62 Brown NA, Sumaya CV, Liu CR, et al. Fall in human herpesvirus 6 seropositivity with age (letter). *Lancet* 1988;2:396.

63 Takahashi K, Sonoda S, Kawakami K, et al. Human herpesvirus 6 and exanthem subitum. *Lancet* 1988;1:1463.

64 Bernstein DI. Human herpesvirus-6 and exanthem subitum. *Adv Pediatr Infect Dis* 1991;6:179–192.

65 Yamanishi K, Okuno T, Shiraki K, et al. Identification of human herpesvirus-6 as a causal agent for exanthem subitum. *Lancet* 1988;1:1065–1067.

66 Asano Y, Yoshikawa T, Suga S, et al. Viremia and neutralizing antibody response in infants with exanthem subitum. *J Pediatr* 1989; 114:535–539.

67 Suga S, Yoshikawa T, Asano Y, Yazaki T, Ozaki T. Neutralizing antibody assay for human herpesvirus-6. *J Med Virol* 1990;30:14–19.

68 Suga S, Yoshikawa T, Asano Y, Yazaki T, Hirata S. Human herpesvirus-6 infection (exanthem subitum) without rash. *Pediatrics* 1989;83:1003–1006.

69 Portolani M, Cermelli C, Pietrosemoli P, et al. Isolation of HHV-6 related virus from children affected by infectious syndrome. *Arch Virol* 1990;110:143–149.

70 Tajiri H, Nose O, Baba K, Okada S. Human herpesvirus-6 infection with liver injury in neonatal hepatitis. *Lancet* 1990;335:863.

71 Dubedat S, Kappagoda N. Hepatitis due to human herpesvirus-6. *Lancet* 1989;2:1463–1464.

72 Irving WL, Cunningham AL. Serological diagnosis of infection with human herpesvirus type 6. *Br Med J* 1990;300:156–159.

73 Steeper TA, Horwitz CA, Ablashi DV, et al. The spectrum of clinical and laboratory findings resulting from human herpesvirus-6 (HHV-6) in patients with mononucleosis-like illnesses not resulting from Epstein-Barr virus or cytomegalovirus. *Am J Clin Pathol* 1990;93: 776–783.

74 Clark DA, Alexander FE, McKinney PA, et al. The seroepidemiology of human herpesvirus-6 (HHV-6) from a case-control study of leukaemia and lymphoma. *Int J Cancer* 1990;45:829–833.

75 Torelli G, Marasca R, Luppi M, et al. Human herpesvirus-6 in human lymphomas: identification specific sequences in Hodgkin's lymphomas by polymerase chain reaction. *Blood* 1991;77:2251–2258.

76 Balachandran N, Tirwatnapong S, Pfeiffer B, Ablashi DV, Salahuddin SZ. Electrophoretic analysis of human herpesvirus 6 polypeptides immunoprecipitated from infected cells with human sera. *J Infect Dis* 1991;163:29–34.

77 Biberfeld P, Petren AL, Eklund A, et al. Human herpesvirus-6 (HHV-6, HBLV) in sarcoidosis and lymphoproliferative disorders. *J Virol Methods* 1988;21:49–59.

78 Krueger GR, Koch B, Ramon A, et al. Antibody prevalence to HBLV (human herpesvirus-6, HHV-6) and suggestive pathogenicity in the general population and in patients with immune deficiency syndromes. *J Virol Methods* 1988;21:125–131.

79 Irving WL, Cunningham AL, Keogh A, Chapman JR. Antibody to both human herpesvirus 6 and cytomegalovirus. *Lancet* 1988; 2:630–631.

80 Carrigan DR, Drobyski WR, Russler SK, Tapper MA, Knox KK, Ash RC. Interstitial pneumonitis associated with human herpesvirus-6 infection after marrow transplantation. *Lancet* 1991;338:147–149.

81 Horvat RT, Wood C, Josephs SF, Balachandran N. Transactivation of the human immunodeficiency virus promoter by human herpesvirus 6 (HHV-6) strains GS and Z-29 in primary human T lymphocytes and identification of transactivating HHV-6 (GS) gene fragments. *J Virol* 1991;65:2895–2902.

82 Lusso P, Ensoli B, Markham PD, et al. Productive dual infection of human CD4 T lymphocytes by HIV-1 and HHV-6. *Nature* 1989;337:370–373.

83 Ensoli B, Lusso P, Schachter F, et al. Human herpes virus-6 increases HIV-1 expression in co-infected T cells via nuclear factors binding to the HIV-1 enhancer. *EMBO J* 1989;8:3019–3027.

84 Carrigan DR, Knox KK, Tapper MA. Suppression of human immunodeficiency virus type 1 replication by human herpesvirus-6. *J Infect Dis* 1990;162:844–851.

85 Pietroboni G, Harnett G, Farr TJ, Bucens MR. Human herpes virus type6 (HHV-6) and its in vitro effect on human immunodeficiency virus (HIV). *J Clin Pathol* 1988;41:1310–1312.

86 Levy J, Landay A, Lennette E. Human herpesvirus 6 inhibits human immunodeficiency virus type 1 replication in cell culture. *J Clin Microbiol* 1990;28:2362–2364.

87 Lusso P, DeMaria A, Mainati M, et al. Induction of CD4 and susceptibility to HIV-1 infection in human CD8 T lymphocytes by human herpesvirus 6. *Nature* 1991;349:533–555.

88 Brown NA, Kovacs A, Lui CR, Hur C, Zaia JA, Mosley JW. Prevalence of antibody to human herpesvirus 6 among blood donors infected with HIV. *Lancet* 1988;2:1146.

89 Fox J, Briggs M, Tedder RS. Antibody to human herpesvirus 6 in HIV-1 positive and negative homosexual men. *Lancet* 1988; 2:396–397.

90 Spira TJ, Bozeman LH, Sanderlin KC, et al. Lack of correlation between human herpesvirus-6 infection and the course of human

immunodeficiency virus infection. *J Infect Dis* 1990;161:567–570.

91   **Russler SK, Tapper MA, Carrigan DR.** Susceptibility of human herpesvirus 6 to acyclovir and ganciclovir (letter). *Lancet* 1989;2:382.

92   **Shiraki K, Okuno T, Yamanishi K, Takahashi M.** Phosphonoacetic acid inhibits replication of human herpesvirus-6. *Antiviral Res* 1989; 12:311–318.

93   **Burns WH, Sanford GR.** Susceptibility of human herpesvirus 6 to antivirals in vitro. *J Infect Dis* 1990;162:634–637.

94   **Kikuta H, Lu H, Matsumoto S.** Susceptibility of human herpesvirus 6 to acyclovir (letter). *Lancet* 1989;2:861.

95   **Huang LM, Lee CY, Lin KH, et al.** Human herpesvirus-6 associated with fatal heomophagocytic syndrome. *Lancet* 1990;336:60–61.

Methicillin-resistant *Staphylococcus aureus:* the persistent resistant nosocomial pathogen

MICHAEL A. MARTIN

EPIDEMIOLOGY: INTRODUCTION INTO THE HOSPITAL, SPREAD, AND ESTABLISHMENT OF RESERVOIRS

Methicillin-resistant *Staphylococcus aureus* (MRSA) is often introduced into a hospital or long-term care facility by an infected or colonized patient or by a colonized healthcare worker (1–15). Once introduced, the major route of spread is transfer from one patient to another via the contaminated hands of medical personnel (1–11,16). Crossley and colleagues (3) and Thompson and associates (1) found that MRSA could be recovered from the hands of medical personnel who had been changing the dressings of wounds infected with MRSA. MRSA may survive for hours on the hands, creating the opportunity for direct transmission following contact with an infected or colonized patient (1,3,17). Cookson and co-workers (17) quantitated the degree of nurses' contact with patients harboring MRSA and found a highly significant association between close contact (e.g., changing wound dressings or bathing a heavily colonized patient) and the acquisition of finger and nasal carriage of MRSA by the nurses.

Epidemiologic observations (1–11) have shown that MRSA disseminates throughout the hospital. Thompson and associates (1) reviewed data supporting spread from patient to roommate in semiprivate rooms and from bed to adjacent bed in intensive care units. Over a period of weeks to months, MRSA may colonize or infect as many as 5% to 10% of all hospitalized patients in a given facility (1,4).

Airborne transmission is a second potential route of spread. Although airborne transmission of methicillin-susceptible *S. aureus* (MSSA) has been described (18–20), transmission of MRSA by this route is not well documented. MRSA is not commonly recovered in samples of hospital air except in burn units, where patients with large wounds may be heavily colonized (3,13,20,21).

Once entrenched in a healthcare facility, complete eradication of MRSA is unlikely to occur. Boyce (22) reviewed outbreaks of infections due to MRSA occurring in 104 hospitals. Postepidemic surveillance conducted for an average of more than 2 years identified only 13 hospitals that were not continuing to observe new cases. Of 18 hospitals with MRSA outbreaks reviewed by Thompson and associates (1), only 2 reported complete eradication of the organism.

The evolution of nosocomial transmission of MRSA in a 300-bed teaching hospital was elegantly detailed by Locksley and colleagues (11). Introduction occurred when a severely burned patient who was heavily colonized with MRSA was admitted in transfer from another hospital where the organism was endemic. Despite the institution of standard precautions for colonized wounds, the organism spread first to 8 other patients in the burn unit and then into the surgical intensive care unit via intrahospital transfer of a patient with nosocomial MRSA pneumonia. An outbreak next ensued in the surgical unit. A new burn unit was opened with patients who had not had contact with any of the epidemic cases. Nonetheless, the epidemic strain of MRSA appeared in 6 patients in the new unit and was traced to a staff nurse with chronic dermatitis. Five months earlier, she had worked as a student nurse in the old burn unit. Over the 15-month outbreak, 34 patients became colonized, 27 went on to develop infection, and 17 died.

After initial dissemination, MRSA populates human and environmental niches and establishes reservoirs among colonized and infected persons, including patients and healthcare personnel, as well as in the inanimate environment (1–11). The prevalent cohort of colonized and infected patients is generally assumed to be the most significant reservoir from which MRSA is transmitted to other individuals. Clinically uninfected colonized patients account for approximately half the total population of this major reservoir (1).

Common sites of colonization include the anterior nares, skin (especially in areas involved by dermatitis or other loss of normal integrity), the rectum, the perineum, the upper respiratory tract, surgical wounds, burns, decubitus ulcers, and cutaneous areas adjacent to foreign bodies such as tracheostomy tubes, gastrostomy tubes, and orthopedic external fixation devices (1–12). The most frequent sites of infection or colonization during outbreaks are postoperative and other cutaneous wounds, followed by the lower respiratory tract (1). After becoming colonized, patients may harbor MRSA for months (23,24) and presumably for years (8).

A second reservoir exists among healthcare workers who may be colonized with MRSA at various sites, (particularly the nares, or infected), as with a pustule or paronychia. Nasal carriage of MRSA in medical personnel, although usually transient, may persist for weeks or months in a minority of persons (25,26). In a 7-week study of 26 nurses who attended solely to patients in a newly established isolation ward for MRSA, Cookson and colleagues (17) detected carriage in half. In all nurses but one, episodes of nasal or finger carriage were transient (i.e., detected on two consecutive occasions at most). One nurse, who was taking trimethoprim-sulfamethoxazole for a urinary tract infection, was persistently colonized in the throat and the perineum.

During an outbreak, exposed personnel typically acquire nasal carriage of MRSA at a frequency of 0.5% to 8.0% (1,3,4,6–11,13,24). However, some Veterans Administration Hospitals and burn units have reported considerably higher rates (27,28). MRSA carried out in the nares may then be transmitted to patients, presumably via hand contact (1–4, 8–10, 28–35). When MRSA carriage among personnel is identified, the individual is typically a nurse or a physician who has had close contact with an infected or heavily colonized patient (29,30). MRSA carriage is generally not found among other personnel, including phlebotomists, radiology technologists, and housekeepers (3,6,8). However, Boyce and colleagues (31) recently reported an outbreak associated with respiratory therapists. The extent to which nasal carriage by personnel contributes to nosocomial transmission of MRSA is unclear.

Contaminated surfaces in the inanimate environment (24,36) constitute a third potential reservoir from which MRSA may be transmitted, although the importance of this reservoir is controversial (33,34). The greatest magnitude of environmental contamination with MRSA is usually found in burn units (13,21,28). During an outbreak in a burn unit associated with monthly attack rates for colonization of 74% to 100%, Crossley and colleagues (3) found significant contamination with MRSA on environmental surfaces, hydrotherapy equipment, and in the operating room associated with the burn unit. Environmental contamination in other areas of the hospital associated with lower attack rates was distinctly unusual. Similar findings were confirmed by Thompson and associates (1) and Rutala and colleagues (21). However, in most outbreaks that occurred in wards other than burn units in which environmental cultures have been obtained, significant contamination has not been found (2,3,7,9,17,24,29). Other fomites that have been proposed as reservoirs from which MRSA has been transmitted include stethoscopes (24,37), tourniquets (38), and mattresses (39).

SURVEILLANCE OF MRSA

Most studies suggest that MRSA is no more virulent than MSSA (3,4,8,40–43). Although it is often stated that MRSA spreads more rapidly through hospitals than MSSA, there is currently no biologic basis for this statement. Studies comparing the adherence of MRSA and MSSA with nasal epithelial cells (44) show no significant difference in adherence. For these reasons and others, some authors have argued that special measures to control transmission of MRSA are not warranted, especially if they are costly or labor-intensive (40).

The major reason for instituting surveillance and control measures for MRSA, beyond those employed for MSSA, is that most MRSA infections are preventable. Moreover, vancomycin, the treatment of choice, is expensive, potentially toxic, and available only in parenteral form. In addition, given the tendency of MRSA to develop resistance to antibiotics and the recent descriptions of vancomycin-resistant gram-positive cocci (45–47), there is reason for concern about the potential for vancomycin resistance in S. aureus.

To prevent hospital transmission of MRSA, it is first necessary to identify its reservoirs. Because colonized and infected patients are the major source, the most sensitive (and the most labor-intensive) method of detecting cases is prospective screening of all patients on admission and intermittently throughout their stay. Although costly, such active surveillance might be employed in hospitals with a very high prevalence or during an outbreak (1,15,48). There is disagreement over what sites should be cultured. Walsh and colleagues (48) found that wound and tracheostomy cultures provided the greatest yield of detection of new cases. In contrast, Sanford and co-workers

(49) found that cultures from nares and wounds provided optimal detection. Other sites of carriage include the perineum or the rectum, stool, foreign bodies, and, in neonates, the umbilical stump.

Alternatively, a point prevalence survey, either of the entire population of the facility or of those at increased likelihood of harboring MRSA (Table 9-1) might be conducted periodically (1,24,48,50). Bitar and colleagues (24) found that tracing contacts of cases and performing serial weekly cultures from multiple body sites of the identified contacts was an effective case-finding technique.

Passive surveillance conducted by reviewing routine clinical microbiology records involves less expenditure of time and money but will usually detect only those patients with active infections. This type of surveillance identified approximately one third of the total cases of colonization and infection at the University of Virginia (1).

Once the cohort of colonized and infected patients is identified, a registry can be created and maintained as new cases are found. Because identified carriers of MRSA may remain colonized for months to years, they may reintroduce the organism into the hospital on readmission (1,42). The registry may be used to identify these persons, either by labeling the medical record or, as in our hospital, by a computer prompt to the admitting coordinator. The appropriate isolation precautions are then instituted while the results of new cultures are pending. The criteria to delete a patient's record from such a registry are not well established, because screening cultures can be falsely negative and carriage may be intermittent. Bannister (52) followed 38 patients colonized with an epidemic strain of MRSA with weekly screening cultures. The average duration of carriage was 2 months. Five patients had subsequent recovery of MRSA

Table 9-1   Risk factors for nosocomial acquisition of MRSA colonization and infection

---

Advanced age
Male sex
Previous hospitalization
Length of stay
Stay in a burn unit or ICU
Chronic underlying disease
Prior antibiotic therapy
    Number of antibiotics
    Duration of therapy
Exposure to a colonized HCW
Exposure to another colonized or infected patient
Surgical wound
Extent of burn wound
Invasive devices
    Central venous catheter
    Indwelling bladder catheter
    Endotracheal or tracheostomy tube

SOURCE: Data from References 1–17, 23–26, 28, 29, 35, 41, 51.

after 3 negative screening tests, 1 after 4 negative screens, and none after 5 or more negative screens. Most experts recommend 3 negative cultures.

CONTROL MEASURES

Prevention of new acquisition of MRSA is accomplished by blocking its transmission, eradicating it from existing reservoirs, or both. Transmission via direct contact may be interrupted by removal of MRSA from the hands, by the use of barriers, or by segregation of colonized and infected persons (53).

Skin cleansing and antisepsis for patients and personnel

Removal of MRSA from the hands by soaps and antiseptics is considered the cornerstone of infection control. Washing with ordinary detergent soap and water has been effective in removing MRSA in certain instances (1,3). However, several studies have shown that after a 7 to 10 second hand wash with a nonantimicrobial soap, the number of microbes that could be transmitted from the hands increased significantly due to increased shedding of bacteria-laden skin squamous cells (54–58).

Antiseptic soaps are more effective than plain detergent soaps for removing microbes from the hands (3,13,24,29,50,59,60). Numerous studies have confirmed the association between the use of soaps containing antiseptic agents and a reduction in nosocomial infections (61–63). However, the optimal antiseptic agent for MRSA is not clear. Isolates of MRSA may be resistant to antiseptics. Povidone-iodine and chlorhexidine are commonly used antiseptics that are active against MSSA. Haley and colleagues (64) tested the susceptibility of patient isolates of MRSA and MSSA to serial dilutions of 4% chlorhexidine-gluconate-alcohol (Hibiclens), 1% p-chloro-m-xylenol (Acute-Kare), 3% hexachlorophene (Phisohex), and 10% povidone-iodine (Betadine). Povidone-iodine, diluted 1:100, was most rapidly bactericidal against all strains, killing all within 15 seconds. McClure and Gordon (65) found the in vitro activity of povidone-iodine against MRSA to be superior to that of chlorhexidine over a wide range of dilutions. Kobayashi and associates (66) confirmed this finding, and showed that hypochlorite was the most effective agent for disinfection of MRSA on inanimate objects.

Resistance of MRSA to chlorhexidine is encoded on a plasmid (GNAB), which also confers resistance to gentamicin and nucleic acid-binding compounds (33,67). The clinical significance of chlorhexidine resistance has been questioned. Cookson and colleagues (67) performed in vivo skin tests using a MSSA transcipient strain into which they transferred the GNAB plasmid from a strain of MRSA. No significant difference was seen in survival rates between the resistant and parental (susceptible) strains after chlorhexidine was applied, despite the higher minimum inhibitory concentrations (MICs) in strains with the plasmid. In contrast, Reboli and co-workers (60) reported an outbreak in a neonatal intensive care unit that could not be controlled with standard measures (including the use of chlorhexidine) until hand disinfection with hexachlorophene was instituted. When MRSA isolates from 10 neonates were tested for susceptibility to chlorhexidine and hexachlorophene, the mean minimum bactericidal concentrations (MBCs) were 7.7 and 2.2 µg/mL, respectively. Currently, there are insufficient data to make general recommendations about the optimal antiseptic for MRSA.

Barriers

The evidence for transient hand carriage of MRSA, as well as the observation that patients are often colonized at multiple sites and that the inanimate environment of the room may be heavily contaminated, support the recommendation of requiring all persons who enter the room to wear gloves (15).

In contrast, there is little support for the practice of wearing a gown to prevent transmission of MRSA. In a prospective study of nurses caring for patients with MRSA, the microbe was not recovered from the nurses' aprons or clothes (17). Similarly, the value of wearing a mask is not well documented (15).

Ribner and colleagues (68) conducted a crossover study in which patients in each of 2 surgical critical care units were placed in strict isolation (i.e., requiring the use of gloves, mask, and gown by all persons entering the room) or in a modified contact isolation regimen (69), in which barriers appropriate to the patient's site or sites of colonization (or infection) were employed. No difference in the rate of transmission was found.

Segregation of patients and staff

The rationale for isolating patients with MRSA is based on the evidence that transmission, at least during outbreaks, often occurs from a colonized or infected patient to their roommate or other close contacts (4,24,34,70). Isolation measures have included placing patients with MRSA in a private room (6,24) or placing cohorts of 2 or more patients in the same room (8,34). An extension of this approach that has been used to contain outbreaks involves transferring all patients colonized or infected with MRSA to 1 or more designated isolation wards (6,7,14,24,25,34,71,72). In addition, a cohort of nurses may be assigned to provide care only to patients with MRSA (8,19,24, 25,36,48). The cohort of patients (and personnel) is maintained until all colonized patients are either discharged from the facility or successfully decolonized, or until the outbreak abates and remaining patients can be transferred back to their ward of origin. One of the major drawbacks to this approach is the revenue lost when beds or rooms cannot be used for new patients admitted to the hospital (24). Some authors have recommended placing patients with MRSA in rooms that are at negative pressure with respect to the hallway (72–77). This type of isolation might be appropriate if clinical data strongly suggest that airborne transmission is occurring.

Although there are no controlled trials of use of segregation as an infection control measure, reports of the failure to contain outbreaks in hospitals with inadequate isolation facilities suggest its efficacy (73,78). At a 600-bed hospital in Melbourne, the opening of a 9-bed isolation ward produced a "gratifying decrease" in the incidence of MRSA acquisition (73). When the capacity of the ward was exceeded and patients with MRSA were isolated in private rooms throughout the hospital, the incidence increased dramatically (Figure 9-1). In general, a reasonable approach is to employ contact

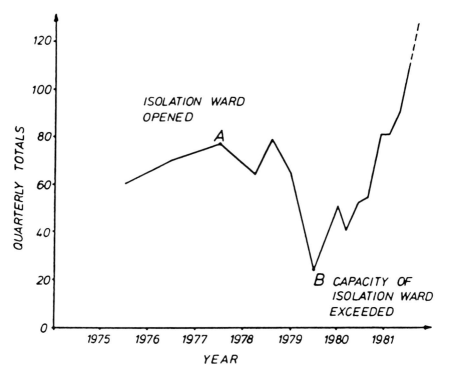

Figure 9-1 The opening of a 9-bed isolation ward resulted in a decrease in the incidence of nosocomial MRSA acquisition until the capacity of the ward was exceeded, resulting in rapid spread throughout the hospital.

isolation during endemic periods and to reserve strict isolation for major outbreaks (72,79,80).

Elimination of MRSA carriage

Attempts at eradication of MRSA carriage may be warranted in certain circumstances, such as during an epidemic or when epidemiologic data suggest that one particular carrier is transmitting MRSA to multiple individuals.

Chemotherapeutic agents for elimination of carriage include (a) topical antimicro-bials and antiseptics applied directly to the nares or other sites of carriage, (b) systemic agents that achieve adequate concentrations in these sites, and (c) antiseptic soaps for bathing.

Topical antimicrobials Various topical antimicrobials, including bacitracin, vanco-mycin, and gentamicin (81), have been employed to eliminate nasal staphylococcal carriage. Some have been effective in the short term, but recolonization occurs fre-quently when these agents are used (82).

Currently, it appears that the topical agent of choice for eradication of nasal carriage of MRSA is mupirocin applied to the anterior nares 2 to 4 times daily for 5 days. This naturally occurring antibiotic produced by *Pseudomonas fluorescens* acts by binding to bacterial iso-leucyl-t RNA synthetase, arresting protein synthesis (82). It is highly active against staphylococci and most streptococci, but considerably less active against gram-negative bacilli (82). Although unsuitable for systemic use due to rapid hydrolysis in plasma, it is useful as a topical 2% preparation in either a lanolin or a polyethylene glycol base. Because the latter drug is an irritant, the lanolin base is preferred for intranasal application.

Hill and associates (83) treated 32 patients who had nasal staphylococcal carriage with mupirocin ointment applied to the anterior nares 4 times daily for 5 days. Initial success in eradicating nasal carriage was uniformly observed. Skin carriage at the wrist or the perineum was also eliminated immediately after treatment, and there was a dramatic reduction of the normal nasal flora without overgrowth of gram-negative bacilli. At 22 weeks, 56% of the cohort remained free of colonization.

Reagan and colleagues (32) conducted a randomized, placebo-controlled trial of the efficacy of mupirocin in eliminating nasal as well as hand carriage of S. *aureus*. Mupirocin therapy eliminated nasal carriage in almost all patients immediately after treatment. Twelve weeks later, only 29% of treated patients had nasal carriage compared with 82% of control subjects. Hand carriage of S. *aureus* 3 days after treatment decreased from 58% to 3%. Mupirocin treatment was associated with nasal itching in 15% of patients, and less frequently with rhinorrhea, dryness, or burning. In a similar study involving 339 health volunteers, 88% of mupirocin-treated persons remained free of carriage 4 weeks after treatment, compared with 12% of placebo recipients (84). Most treatment failures were due to recolonization with the original strain.

Although most of the controlled studies cited involved few subjects with MRSA carriage, intranasal mupirocin was effective in eradicating MRSA during epidemics (25,77,85–90). In outbreaks involving neonates, mupirocin was also applied to the umbilicus, because this may be a reservoir of MRSA even after eradication from the anterior nares (86,91).

Resistance to mupirocin has occurred in patients colonized with MRSA (84,85). Scully and colleagues (92) found that colonization with MRSA developed in 6 of 34 mupirocin-treated subjects but in none of 36 placebo-treated subjects. Because of concerns about emergence of mupirocin resistance, Casewell and Hill (93) studied the efficacy of "minimal-dose" regimens. Single-dose and 2-day treatments resulted in eradication of S. *aureus*, including MRSA; 92% and 96% of subjects were free of carriage 7 days after treatment, respectively (93). Whether mupirocin resistance will become a widespread problem and whether short-course therapy will prevent it remain to be seen.

Systemic antimicrobials   Topical intranasal mupirocin has effected eradication of extranasal carriage of S. *aureus*, presumably because the nares are the reservoir for carriage at other sites. However, it may be necessary to add a systemic agent, particularly if the patient has a large colonized wound or another extranasal site (15). Rifampin is often used because of its penetration into nasal secretions (94), but resistance emerges if it is used alone. Ward and colleagues (7) documented the effectiveness of combined topical bacitracin and oral rifampin given for 5 days in eliminating nasal carriage of MRSA in all persons in whom this was the only site of involvement. When 16 persons with extranasal sites of colonization were treated with oral trimethoprim-sulfamethoxazole (TMP/SMZ) for 5 days and hexachlorophene baths for 2 days (in addition to the described regimen), decolonization was achieved in 13 (81%). In both regimens, failure occurred in patients with colonized surgical wounds.

The combination of rifampin (600 mg daily) and TMP/SMZ (80 mg/400 mg orally twice daily for 5 days) (68,87) has been used with success rates of 50% to 75% in eliminating MRSA nasal carriage. Other systemic agents that have been employed, usually in combination with rifampin, include ciprofloxacin, novobiocin, and fusidic acid. The results with ciprofloxacin therapy have been disappointing. Many isolates of MRSA demonstrate de novo resistance and others developed resistance during therapy, even when ciprofloxacin is combined with rifampin (88,95).

Walsh and colleagues (96) reported eradication of MRSA carriage with a combination of novobiocin, a coumarin derivative, and rifampin in 30 of 45 patients (67%) compared with 26 of 49 (53%) treated with TMP/SMX and rifampin. Rifampin resistance developed in 14% of patients receiving TMP/SM7, but in only one of 45 patients (2%) receiving Novobiocin. In an uncontrolled study (97), novobiocin was given in a daily dose of 500 mg orally in combination with rifampin (600 mg) to 12 patients in a rehabilitation ward who were colonized with MRSA. Successful eradication of carriage was achieved in 11 of 14 courses of treatment. Pearman and co-workers (72) reported success with rifampin (600 mg daily) and sodium fusidate, a steroid-like antibiotic (500 mg 3 times a day), in 17 of 22 (77%) hospital personnel with persistent MRSA carriage who failed to respond to topical chlorhexidine.

Antiseptics Efforts to eradicate MRSA colonization have often included bathing patients with antiseptic soaps containing povidone-iodine, chlorhexidine, hexachlorophene, or triclosan, often in conjunction with a topical or systemic antibiotic (9,35,34,42,50,71,72,77,98). The extent to which these measures contribute to eradication of MRSA is not clear (15).

Disinfection of the inanimate environment

Quaternary ammonium compounds are commonly used for disinfection of surfaces in patients' rooms. However, some isolates of MRSA display in vivo resistance to quaternary ammonium compounds (99). For this reason, some authors have suggested that phenolics should be used, particularly for disinfecting hydrotherapy equipment in burn units (28). Currently, there are insufficient data to determine the efficacy of phenolics over quaternary ammonium compounds. Moreover, the concentrations of quaternary ammonium compounds used in most hospitals are significantly higher than the reported MICs of resistant strains (15).

Education and feedback

One of the major goals of performing surveillance is to report the data collected back to the medical and nursing personnel caring for the patients, often with the intent of effecting some change in practices and procedures. Feedback used in combination with education was associated with a reduction in the incidence of MRSA acquisition at the Iowa City Veterans Administration Medical Center (100). When a new case was identified, a letter mentioning the case, recent infection rates, modes of transmission, and the importance of hand washing was sent to the resident physician responsible for the patient.

Identification of epidemiologically significant strains of MRSA

A number of reports have identified an MRSA carrier, often a nurse or a physician, as the presumed source of the outbreak (1,6,7,11,29). Such individuals often carry MRSA in the nares as well as at other sites, often for prolonged periods (30). They may also be more apt to transmit their carried strain due to shedding of large amounts of staphylococci or to the presence of skin lesion (5,101). Control measures have included suspending such persons from patient care activities while efforts to eradicate carriage are carried out. To implicate an individual as the source of an outbreak, it is useful to identify the epidemic strain beyond the species level with some phenotypic or genotypic characteristic. However, although these techniques are important tools in determining the genetic relatedness of 2 or more strains of MRSA, the information supplied by the laboratory must be thoughtfully used in conjunction with clinical and epidemiologic data before concluding that an individual is the source of an outbreak.

In the past, phenotypic characteristics such as bacteriophage type were used (3,4,6,13). However, the expression of phenotypic characteristics may vary with conditions, and isolates may not be typeable (10). Typing methods that involve plasmid or chromosomal DNA or ribosomal RNA of isolates are superior in their ability to distinguish among different strains (102). Still greater discriminatory power can be achieved by the use of restriction enzymes (endonucleases), which digest plasmid or chromosomal DNA into "restriction" fragments (103). The resulting fragments can then be separated by conventional constant voltage agarose-gel electrophoresis or by newer techniques that give greater resolution, such as pulsed-field gel electrophoresis (104,105). Nucleic acid fragments separated by these methods may be electrophoretically transferred to a nitrocellulose membrane and then hybridized with complimentary DNA or RNA probes (102,104).

MRSA IN SPECIAL SETTINGS

MRSA in long-term care facilities

The prevalence of MRSA in long-term care facilities often equals or exceeds that observed in acute care hospitals (27,106–112). Risk factors for acquisition of MRSA in long-term care facilities include open wounds, gastrostomy tubes, bladder catheters, and multiple functional disabilities (106–108). Roommate-to-roommate transmission appears to occur less frequently than in acute care hospitals (107,112). Patients transferred from long-term care facilities commonly introduce MRSA into acute care hospitals; likewise, those discharged from large teaching hospitals often carry MRSA into chronic care facilities (7,12,106,107,112). Despite evidence for this interfacility transfer, patients colonized with MRSA should not be refused admission to long-term care facilities. Such exclusion policies lead to inappropriate utilization of acute care beds. Instead, persons responsible for transferring the patient should notify the receiving facility that the patient is colonized with MRSA so that appropriate precautions can be instituted. As suggested by Mulligan and associates (113), infection control practitioners at the acute care hospital should educate caregivers in institutions unfamiliar with MRSA about management of the colonized patient.

MRSA in the community

Hsu (112) reported that 10% to 15% of S. aureus isolates obtained from patients admitted directly from the community were methicillin-resistant. Community-acquired MRSA infections have occurred in intravenous drug users (114), as well as in patients chronically taking antibiotics and in hemodialysis patients (113). Hospital personnel (14) and their household contacts (115) may carry MRSA into the community.

Community outbreaks of MRSA have led to hospital admissions (116). In a 1987 MRSA outbreak involving 223 patients at the University of Cincinnati Hospital, 63 (28%) of the cases were community-acquired (117). Of these 63, 21 were nursing home patients. In addition, 27 patients with MRSA were seen in the outpatient clinics but were not admitted, emphasizing the need for infection control in the clinic setting.

ANTIBIOTIC THERAPY OF INFECTIONS CAUSED BY MRSA

Vancomycin

Vancomycin, a glycopeptide, is the drug of choice for treatment of infections due to MRSA (118–121). Glycopeptide antibiotics are large, rigid molecules that inhibit a late step in bacterial cell wall synthesis by forming hydrogen bonds with the D-alanyl-D-alanine terminus of the peptidoglycan side chains (122). Resistance to vancomycin has not been observed in clinical isolates of S. aureus, although it has been detected in S. haemolyticus (46,123,124). In both instances, tolerant strains were recovered from patients who had prolonged exposure to vancomycin, sometimes at subinhibitory concentrations. Tolerance of MRSA to vancomycin occurs and has been associated with therapeutic failure (118). When failure is suspected, a second drug, such as rifampin (125,128), an aminoglycoside (127,128), or fusidic acid (129) should be added.

The usual daily intravenous dose of vancomycin in adults with normal renal function is 30 mg/kg. It may be given by continuous infusion or more commonly by intermittent doses given every 6 to 12 hours. Doses for neonates are adjusted for chronologic and gestational age (130,131). For older children, the recommended dose is 40 mg/kg (131). Intermittent doses should be given over 1 hour to avoid infusion-related adverse events

(132). These events include hypotension (133), muscle pain and spasm in the chest and lower back (134), and the so called red man's syndrome (135). The latter syndrome is due to histamine release and is related to rapid infusion of vancomycin (136). Increasing the infusion time to 1 hour or longer and pretreating the patient with an antihistamine such as hydroxyzine will usually prevent this reaction (137).

Peak and trough serum concentrations should be monitored to ensure effective dosing and to avoid ototoxicity and nephrotoxicity. There is a lack of adequate data correlating serum vancomycin levels with outcome. Recommended peak levels (drawn 1 hour after completion of the infusion) and trough levels are 20 to 40 μg/mL and 5 to 10 μg/mL, respectively. These often quoted dose recommendations are based on an assumption made decades ago. that trough levels should remain above 2 μg/mL, higher than the MICs of most staphylococci. Vancomycin in cleared primarily by glomerular filtration. Hence, the dose should be adjusted for renal insufficiency in accordance with a published nomogram (138). The drug is not removed by hemodialysis (139). Anuric patients may be safely and effectively treated with a dose of 1 gram given every 7 to 10 days (140). Topical vancomycin has been used for conjunctivitis due to MRSA (141). Meningitis and Ommaya reservoir infections due to MRSA may require the use of small (5–20 mg) doses of vancomycin administered intraventricularly as well as larger systemic doses (142).

Other glycopeptide antibiotics

Teicoplanin, a glycopeptide structurally related to vancomycin, has a longer half-life than vancomycin (40–100 hr) (143). It is at least as active against MRSA and MSSA in vitro as is vancomycin and appears to be less ototoxic and nephrotoxic (143,144). Clinical failures have occurred in patients with *S. aureus* bacteremia when lower doses were used (145). The currently recommended dose is 12 mg/kg daily for the first several days, followed by 6 mg/kg daily after blood cultures are no longer positive (143). The drug is currently available in Europe but not in the United States. Its potential role may be as a substitute in patients unable to tolerate vancomycin.

Daptomycin (LY 146032) is an acidic lipopeptide that inhibits the synthesis of lipoteichoic acid. Its in vitro activity is comparable to vancomycin and teicoplanin (143). Few clinical studies have been published to date (119). Its usefulness is limited by its toxicity.

Beta-lactam antibiotics

In vitro, penems and other beta-lactams appear to be active against MRSA (146). However, in experimental models of endocarditis, they have been ineffective (147). Moreover, there are numerous reports of clinical failures when beta-lactams have been used to treat serious MRSA infections (1,2). Currently, use of beta-lactam and penem antibiotics for MRSA cannot be recommended. Whether new cephalosporins, such as cefpirome (HR 810), with activity against MRSA will be clinically effective remains to be determined.

Quinolones

As mentioned earlier, ciprofloxacin resistance in MRSA has developed rapidly (88,95,148). Among ciprofloxacin-resistant strains, cross resistance to other fluoroquinolones, including oxfloxacin, pefloxacin, enoxacin, and fleroxacin, is common (149). Currently available quinolones are not recommended for therapy of MRSA infections.

Trimethoprim-sulfamethoxazole

The combination of trimethoprim and sulfamethoxazole (TMP/SMX) is active in vitro against many strains of S. *aureus* (150). When intravenous TMP/SMX was compared with vancomycin for treatment of endocarditis and other severe infections in intravenous drug users, patients with MSSA had a lower success rate with TMP/SMX (73%) than with vancomycin (97%). Among the 47 with MRSA, however, both TMP/SMX and vancomycin exhibited a 100% success rate (151). Some strains of MRSA are resistant to TMP/SMX (152), and susceptibilities should be determined before this combination is used.

Rifampin

Rifampin has a large volume of distribution and enters tears, nasal secretions, and cerebrospinal fluid (94). Although monotherapy with rifampin selects out resistant mutants (153), this drug is synergistic with many antistaphylococcal antibiotics and has been used effectively in combination with vancomycin (125,154), teichoplanin (155), ciprofloxacin (156), TMP/SMX (7), novobiocin (96,97), fusidic acid (129), and minocycline (157). Resistance will also emerge if rifampin is used in combination with a drug to which the infecting strain is resistant (156).

Clindamycin

In one report, clindamycin was used successfully in the treatment of 5 patients infected or colonized with susceptible strains of MRSA (158). However, resistance to clindamycin is common in MRSA (159). Clindamycin is not the drug of choice, even for susceptible isolates.

Aminoglycosides

Resistance to aminoglycosides is common among isolates of MRSA (3). Even when the infecting strain is susceptible in vitro, single-agent therapy with aminoglycosides has been associated with an unacceptably high mortality rate (160). The combination of vancomycin and an aminoglycoside is synergistic against some strains of MRSA (125). However, there are only sparse data available from clinical reports, and the combination may be more nephrotoxic than either drug alone (132).

Fusidic acid

Fusidic acid is a steroid-like antibiotic that interferes with protein synthesis. It is bacteriocidal at high concentrations against coagulase-positive and -negative staphylococci (129). Oral, intravenous, and topical preparations are available in the United Kingdom and Canada. Adverse reactions to fusidic acid include granulocytopenia, rash, hepatotoxicity, and thrombophlebitis with venospasm during intravenous infusion (161). Because resistance develops rapidly (162), combination therapy has been recommended (129). Strains of MRSA have developed resistance to fusidic acid during concomitant vancomycin therapy (163) and to both gentamicin and fusidic acid during combination (164) therapy (163).

In an uncontrolled study of 49 severe infections due to *S. aureus* treated with fusidic acid, cure rates for infections due to MSSA and MRSA were 75% and 67%, respectively (165). Fusidic acid was used alone in only 3 patients. Drugs used in combination with fusidate included aminoglycosides, vancomycin, quinolones, and rifampin.

Minocycline

In vitro, minocycline is active against MRSA and interacts synergistically with rifampin (157,166). There are anecdotal reports of the successful use of minocycline to treat staphyloccal infections, including MRSA endocarditis (167,168).

Novobiocin and coumermycin

Novobiocin is a bis-hydroxycoumarin compound with in vitro activity against MRSA (48). Its use has resulted in hypersensitivity reactions, hepatotoxicity, and bone marrow suppression. It has been used effectively in the past at doses up to 2 grams daily to treat infections due to *S. aureus* (92). It inhibits DNA gyrase activity (169), and resistance emerges with single-drug use. Coumermycin, another coumarin derivative with affinity for DNA gyrase, has in vitro activity against MRSA (169). An intravenous preparation has recently been developed.

Fosfomycin

Fosfomycin inhibits staphyloccal cell wall synthesis at an early stage and is active in vitro against MRSA. Lau and colleagues (170) reported successful treatment of 3 patients with bacteremia. Resistance emerges when the drug is used alone.

Streptogramins

Synergimycins (or streptogramins) are mixtures of components with synergistic inhibitory activity on microbes, including MRSA (143,171). Type A streptogramins (e.g., virginiamycin M) and type B components (e.g., virginiamycin S) both inhibit protein synthesis by binding to the 50S ribosomal subunit and are bactericidal in combination (143,171). Macrolide and lincosamide antibiotics share common mechanisms of action and bacterial resistance with type B streptogramins. Collectively, these agents are referred to as MLS antibiotics (172). Clinical trials of streptogramins for staphylococcal bacteremia in humans are under way.

SUMMARY

Since the first reports of outbreaks in hospitals in the United States, the prevalence of MRSA colonization and infection has increased in acute-care and chronic-care facilities, outpatient clinics, and in the community. Because of the morbidity and mortality associated with MRSA infections, their preventable nature, and the current requirement for treatment with vancomycin, it is reasonable to invest resources into controlling the transmission of MRSA. Transmission occurs primarily from colonized or infected patients to others via the hands of health care personnel. Efforts to prevent the occurrence of new cases are centered around active or passive surveillance to identify the existing patient reservoir of MRSA and the institution of control measures to block transmission from this reservoir. These measures include hand disinfection, barrier precautions, and segregation of colonized patients. Education and feedback of data to medical personnel are also of value.

Health care workers with MRSA colonization are associated with transmission only in a minority of instances. Generally, no treatment is indicated. When eradication of the carrier state is warranted, in personnel or in patients, topical mupirocin ointment appears to be the most effective agent for eliminating nasal carriage. When systemic therapy is required for carriage, rifampin in combination with TMP/SMX or may possibly with Novobiocin be used if the isolate is susceptible.

Vancomycin is currently the drug of choice to treat infections due to MRSA, but it does not eradicate carriage. New agents to treat MRSA infections are in various phases of clinical trials.

REFERENCES

1   Thompson RL, Cabezudo I, Wenzel RP. Epidemiology of nosocomial infections caused by methicillin-resistant *Staphylococcus aureus*. *Ann Intern Med* 1982;97:309–317.

2   Klimek JJ, Marsik FJ, Bartlett RC, Weir B, Shea P, Quintilliani R. Clinical, epidemiologic and bacteriologic observations of an outbreak of methicillin-resistant *Staphylococcus aureus* at a large community hospital. *Am J Med* 1976;61:340–345.

3   Crossley K, Landesman B, Zaske D. An outbreak of infections caused by strains of *Staphylococcus aureus* resistant to methicillin and aminoglycosides. II: epidemiologic studies. *J Infect Dis* 1979;139:280–287.

4   Peacock JE, Marsik FJ, Wenzel RP. Methicillin-resistant *Staphylococcus aureus*: introduc-

tion and spread within a hospital. *Ann Intern Med* 1980;93:526–532.

5   Shanson DC, McSwiggan DA. Operating theatre acquired infection with a gentamicin-resistant strain of *Staphylococcus aureus*: outbreak in two hospitals attributable to one surgeon. *J Hosp Infect* 1980;1:171–172.

6   Linnemann CC Jr, Mason M, Moore P, et al. Methicillin-resistant *Staphylococcus aureus*: experience in a general hospital over four years. *Am J Epidemiol* 1982;115:941–950.

7   Ward TT, Winn RE, Hartstein AI, Sewell DL. Observations relating to an inter-hospital outbreak of methicillin-resistant *Staphylococcus aureus*: role of antimicrobial therapy in infection control. *Infect Control* 1981;2:453–459.

8 Boyce JM, Landry M, Deetz TR, DuPont HL. Epidemiologic studies of an outbreak of nosocomial methicillin-resistant *Staphylococcus aureus* infections. *Infect Control* 1981; 2:110–116.

9 Craven DE, Reed C, Kollisch N, et al. A large outbreak of infections caused by a strain of *Staphylococcus aureus* resistant to oxacillin and aminoglycosides. *Am J Med* 1981;71:53–58.

10 Barrett FF, McGehee RJ Jr, Finland M. Methicillin-resistant *Staphylococcus aureus* at Boston City Hospital: bacteriologic and epidemiologic observations. *N Engl J Med* 1968; 279:441–448.

11 Locksley RM, Cohen ML, Quinn TC, et al. Multiply antibiotic-resistant *Staphylococcus aureus*: introduction, transmission, and evolution of nosocomial infection. *Ann Intern Med* 1982;97:317–324.

12 Haley RW, Hightower AW, Khabbaz RF, et al. The emergence of methicillin-resistant *Staphylococcus aureus* infections in United States hospitals. Possible role of the house staff-patient transfer circuit. *Ann Intern Med* 1982;97:297–308.

13 Bartzokas CA, Paton JH, Gibson MF, Graham F, McLoughlin GA, Croton RS. Control and eradication of methicillin-resistant *Staphylococcus aureus* on a surgical unit. *N Engl J Med* 1984;311:1422–1425.

14 Reboli AC, John JF Jr, Platt CG, Cantey JR. Methicillin-resistant *Staphylococcus aureus* outbreak at a Veteran's Affairs Medical Center: importance of carriage of the organism by hospital personnel. *Infect Control Hosp Epidemiol* 1990;11:291–296.

15 Boyce JM. MRSA in hospitals and long-term care facilities: microbiology, epidemiology and preventive measures. *Infect Control Hosp Epidemiol* 1992;13:725–737.

16 Crossley K, Loesch D, Landesman B, Mead K, Chern M, Strate R. An outbreak of infections caused by strains of *Staphylococcus aureus* resistant to methicillin and aminoglycosides. I: clinical studies. *J Infect Dis* 1979; 139:273–279.

17 Cookson B, Peters B, Webster M, Phillips I, Rahman M, Noble W. Staff carriage of epidemic methicillin-resistant *Staphylococcus aureus*. *J Clin Microbiol* 1989;27:1471–1476.

18 Mortimer EA Jr, Wolinsky E, Gonzaga AJ, Rammelkamp CH Jr. Role of airborne transmission in staphylococcal infections. *Br Med J* 1966;1:319–322.

19 Williams REO. Epidemiology of airborne staphylococcal infection. *Bacteriol Rev* 1966; 30:660–672.

20 Hambraeus A. Studies on transmission of *Staphylococcus aureus* in an isolation ward for burned patients. *J Hyg Camb* 1973;71:171–183.

21 Rutala WA, Katz EBS, Sherertz RJ, Sarubbi FA Jr. Environmental study of a methicillin-resistant *Staphylococcus aureus* epidemic in a burn unit. *J Clin Microbiol* 1983;18:683–688.

22 Boyce JM. Nosocomial staphylococcal infections (letter). *Ann Intern Med* 1981;95:241–242.

23 McNeil JJ, Proudfoot AD, Tosolini FA, et al. Methicillin-resistant *Staphylococcus aureus* in an Australian teaching hospital. *J Hosp Infect* 1984;5:18–28.

24 Bitar CM, Mayhall CG, Lamb Veterans Affairs, Bradshaw TJ, Spadora AC, Dalton HP. Outbreak due to methicillin- and rifampin-resistant *Staphylococcus aureus*: epidemiology and eradication of the resistant strain from the hospital. *Infect Control* 1987;8:15–23.

25 Duckworth GJ, Lothian JL, Williams JD. Methicillin-resistant *Staphylococcus aureus*: report of an outbreak in a London teaching hospital. *J Hosp Infect* 1988;11:1–15.

26 Cafferkey MT, Hone R, Keane CT. Sources and outcome for methicillin-resistant *Staphylococcus aureus* bacteraemia. *J Hosp Infect* 1988;11:136–143.

27 Hsu CCS, Macaluso CP, Special L, Hubble RH. High rate of methicillin resistance of *Staphylococcus aureus* isolated from hospitalized nursing home patients. *Arch Intern Med* 1988;148:569–570.

28 Arnow PM, Allyn PA, Nichols EM, Hill DL, Pezzlo M, Bartlett RH. Control of methicillin-resistant *Staphylococcus aureus* in a burn unit: role of nurse staffing. *J Trauma* 1982;22: 954–959.

29 Coovadia YM, Bhana RH, Johnson AP, Haffejee I, Marples RR. A laboratory-confirmed outbreak of rifampin-methicillin-resistant *Staphylococcus aureus* (RMRSA) in a newborn nursery. *J Hosp Infect* 1989;14:303–312.

30 Gaynes R, Marosok R, Mowry-Hanley J, et al. Mediastinitis following coronary artery bypass surgery: a 3-year review. *J Infect Dis* 1991; 163:117–121.

31 Boyce JM, Potter-Bynoe G, Opal SM, Medeiros AA. Common source outbreak of methicillin-resistant *S. aureus* associated with respiratory therapy and nursing personnel. Presented at the 2nd Annual Meeting of the Society for Hospital Epidemiology of America, Baltimore, MD, April 12–14, 1992.

32 Reagan DR, Doebbeling BN, Pfaller MA, et al. Elimination of coincident *Staphylococcus aureus* nasal and hand carriage with intranasal

application of mupirocin calcium ointment. *Ann Intern Med* 1991;114:101–106.

33 **Brumfitt W, Hamilton-Miller J.** Methicillin-resistant *Staphylococcus aureus*. *N Engl J Med* 1989;320:1188–1196.

34 **Bradley JM, Noone P, Townsend DE, Grubb WB.** Methicillin-resistant *Staphylococcus aureus* in a London hospital. *Lancet* 1985; 1:1493–1495.

35 **Rhinehart E, Shlaes DM, Keys TF, et al.** Nosocomial clonal dissemination of methicillin-resistant *Staphylococcus aureus*. Elucidation by plasmid analysis. *Arch Intern Med* 1987;147:521–524.

36 **Maki DG, McCormick RD, Zilz MA, Stolz SM, Alvarado CJ.** An MRSA outbreak in a SICU during universal precautions: new epidemiology for nosocomial MRSA: downside of universal precautions. Program and Abstracts of the 30th Interscience Congress on Antimicrobial Agents and Chemotherapy, American Society for Microbiology, Atlanta, GA, October 21–24, 1990.

37 **Redington JJ, North DS, Laxson L, et al.** The stethoscope—a forgotten MRSA fomite? Program and abstracts of the 32nd Interscience Congress on Antimicrobial Agents and Chemotherapy, American Society for Microbiology, Anaheim, CA, October 11–14, 1992.

38 **Berman DS, Schaefler S, Simberkoff MS, Rahal JJ.** Tourniquets and nosocomial methicillin-resistant *Staphylococcus aureus* infections. *N Engl J Med* 1986;315:514–515.

39 **Ndawula EM, Brown L.** Mattresses as reservoirs of epidemic MRSA. *Lancet* 1991; 337:488.

40 **McManus AT, Mason AD Jr, McManus WF, Pruitt BA Jr.** What's in a name? Is methicillin-resistant *Staphylococcus aureus* just another *S. aureus* when treated with vancomycin? *Arch Surg* 1989;124:1456–1459.

41 **Peacock JE Jr, Moorman DR, Wenzel RP, Mandell GL.** Methicillin-resistant *Staphylococcus aureus*: microbiologic characteristics, antimicrobial susceptibilities, and assessment of virulence of an epidemic. *J Infect Dis* 1981; 144:575–582.

42 **Law MR, Gill ON, Turner A.** Methicillin-resistant *Staphylococcus aureus*: associated morbidity and effectiveness of control measures. *Epidemiol Infect* 1988;101:301–309.

43 **Hershow RC, Khayr WF, Smith NL.** A comparison of the clinical virulence of nosocomially acquired methicillin resistant-and methicillin susceptible *Staphylococcus aureus* infections in a university hospital. *Infect Control Hosp Epidemiol* 1992;13:587–593.

44 **Ward TT.** Comparison of in vitro adherence of methicillin susceptible *Staphylococcus aureus* and methicillin-resistant *Staphylococcus aureus* to human nasal epithelial cells. *J Infect Dis* 1992;166:400–404.

45 **Veach LA, Pfaller MA, Barrett M, et al.** Vancomycin resistance in *Staphylococcus haemolyticus* causing colonization and bloodstream infection. *J Clin Microbiol* 1990;28:2064–2068.

46 **Schwalbe RS, Ritz WJ, Verma PR, Barranco EA, Gilligan PH.** Selection for vancomycin resistance in clinical isolates of *Staphylococcus haemolyticus*. *J Infect Dis* 1990;161:45–51.

47 **Karanfil LV, Murphy M, Josephson A, et al.** A cluster of vancomycin-resistant *Enterococcus faecium* in an intensive care unit. *Infect Control Hosp Epidemiol* 1992;13:195–200.

48 **Walsh TJ, Vlahov D, Hansen SL, et al.** Prospective microbiologic surveillance in control of nosocomial methicillin-resistant *Staphylococcus aureus*. *Infect Control* 1987;8:7–14.

49 **Sanford MD, Widmer AF, Bale MJ, Jones RN, Wenzel RP.** Evaluation of culture screening methods for detecting patients colonized with methicillin-resistant *Staphylococcus aureus* (MRSA). Program and abstracts of the 32nd Interscience Congress on Antimicrobial Agents and Chemotherapy, American Society for Microbiology, Anaheim, CA, October 11–14, 1992.

50 **Tuffnell DJ, Croton RS, Hemingway DM, Hartley MN, Wake PN, Garvey RJP.** Methicillin-resistant *Staphylococcus aureus*; the role of antisepsis in the control of an outbreak. *J Hosp Infect* 1987;10:255–259.

51 **Bernstein CA, McDermott W.** Increased transmissibility of staphylococci to patients receiving an antimicrobial drug. *N Engl J Med* 1960; 262:637–642.

52 **Bannister BA.** Management of patients with epidemic methicillin-resistant *Staphylococcus aureus*: experience at an infectious diseases unit. *J Hosp Infect* 1987;9:126–131.

53 **Goetz AM, Muder RR.** The problem of MRSA: a critical appraisal of the efficacy of infection control procedures with a suggested approach for infection control programs. *Am J Infect Control* 1992;20:80–84.

54 **Dineen P, Hildick-Smith G.** Antiseptic care of hands. In: Maibach HI, Hildick-Smith G, eds. *Skin Bacteria and Their Role in Infection*. New York: McGraw-Hill, 1965:291–310.

55 **Lowbury EJL, Lilly HA, Bull JP.** Disinfection of hands: removal of transient organisms. *Br Med J* 1964;2:230–233.

56 **Meers PD, Yeo GA.** Shedding of bacteria and

skin squames after handwashing. *J Hyg (Lond)* 1978;81:99–105.

57 Maki DG, Zilz MA, Alvarado CJ. Evaluation of the antibacterial efficacy of four agents for handwashing. Proceedings and Abstracts of the 19th Interscience Congress on Antimicrobial Agents and Chemotherapy, American Society for Microbiology 1980.

58 Maki DG. Skin as a source of nosocomial infection: directions for future research. *Infect Control* 1986;7:113–116.

59 Onesko KM, Wienke EC. The analysis of the impact of a mild, low-iodine, lotion soap on the reduction of nosocomial methicillin-resistant *Staphylococcus aureus*: a new opportunity for surveillance by objectives. *Infect Control* 1987;8:284–288.

60 Reboli AC, John JF Jr, Levkoff AH. Epidemic methicillin-gentamicin-resistant *Staphylococcus aureus* in a neonatal intensive care unit. *Am J Dis Child* 1989;143:34–39.

61 Doebbeling BN, Stanley GL, Sheetz CT, et al. Comparative efficacy of alternative handwashing agents in reducing nosocomial infections in intensive care units. *New Engl J Med* 1992;327:88–93.

62 Maki D, Hecht J. Antiseptic containing handwashing agents reduce nosocomial infections: a prospective study. Program and abstracts of the 22nd Interscience Conference on Antimicrobial Agents and Chemotherapy, American Society for Microbiology, Miami Beach, Oct 4–6, 1982.

63 Massanari RM. Hierholzer WJ Jr. A crossover comparison of antiseptic soaps on nosocomial infection rates in intensive care units (abstract). *Am J Infect Control* 1984;12:247–248.

64 Haley CE, Marlin-Cason M, Smith JW, Luby JP, Mackowiak PA. Bactericidal activity of antiseptics against methicillin-resistant *Staphylococcus aureus*. *J Clin Microbiol* 1985;21:991–992.

65 McLure AR, Gordon J. In vitro evaluation of povidone-iodine and chlorhexidine against methicillin-resistant *Staphylococcus aureus*. *J Hosp Infect* 1992;21:291–299.

66 Kobayashi H, Tsuzuki M, Hosobuchi K. Brief report: bactericidal effects of antiseptics and disinfectants against methicillin-resistant *Staphylococcus aureus*. *Infect Control Hosp Epidemiol* 1989;10:562–564.

67 Cookson BD, Bolton MC, Platt JH. Chlorhexidine resistance in methicillin-resistant *Staphylococcus aureus* or just an elevated MIC? An in vitro and in vivo assessment. *Antimicrob Agent Chemother* 1991;35:1997–2002.

68 Ribner BS, Landry MN, Gholson GI. Strict versus modified isolation for prevention of nosocomial transmission of methicillin-resistant *Staphylococcus aureus*. *Infect Control* 1986;7:317–320.

69 Garner JS, Simmons BP. CDC guideline for isolation precautions in hospitals. *Infect Control* 1983;4(suppl):245–325.

70 Ellison RT III, Judson FN, Peterson LC, Cohn DL, Ehret JM. Oral rifampin and trimethoprim/sulfamethoxazole therapy in asymptomatic carriers of methicillin-resistant *Staphylococcus aureus* infections. *West J Med* 1984; 140:735–740.

71 Murray-Leisure KA, Geib S, Graceley D, et al. Control of epidemic methicillin-resistant *Staphylococcus aureus*. *Infect Control Hosp Epidemiol* 1990;11:343–350.

72 Pearman JW, Christiansen KJ, Annear DI, et al. Control of methicillin-resistant *Staphylococcus aureus* (MRSA) in an Australian metropolitan teaching hospital complex. *Med J Aust* 1985;142:103–108.

73 Pavillard R, Harvey K, Douglas D, et al. Epidemic of hospital-acquired infection due to methicillin-resistant *Staphylococcus aureus* in major Victorian hospitals. *Med J Aust* 1982; 1:451–454.

74 Seldon JB, Stokes ER, Ingham HR. The role of an isolation unit in the control of hospital infection with methicillin-resistant staphylococci. *J Hosp Infect* 1980;1:41–46.

75 Spicer WJ. Three strategies in the control of staphylococci including methicillin-resistant *Staphylococcus aureus*. *J Hosp Infect* 1984; 5:45–49.

76 Shanson DC, Johnstone D, Midgley J. Control of a hospital outbreak of methicillin-resistant *Staphylococcus aureus* infections: value of an isolation unit. *J Hosp Infect* 1985;6:285–292.

77 Dacre J, Emmerson AM, Jenner EA. Gentamicin-methicillin-resistant *Staphylococcus aureus*: epidemiology and containment of an outbreak. *J Hosp Infect* 1986;7:130–136.

78 Melo Cristino JAG, Pereira AT. MRSA: a six-month survey in a Lisbon paediatric hospital. *J Hyg (Camb)* 1986;97:265–272.

79 Cohen SH, Morita MM, Bradford M. A seven year experience with methicillin-resistant staphylococcus aureus. *Am J Med* 1992;91(suppl 3B):233–237.

80 Garner S, Simmons P. CDC guideline for prevention and control of nosocomial infections. *Am J Infect Control* 1984;12:103–163.

81 Bryan CS, Wilson RS, Meade P, Sill LG. Topical antibiotic ointments for staphylococcal nasal carriers: survey of current practices and

comparison of bacitracin and vancomycin ointments. *Infect Control* 1980;1:153–156.

82 **Casewell MW, Hill RCR.** Mupirocin ('pseudomonic acid')—a promising new topical antimicrobial agent. *J Antimicrob Chemother* 1987; 19:1–5.

83 **Hill RL, Duckworth GJ, Casewell MW.** Elimination of nasal carriage of MRSA with mupirocin during a hospital outbreak. *J Antimicrob Chemother* 1988;22:377–384.

84 **Doebbeling B, Brennemann D, Marsh R, Reagan D, Wenzel R.** Multi-center study of elimination of *Staphylococcus aureus* carriage with calcium mupirocin ointment in healthy subjects. Program and abstracts of the 32nd Interscience Congress on Antimicrobia Agents and Chemotherapy, American Society for Microbiology, Anaheim, CA, October 10–14, 1992.

85 **Frank U, Lenz W, Damrath E, Kappstein I, Daschner FD.** Nasal carriage of *Staphylococcus aureus* treated with topical mupirocin (pseudomonic acid) in a children's hospital. *J Hosp Infect* 1989;13:117–120.

86 **Davies EA, Emmerson AM, Hogg GM, Patterson MF, Shields MD.** An outbreak of infection with a MRSA in a special care baby unit: value of topical mupirocin and of traditional methods of infection control. *J Hosp Infect* 1987; 10:120–128.

87 **Bacon AE, Jorgensen KA, Wilson KH, Kauffman CA.** Emergence of nosocomial methicillin-resistant *Staphylococcus aureus* and therapy of colonized personnel during a hospital-wide outbreak. *Infect Control* 1987;8:145–150.

88 **Peterson L, Quick J, Jensen B, et al.** Emergence of ciprofloxacin resistance in nosocomial methicillin-resistant *Staphylococcus aureus* isolates. Resistance during ciprofloxacin plus rifampin therapy for methicillin-resistant *S. aureus* colonization. *Arch Intern Med* 1990; 150:2151–2155.

89 **Reagan DR, Dula RT, Palmer BH, Gutierrez CN, Franzus BF, Sarubbi FA.** Control of MRSA in a VAMC with limited resources. Program and Abstracts of the 31st Interscience Conference on Antimicrobial Agents and Chemotherapy, American Society for Microbiology, Chicago, IL, September 29–October 2, 1991.

90 **Kauffman C, Terpenning M, HE X, Ramsey M, Zarins L, Bradley S.** Use of mupirocin to decrease MRSA colonization in a long-term care facility. Program of the 31st Interscience Conference on Antimicrobial Agents and Chemotherapy, American Society for Microbiology, Chicago, IL, September 29–October 2, 1991.

91 **Sanchez PJ, Shelton S, Threlkelb N, Fisher L,**

Sumner J, Grier CE. Randomized double-blind placebo-controlled evaluation of mupirocin ointment for eradication of MRSA colonization in pre-term infants. Program of the 31st Interscience Conference on Antimicrobial Agents and Chemotherapy, American Society for Microbiology, Chicago, IL, September 29–October 2, 1991.

92 **Scully BE, Briones F, Gu J-W, Neu HC.** Mupirocin treatment of nasal staphylococcal colonization. *Arch Intern Med* 1992;152:353–356.

93 **Casewell MW, Hill RL.** Minimal dose requirements for nasal mupirocin and its role in the control of epidemic MRSA. *J Hospital Infect* 1991;19(suppl B):35–40.

94 **Darouiche R, Perkins B, Musher D, Hamill R, Tsai S.** Levels of rifampin and ciprofloxacin in nasal secretions: correlation with MIC_{90} and eradication of nasopharyngeal carriage of bacteria. *J Infect Dis* 1990;162:1124–1127.

95 **Aboukasm AG, Buu-Hoi AY, El Solh N, et al.** Epidemiological study of *Staphylococcus aureus* resistance to new quinolones in a university hospital. *J Hosp Infect* 1991;17:25–33.

96 **Walsh TJ, Reboli AC, et al.** Randomized double–blinded trial of rifampin or trimethoprim-sulfa methoxazole against methicillin-resistant *Staphylococcus aureus* colonization prevention at antimicrobial resistance and effect of host factors on outcome. *Antimicrob Agents Chemother* 1993; 37:1334–1342.

97 **Arathoon EG, Hamilton JR, Hench CE, Stevens DA.** Efficacy of short courses of oral novobiocin-rifampin in eradicating carrier state of methicillin-resistant *Staphylococcus aureus* and in vitro killing studies of clinical isolates. *Antimicrob Agents Chemother* 1990; 34:1655–1659.

98 **Gezon HM, Thompson DJ, Rogers KD, Hatch TF, Rycheck RR, Yee RB.** Control of staphylococcal infections and diseases in the newborn through the use of hexachlorophene bathing. *Pediatrics* 1973;51:331–344.

99 **Al-Masaudi SB, Day JM, Russell AD.** Sensitivity of methicillin-resistant *Staphylococcus aureus* strains to some antibiotics, antiseptics and disinfectants. *J Appl Bacteriol* 1988;65: 329–337.

100 **Nettleman MD, Trilla A, Fredrickson M, Pfaller M.** Assigning responsibility: using feedback to achieve sustained control of methicillin-resistant *Staphylococcus aureus*. *Am J Med* 1991;91(suppl 3B):228S–232S.

101 **Nakashima AK, Allen JR, Martone WJ, et al.** Epidemic bullous impetigo in a nursery due to a nasal carrier of *Staphylococcus aureus*:

role of epidemiology and control measures. *Infect Control* 1984;5:326–331.

102 **Pfaller MA, Wakefield DS, Hollis R, Frederickson M, Evans E, Massanari RM.** The clinical microbiology lab as an aid in infection control: the application of molecular techniques in epidemiologic studies of MRSA. *Diagn Microbiol Infect Dis* 1991;14:209–217.

103 **Pignatari A, Boyken LD, Herwald LA, et al.** Application of restriction endonuclease analysis of chromosomal DNA in the study of *Staphylococcus aureus* colonization in continuous ambulatory peritoneal dialysis patients. *Diagn Microbiol Infect Dis* 1992; 15:195–199.

104 **Goering RV, Duensing TD.** Rapid field inversion gel electrophoresis in combination with an rRNA gene probe in the epidemiologic evaluation of staphylococci. *J Clin Microbiol* 1990;28:426–429.

105 **Saulnier P, Bourneix C, Prevost G, Andremont A.** Random amplified polymorphic DNA assay is less discriminant than pulsed-field gel electrophoresis for typing strains of MRSA. *J Clin Microbiol* 1993;31:982–985.

106 **Strausbaugh LJ, Jacobson C, Sewell DL, Potter S, Ward TT.** Methicillin-resistant *Staphylococcus aureus* in extended-care facilities. *Infect Control Hosp Epidemiol* 1991; 12:36–45.

107 **Bradley SF, Terpenning MS, Ramsey MA, et al.** Methicillin-resistant *Staphylococcus aureus:* colonization and infection in a long-term care facility. *Ann Intern Med* 1991; 115:417–422.

108 **Thomas JC, Bridge J, Waterman S, et al.** Transmission and control of methicillin-resistant *Staphylococcus aureus* in a skilled nursing facility. *Infect Control Hosp Epidemiol* 1989;10:106–110.

109 **Storch GA, Radcliff JL, Meyer PL, Hinrichs JH.** Methicillin-resistant *Staphylococcus aureus* in a nursing home. *Infect Control* 1987;8:24–29.

110 **Muder RR, Brennen C, Wagener MM, et al.** Methicillin-resistant staphylococcal colonization and infection in a long-term care facility. *Ann Intern Med* 1991;114:107–112.

111 **Budnick LD, Schaefler S.** Ciprofloxacin-resistant methicillin-resistant *Staphylococcus aureus* in New York health care facilities, 1988. The New York MRSA Study Group. *Am J Public Health* 1990;80:810–813.

112 **Hsu CCS.** Serial survey of methicillin-resistant *Staphylococcus aureus* nasal carriage among residents in a nursing home. *Infect Control Hosp Epidemiol* 1991;12:416–421.

113 **Mulligan ME, Murray-Leisure KA, Ribner BS, et al.** MRSA: a consensus review of the microbiology, pathogenesis, and epidemiology with implications for prevention and management. *Am J Med* 1993;94:313–328.

114 **Saravolatz LD, Pohlod DJ, Arking LM.** Community-acquired MRSA infections: a new source for nosocomial outbreaks. *Ann Intern Med* 1982;97:325–329.

115 **Widmer AF, Doebbeling BN, Costigan M, et al.** Source of recolonization following elimination of *S. aureus* nasal carriage from chronic carriers. Program and abstracts of the 32nd Interscience Congress on Antimicrobial Agents and Chemotherapy, American Society for Microbiology, Anaheim, CA, October 11–14, 1992.

116 **Dammann TA, Wiens RM, Taylor GD.** Methicillin-resistant *Staphylococcus aureus:* identification of a community outbreak by monitoring of hospital isolates. *Can J Public Health* 1988;79:312–314.

117 **Linnemann CC Jr, Moore P, Stanebeck JL, Pfaller MA.** Reemergence of epidemic Methicillin-resistant *Staphylococcus aureus* in a general hospital associated with changing staphylococcal strains. *Am J Med* 1991; 91(suppl 3B):238–244.

118 **Sorrell TC, Packham DR, Shanker S, et al.** Vancomycin therapy for methicillin-resistant *Staphylococcus aureus. Ann Intern Med* 1982;97:344–350.

119 **Hackbarth CJ, Chambers HF.** Methicillin-resistant staphylococci: detection methods and treatment of infections. *Antimicrob Agents Chemother* 1989;33:995–999.

120 **Watanakunakorn C.** Treatment of infections due to methicillin-resistant *Staphylococcus aureus. Ann Intern Med* 1982;97:376–378.

121 **Levine JF.** Vancomycin: a review. *Med Clin North Am* 1987;71:1135–1145.

122 **Reynolds PE.** Structure, biochemistry and mechanism of action of glycopeptide antibiotics. *Eur J Clin Microbiol Infect Dis* 1989; 8:943–950.

123 **Schwalbe RS, Stapleton JT, Gilligan PH.** Emergence of vancomycin resistance in coagulase-negative staphylococci. *N Engl J Med* 1987;316:927–931.

124 **Veach LA, Pfaller MA, Barrett M, Koontz FP, Wenzel RP.** Vancomycin resistance in *Staphylococcus hemolyticus* causing colonization and bloodstream infection. *J Clin Microbiol* 1990;28:2064–2068.

125 **Faville RJ Jr, Zaske DE, Kaplan EL, et al.** *Staphylococcus aureus* endocarditis: combined

therapy with vancomycin and rifampin. *J Am Med Assoc* 1978;240:1963–1965.

126 **Watanakunakorn C, Guerriero JC.** Interaction between vancomycin and rifampin against *Staphylococcus aureus. Antimicrob Agents Chemother* 1981;19:1089–1091.

127 **Watanakunakorn C, Tisone JC.** Synergism between vancomycin and gentamicin or tobramycin for methicillin-susceptible and methicillin-resistant *Staphylococcus aureus* strains. *Antimicrob Agents Chemother* 1982; 22:903–905.

128 **Watanakunakorn C.** Mode of action and in vitro activity of vancomycin. *J Antimicrob Chemother* 1984;14(suppl D):7.

129 **Verbist L.** The antimicrobial activity of fusidic acid. *J Antimicrob Chemother* 1990; 25(suppl B):1–5.

130 **Schaad UB, Nelson JD, McCracken GH Jr.** Pharmacology and efficacy of vancomycin for staphylococcal infections in children. *Rev Infect Dis* 1981;3(suppl):282.

131 **Kaplan EL.** Vancomycin in infants and children: a review of pharmacology and indications for therapy and prophylaxis. *J Antimicrob Chemother* 1984;14(suppl):59.

132 **Sorrell TC, Collingnon PJ.** A prospective study of adverse reactions associated with vancomycin therapy. *J Antimicrob* 1985; 16:235–241.

133 **Southorn PA, Plevak DJ, Wright AJ, et al.** Adverse effects of vancomycin administered in the perioperative period. *Mayo Clin Proc* 1986;61:721.

134 **Gatterer G.** Spasmatic low back pain in a patient receiving intravenous vancomycin during continuous ambulatory peritoneal dialysis. *Clin Pharmacol* 1984;3:87.

135 **Garrelts JL, Peterie JD.** Vancomycin and the "red man's syndrome." *N Engl J Med* 1985;312:245.

136 **David RL, Smith AL, Koup JR.** The "red man's syndrome" and slow infusion of vancomycin (letter). *Ann Intern Med* 1986; 104:285–286.

137 **Sahai J, Healy DB, Garris R, Berry A, Polk RE.** Influence of antihistamine pretreatment of vancomycin-induced red man's syndrome. *J Infect Dis* 1989;160:876–881.

138 **Mollering RC Jr, Krogstand DJ, Greenblatt DJ.** Vancomycin therapy in patients with impaired renal function: a nomogram for dosage. *Ann Intern Med* 1981;94:343.

139 **Lindholm PD, Murray JS.** Persistence of vancomycin in the blood during renal failure and its treatment by hemodialysis. *N Engl J Med* 1966;274:1047.

140 **Barcenas CG, Fuller TJ, Elms J, et al.** Staphylococcal sepsis in patients on chronic hemodialysis regimens. Intravenous treatment with vancomycin given once weekly. *Arch Intern Med* 1976;136:1131.

141 **Ross J, Abate MA.** Topical vancomycin for the treatment of *Staphylococcus epidermidis* and methicillin-resistant *Staphylococcus aureus* conjunctivitis. *DICP* 1990;24:1050–1053.

142 **Hirsch BE, Amodio M, Einzig AI, Halevy R, Soeiro R.** Instillation of vancomycin into a cerebrospinal fluid reservoir to clear infection: pharmacokinetic considerations. *J Infect Dis* 1991;163:197–200.

143 **Neu HC.** Glycopeptides and lipopeptides: agents trying to meet the demands of the future. *Antimicrobic Newsletter* 1988;5:77–84.

144 **Greenwood D.** Microbiological properties of teicoplanin. *J Antimicrob Chemother* 1988; 21(suppl A):1–13.

145 **Gilbert DN, Wood CA, Kimbrough RC.** Infectious Diseases Consortium of Oregon. Failure of treatment with teicoplanin at 6 milligrams/kilogram/day in patients with *Staphylococcus aureus* intravascular infection. *Antimicrob Agents Chemother* 1991;35:79–87.

146 **Sachdeva M, Hackbarth C, Stella FB, Chambers HF.** Comparative activity of CGP 31608, nafcillin, cefamandole, imipenem, and vancomycin against methicillin-susceptible and methicillin-resistant staphylococci. *Antimicrob Agents Chemother* 1987;31:1549–1552.

147 **Berry AJ, Johnston JL, Archer GL.** Imipenem therapy of experimental *Staphylococcus epidermidis* endocarditis. *Antimicrob Agents Chemother* 1986;29:748–752.

148 **Blumberg HM, Rimland D, Carroll DJ, Terry P, Wachsmuth IK.** Rapid development of ciprofloxacin resistance in methicillin-susceptible and resistant *Staphylococcus aureus. J Infect Dis* 1991;163:1279–1285.

149 **Sader HS, Pignatori AL, Hollis RJ, Leme I, Janes, RN.** Oxacillin—and quinolone-resistant Staphylococcus Aureus in Sao Paulo, Brazil: a multicenter molecular epidemiology study. *Infect Control Hosp Epidemiol* 1993;14:260–264.

150 **Elwell LP, Wilson HR, Knick VB, Keith BR.** In vitro and in vivo efficacy of the combination trimethoprim-sulfamethoxazole against clinical isolates of methicillin-resistant *Staphylococcus aureus. Antimicrob Agents Chemother* 1986;29:1092–1094.

151 **Markowitz N, Quinn EL, Saravolatz LD.** Trimethoprim-sulfamethoxazole compared with

vancomycin for the treatment of *Staphylococcal aureus* infection. *Ann Intern Med* 1992;117:390–398.

152 Schaefler SD, Jones W, Perry L, et al. Emergence of gentamicin- and methicillin-resistant *Staphylococcus aureus* strains in New York City hospitals. *J Clin Microbiol* 1981; 13:754–759.

153 Sande MA, Mandell GL. Effect of rifampin on carriage of nasal *Staphylococcus aureus*. *Antimicrob Agents Chemother* 1975;7:294–297.

154 Massanari RM,Donta ST. The efficacy of rifampin as adjunctive therapy in selected cases of staphylococcal endocarditis. *Chest* 1978;73:375–377.

155 Simon UC, Simon M. Antibacterial activity of teicoplanin and vancomycin in combination with rifampicin, fusidic acid or foscomycin against staphylococci on vein catheters. *Scand J Infect Dis* 1990;72(suppl):14–19.

156 Smith SM, Eng RHK, Tecson-Tumang F. Ciprofloxacin therapy for methicillin-resistant *Staphylococcus aureus* infections or colonizations. *Antimicrob Agents Chemother* 1989; 33:181–184.

157 Darouiche R, Wright C, Hamill R, et al. Eradication of colonization by methicillin-resistant *Staphylococcus aureus* by using oral minocycline-rifampin and topical mupirocin. *Antimicrob Agents Chemother* 1991;1612.

158 Smith SM, Mangia A, Eng RH, Rugeri P, Koza M, Lewis D, Markowski J. Clindamycin for colonization and infected by MRSA. *Infection* 1988;16:95–97.

159 Reeves DS, Holt HA, Phillips I, et al. Activity of clindamycin against *Staphylococcus aureus* and *Staphylococcus epidermidis* from four UK centres. *J Antimicrob Chemother* 1991;27:469–474.

160 Cafferkey MT, Hone R, Keane CT. Antimicrobial therapy of septicemia due to MRSA. *Antimicrob Agents Chemother* 1985;28:819–823.

161 Iwarson S, Fasth S, Olaison L, et al. Adverse reactions to intravenous administration of fusidic acid. *Scand J Infect Dis* 1981;13:65–67.

162 Lowbury JL, Cason JS, Jackson DM, et al. Fucidin for staphyloccal infection of burns. *Lancet* 1962;1:478–480.

163 Amirak ID, Li AKC, Williams RJ, et al. A fatal infection caused by MRSA acquiring resistance to gentamicin and fusidic acid during therapy. *J Infect* 1981;3:50–58.

164 Besnier JM, Kanoun F, Martin C, et al. Failure of a combination of vancomycin and fusidic acid in a patient with staphylococcal infection. *J Antimicrob Chemother* 1991; 27:560–562.

165 Portier H. A multicentre, open, clinical trial of a new intravenous formulation of fusidic acid in severe staphylococcal infection. *J Antimicrob Chemother* 1990;25(suppl B):39–44.

166 Chow JW, Hilf M, Yu VL. Synergistic interaction of antibiotics with nasal penetration to methicillin-sensitive and methicillin-resistant *Staphylococcus aureus*. *J Antimicrob Chemother* 1991;27:558–560.

167 Kuwabara K, Shigeoka H, Ontonari T, et al. Successful treatment with minocycline of two cases of endocarditis caused by Staphylococcus. *Chemotherapy* 1985;33:904–905.

168 Lawlor M, Sullivan M, Levitz R, et al. Treatment of prosthetic valve endocarditis due to MRSA with minocycline. *J Infect Dis* 1990;161:812–814.

169 Hooper DC, Wolfson JS, McHugh GL, et al. Effects of novobiocin, coumermycin A1, clorobiocin and their analogs on *Escherichia coli* DNA gyrase and bacterial growth. *Antimicrob Agents Chemother* 1982;22:662–671.

170 Lau WY, Teoh-Chan CH, Fan ST, Lau KF. In vitro and in vivo study of fosfomycin in MRSA septicaemia. *J Hyg* 1986;96:419–423.

171 DiGiambattista M, Chinali G, Cocito C. Review: the molecular basis of the inhibitory activities of type A and type B synergimycins and related antibiotics on ribosomes. *J Antimicrob Chemother* 1989;24:485–507.

172 Thabaut A, Meyran M, Huerre M. Evolution and present situation of *Staphylococcus aureus* sensitivity to MLS in hospitals (1975–83). *J Antimicrob Chemother* 1985;16(suppl A):205–206.

How vaccines are developed

R. GORDON DOUGLAS, JR

INTRODUCTION

Enhancing human health through new and improved vaccines is both a promise and an accomplishment of medical science. Specific advances in the past two decades that have radically changed the prospects for vaccine development include new developments in immunology since the advent of acquired immunodeficiency virus (AIDS); molecular understanding of viruses, bacteria, and other parasites; recombinant DNA technology, including commercially available hepatitis B virus vaccines; discovery of the etiologic infectious agents of several diseases, including Lyme disease and forms of cervical cancer and peptic ulcer disease; improvements in analytic biochemistry and macromolecular purification; development of monoclonal antibodies; and discovery of experimental methods to release antigens slowly over sustained periods. As a result, many new candidate vaccines are in research or in development in both academia and industry, and some of them may become available in the next 10 years.

NEW VACCINES IN RESEARCH AND DEVELOPMENT

Among the diseases or organisms for which vaccines are currently in research or in development are human immunodeficiency virus (HIV), cytomegalovirus, gonococcus, hepatitis C, hepatitis E, herpes simplex virus, nontypeable *Haemophilus influenzae*, malaria, pertussis (acellular), pneumococcus, polyvalent bacterial urinary tract infections, rotavirus, respiratory syncytial virus (RSV), varicella, staphylococcus, Lyme disease, dengue, meningococcus B, tuberculosis, *Helicobacter pylori*, human papillomavirus, Epstein-Barr virus, schistosomiasis, and streptococcus group B (1). This list is in no particular order except that HIV is listed first because it is the area that necessarily attracts the greatest effort. Vaccines against most of these diseases or organisms will be developed (a) when technical feasibility is established, and (b) if the potential medical

192

interest and market size is sufficient. Conversely, when one of these two criteria is not met, scientific effort will be directed elsewhere.

How are vaccines discovered and developed? First, we must understand what they are. *Biologics* are pharmaceutical products that are derived from living matter. This attribute generally distinguishes them from *drugs*, which are usually chemicals of defined structure produced by synthetic or fermentation processes. Biologic products generally include vaccines, therapeutic proteins, blood fractions, and antibodies. *Antibodies*, such as human immune globulins, provide immediate *passive* and short-term protection against infection by micro-organisms when given before or soon following exposure (e.g., measles, varicella, rabies, cytomegalovirus, hepatitis A, and hepatitis B immune globulins). *Vaccines*, in contrast, are designed for *active* prevention of long-term duration. Usually given well in advance of exposure, they stimulate appropriate humoral and cellular immune responses in the recipient host; some may be effective even when administered near the time of exposure. Vaccines may consist of whole live attenuated or killed micro-organisms or of polysaccharide or polypeptide subunits of the micro-organisms.

RESEARCH LEADING TO VACCINE DEVELOPMENT

Exploratory research

Vaccine development is a long and complicated process that best emerges from a continuing program in basic research in the immunology and microbiology of a number of infectious disease agents. Knowledge evolves at different rates for different agents, and vaccine research and development can begin only when there is a sufficient technologic and biologic data base to permit a reasonable chance for success. Such basic information may come from research programs of vaccine companies, academia, government laboratories, or biotechnology companies.

Developmental research

All serious candidate vaccines must fulfill at least two major criteria for the transition from exploratory to developmental research. First, the disease to be prevented must be of sufficient importance to public health to justify the commitment of resources. Second, there must be a technologic data base that indicates, but does not need to establish, feasibility.

Development of a new vaccine requires a body of knowledge, adequate modern facilities, organizational commitment, and a critically large enough group of scientific workers of diverse disciplines who are trained to provide the technical support. The elements that need to be resolved before a vaccine can be considered for candidate status are several. (a) The disease-producing agent must be discovered, isolated, and defined. (b) The number and relative immunologic importance of serotypes of the organism must be determined. (c) There must be means either for propagating the agent as a whole organism in culture or for a recombinant system to express a subunit antigen. (d) The pathogenesis of the disease needs to be understoood so that meaning-ful points for immunologic intervention can be targeted. (e) Surrogate markers for protective immunity should be identified. (f) Inherent safety assurance of the compo-nents of the vaccine must be proven. (g) Animal models for tests of safety and protective efficacy should be established, if feasible. Attention must be paid to methods and systems for propagation and processing of the agent to make a reproducible vaccine for which an acceptable safety profile can be confidently developed.

Preclinical testing

A candidate experimental vaccine is one that will induce an immune response in an animal model that is believed to have relevance to protective immunity in people. This vaccine may involve a well-characterized live or killed micro-organism, a subunit, or a recombinant vector bearing added gene sequences of the pathogen that demonstrates the ability to express an antigen or antigens. Some live virus vaccines—as was the case for measles, mumps, and rubella—needed to be tested directly in humans because no experimental animal model relevant to the human infection existed.

In vitro and *in vivo* testing are extensive. *In vitro* tests measure vaccine composition, quantity of antigen (i.e., amount, or infectivity titer), absence of foreign infectious agents (i.e., contaminating viruses or other microbes), purity, potency, and stability on storage. *In vivo* tests in animals are used to ensure, insofar as is possible, immunogeni-city, potency, and efficacy of vaccines. Animal testing is also employed to identify the safety profile, tolerance (toxicity), and, when possible, lack of immunologic interfer-ence between competing antigens or viruses.

All lots of vaccine intended for tests in humans are required by governmental regulation to be prepared by good manufacturing procedures. The product must be examined exhaustively by chemical, microbiologic, and *in vitro* and *in vivo* testing that, collectively, will provide an acceptable level of product safety and will form the basis for expectation that it will be efficacious for its intended use in humans. Hence, each lot of experimental vaccine is as complicated and requires as long to manufacture as does a lot of licensed vaccine destined for commercial distribution. All animal testing and all quality control procedures are carried out by the same general methods and by the same well-trained personnel as those used for release of vaccines for sale.

The time required between conceptualization and demonstration of feasibility for a vaccine is extensive. Preclinical research to bring a candidate vaccine to the point of clinical tests requires 2 years or more.

Clinical testing

Clinical research provides the data that take a candidate vaccine from completion of preclinical testing to the end stage of clinical evaluation, at which time a license for marketing and distribution of the vaccine can be granted by governmental licensing authorities. This can require 4 to 5 years or longer.

There is a vast difference in complexity between the development of biologics, especially vaccines, and that of drugs. Biologics, inherently, are diverse and antigenically indefinable; they therefore require a very large group of technical disciplines to support work on them. These disciplines may include virology, bacteriology, cell culture, biochemistry, organic chemistry, process chemistry, formulations preparation, analytic chemistry, biology, immunology, and animal experimentation, among others. Production of vaccines is controlled as much by adherence to a rigorously defined procedure as by measurement of the attributes of the final product. In conventional drug research and development, a drug, unlike a biologic, is completely definable from the start as a unique chemical entity, and manufacturing can be controlled on a technically simple and orderly basis.

Regulatory control of clinical research and licensure of biologics are conducted by the Food and Drug Administration (FDA), Center for Biologics Evaluation and Research (CBER). Licensure is based on the content of a Product License Application (PLA). Unlike for drugs, CBER also grants a license for the facilities (establishment) used to manufacture the product as well as for the product itself.

FROM IND TO PRODUCT LICENSURE

Federal regulatory laws specify a specific flow of information and reporting that begins with filing an Investigative New Drug (IND) application for initiating the conduct of clinical testing of an experimental vaccine. This investigation phase terminates with the granting of a product license for commercial distribution of the product.

IND regulations

Initiation of clinical testing of an experimental vaccine begins with the filing of an IND application. In the conduct of clinical trials under the IND laws, prior approval must be obtained from CBER for clinical test protocols, study plans, and vaccine lot summaries. In addition, the clinical research investigators in academia who conduct the trials must be qualified and approved by CBER, as part of the IND process.

Participation by a subject in a clinical trial must be by voluntary and informed consent of the volunteer or by a parent or guardian where age prevents a voluntary decision. At each study site where a trial is conducted, there must be approval by a local committee that reviews and monitors the conduct of the trials to ensure adherence to the highest ethical standards. Periodic and annual reporting of each study under IND is made to CBER, and immediate reporting of serious adverse reactions is made if and when they occur.

Phase control clinical testing

Clinical testing of biologics, as for drugs, is carried out in progressive steps involving increasing numbers of volunteers. The lines between the successive stages in clinical trials are not distinct and tend to overlap. There must be full compliance with the IND regulations during all phases of clinical testing.

Phase I clinical   Phase I trials are initially conducted in small numbers of adults to establish safety, and then are carried out in children and finally in infants. The purpose is to establish a tolerability profile for the vaccine in a stepwise fashion, testing those less likely to have clinical reactions (i.e., healthy immune adults) first. Dose and regimen studies are conducted, and immunogenicity and tolerability profiles are established for each dose and regimen.

Phase II clinical   Phase II trials are broadly directed and fall into 2 separate subphases. The *first subphase* is usually conducted in approximately 200 to 400 volunteers during a 6- to 18-month period or longer. The purpose is to confirm immunogenicity, safety, tolerability, and the optimal dose in the targeted age groups.

The *second subphase* is conducted in up to 500 to 1,000 or more volunteers during a 6- to 18-month period or longer. Its purpose is definitive establishment of immunogenicity, safety, and tolerability, as well as final definition of the dosage level, formulation, and dosing regimen. Such studies may be blinded and may yield efficacy data.

Phase III clinical   Phase III clinical tests are conducted for the purpose of establishing the protective efficacy of the product, in a blinded and placebo-controlled design, if possible, then performance of the product in its final formulation is proven. For killed vaccines, 2,000 volunteers may suffice for this latter phase. With live virus vaccines, studies in 10,000 to 30,000 volunteers may be required.

As seen, there can be very large variations in numbers of volunteers to be tested clinically and in the time required to complete the tests. With time, the governmental requirements for compliance and for establishing safety and efficacy have expanded. Currently, clinical testing of a new vaccine can be expected to take 4 to 10 years or more and may involve 5,000 to 30,000 volunteers.

It may be instructive to note that it took 6 years of clinical testing to bring the first *plasma-derived* hepatitis B vaccine to licensure in 1981; this period was preceded by 7 years of intensive basic research discovery and preclinical development, for a total of 13 years. *Recombinant-produced* hepatitis B vaccine, which represented a modification in the source of antigen for the vaccine, required a total time of 9 years to bring to licensure. Varicella vaccine will have taken 24 years or more from IND to licensure.

Process research and development

At the appropriate time during early clinical testing and prior to licensure, establishment of a process for making vaccine in scaled-up volume is essential. The process must be consistent, rugged. reproducible, reliable, efficient, and capable of large-volume production. The physical plant must be completed and operational. In the end stage, at least 3 to 5 lots of vaccine must be manufactured by the exact process intended for routine commercial production. All lots must meet FDA (CBER) specifications with regard to purity, potency, sterility, storage stability, consistency in antigen content, and safety and antibody production in human subjects, at least 200 per lot. Any significant revision or modification in process may require additional testing of 3 to 5 lots in 25 to 50 or more volunteers per lot. Release standards for each batch must be developed that assure potency and sterility. To provide vaccine to the market in a timely fashion, the Establishment License Application (ELA), which requests approval of the production facilities, must be ready for submission at the same time as the PLA.

After licensure, continuing technical surveillance of the product and the process is required to keep the product at state-of-the-art levels, to meet competition, and to improve purity, potency, and tolerability.

LICENSURE AND POSTLICENSURE

Product license application

The final step in bringing a biologic product to approval for licensing and commercial distribution is submission of a PLA and an ELA to CBER. These documents are voluminous and include all background research, details of product preparation, findings in clinical tests of the product that justify its general commercial distribution, and an exhaustive description of the production facility. Extensive data must be submitted showing proof of stability for the designated period that the product would be stored in the field. The contents of the package circular—which describes preparation, clinical trials, indications, contraindications, precautions, warnings and adverse reactions, dosage, and administration of the product—and the labels that are affixed to the vial are, collectively, called "labeling" and are subject to review and approval by the FDA.

The time required to obtain a license for distribution of a new vaccine following license application may be 6 months to 2 or more years.

Postlicense control

Recommendations for use   Although the FDA grants licenses for sale of products, the Advisory Committee for Immunization Practices of the Centers for Disease Control and Prevention (CDC) of the United States Public Health Service, the Committee on Infectious Diseases of the American Academy of Pediatrics (AAP), and the Task Force on Adult Immunization of the American College of Physicians with the Infectious Diseases Society of America review and formulate recommendations and regimens for the use of vaccines. Although these prestigious professional organizations have no direct legal authority, their advice is generally heeded by manufacturers and the labeling of the product may incorporate their recommendations, provided they are acceptable to the licensing authority (CBER). The Armed Forces Epidemiological Board develops recommendations for use of vaccines in military personnel. Clinical trials are often designed based on anticipated recommendations by these groups.

Lot release and surveillance   CBER tests, reviews, and approves the release for sale of each individual lot of a biologic product. Furthermore, it serves as an information collection agency that receives and acts on reports of significant adverse reactions that may require investigation. The CDC shares this responsibility with the FDA, and systems are being developed and automated to increase and improve the conduct of postmarketing surveillance. With the more recently licensed vaccines, pharmaceutical companies have been required by CBER to conduct surveillance in 10,000 to 30,000 vaccine recipients after licensure.

Foreign licensure and the roles of WHO and the European community

Individual nations   Vaccines are used worldwide; virtually all nations have their own licensing agencies that must be satisfied before marketing is permitted in a particular country. Many nations rely on licensure by the United States government or other qualified government, such as the United Kingdom, either as a guide or for automatic product approval.

European Community   Integration of standards for drugs and biologics within the European Community poses special problems because all existing licensed vaccines must be reregistered to meet a single standard for all nations.

The World Health Organization (WHO), a branch of the United Nations, has a biologics section that prepares detailed guidelines for content and quality assessment of vaccines for member nations to follow. These are "global standards" for many parts of the world, but the regulatory authorities in individual nations are not bound by WHO recommendations and are given the responsibility for making all determinations.

VACCINES AS A BUSINESS VENTURE

Marketing of vaccines is indispensable to vaccine manufacturers, because this is the necessary device by which the costs of research and development and manufacturing can be recovered and a profit can be realized.

Roughly, only 1 in 3 choices made for vaccine development actually sees its way to a product, perhaps after 7 to 15 years of work. Historically, approximately one fifth of all candidate vaccines taken to clinical trial have become licensed products. Some have had only limited application, such as the vaccines against pneumococcal and meningococcal infections. Collectively, all of these factors make vaccine research and development investment more risky than that for drugs.

Although flourishing at one time, most of the vaccine manufacturers in the United States gradually abandoned the field during the 1970s and the 1980s due to low profitability and rising liability risks, especially for pertussis.

Product liability claims involving biologics

The expanding actions of a litigious society during the 1970s and the 1980s led to a profusion of lawsuits against vaccine providers, usually physicians and nurses, as well as vaccine manufacturers. Lawsuits were brought for real or perceived damages believed to have been caused by administration of vaccines. Most lawsuits were based on temporal association of the injury to the vaccination. Actual causation was often difficult, if not impossible, to prove in lawsuits. However, these lawsuits were decided for the most part by a jury sympathetic to the plaintiff; these juries would award large monetary settlements despite lack of association or causation of the injury to the vaccine administered.

The product liability lawsuits, for the most part, involved diphtheria, pertussis, and tetanus (DPT) and polio vaccines, although litigation against measles, mumps, and rubella vaccines was also prominent. By 1985, there was a serious concern that continued vaccine litigation would interrupt the supply of mandated vaccines to the serious detriment of national immunization goals. During this period, the cost of DPT vaccine increased as a consequence of the high liability costs for which there was no commercial insurance.

To meet the crisis, the American Academy of Pediatrics, vaccine manufacturers, and concerned consumers and lawmakers joined together to draft legislation to ameliorate the vaccine liability problem. The result was passage of the National Childhood Vaccine Injury Act of 1986 (NCVIA), which created the Federal Vaccine Injury Compensation Program. The program provides review and consideration for compensation to all those who claim injury from vaccines covered by the NCVIA—namely measles, mumps, and rubella; diphtheria, pertussis, and tetanus; and polio vaccines. Following review, the claimant may be denied an award, or an award of a prespecified amount is offered. The claimant may accept and forego all further rights of legal action. Alternatively, the claimant may reject the award and file for damages under the traditional tort system.

In general, funds to pay for the awards made to injured parties under the federal compensation programs are derived from an excise tax imposed on all sales from mandated vaccines.

The federal compensation program has dramatically reduced litigation against health care providers and vaccine manufacturers from lawsuits arising from the covered vaccines. This stability, together with vaccine prices increasing with inflation and new scientific discoveries, has begun to attract new pharmaceutical as well as biotechnical companies to the market, making it a promisingly vigorous and healthy industry.

Although the federal compensation program has been eminently successful, there are several limitations and concerns. The NCVIA covers only the mandated vaccines: measles, mumps, rubella, DPT, and poliomyelitis. Nonmandated vaccines, such as those against hepatitis B, influenza, *Haemophilus influenzae* type B, pneumococcal pneumonia, and meningococcal meningitis, are not covered. Health care providers and manufacturers of noncovered vaccines continue to face the threat of litigation involving administration of those products. Clearly, with the increasingly broad use of these nonmandated vaccines, Congress should be encouraged to add them to the list of vaccines covered under the NCVIA. Protection against perceived damage by these vaccines would not only encourage immunization compliance by potential vaccinees but would also generate continued research, development, and manufacture of more effective and innovative new vaccine products.

Patents

Worldwide patent laws have allowed individuals and companies to exclude others from making, using, and selling an invention for a specified time. Because research is both time-consuming and expensive, this period of exclusivity allows the patent owner to exploit the invention.

Vaccines and biologics, although patentable, have been more difficult to define than pharmaceutical drugs, which are simple chemicals. Patentability of vaccines, as well as other pharmaceutical inventions, is dependent on the vaccine substance being novel, being useful as a vaccine, and not being obvious. Whole cell or whole virus vaccines are patentable because the micro-organism or virus has been purified and induces protective immunity. Subunit vaccines, either protein or nucleic acids in pure form, may also be patented. Patents may also be obtained on vaccine compositions and processes of making the vaccines.

The biotechnology explosion that began in the mid-1970s has resulted in patenting of a wide array of biotechnological products. These products, including new vectors for delivery of genetic information, genetic alternation of existing life forms, and creation of polypeptide expression systems, have created problems regarding what is patentable and what constitutes infringement.

Whatever the problems, valid patents are the lifeblood of the pharmaceutical industry. Without patents, few vaccines would be developed and marketed. Proliferation of smaller biotechnology companies is directly related to the ability of the company to obtain patents for their novel inventions. In many instances, the ability to raise money is dependent on a strong patent portfolio. By such device, combinations of patented subject matter can be assembled and joined to create new and useful biologics for the future.

Incentives to vaccine development

Having considered risks, costs, and disincentives, it is worth asking whether there are any incentives at all. Clearly, there are. They lie mainly in the increasing participation of the private sector and of governments in ensuring widespread use of pediatric vaccines in all children in the developed and developing world, thus creating a stable and predictable demand for vaccines.

Although some government-owned companies manufacture older vaccines, research, development, manufacture, and distribution of newer vaccines is primarily the province of vaccine companies in the private sector. For them to be successful, and to achieve the promise for the future of prevention through new vaccines, a fair and adequate return for their risk and investment is critical (i.e., prices of vaccines must be sufficient so that companies will take risks on new products and make investments in research and development and in manufacturing facilities). When these prices are not affordable in certain countries or to certain populations, governments and agencies must purchase vaccines and provide them free or at affordable prices.

Vaccine initiatives in the United States

It has become increasingly evident that the prevention of disease through vaccination is a highly cost-effective tool for health maintenance. In support of this finding, there has been a literal explosion of public and private initiatives to promote and expand vaccine use in the United States (Table 10-1). Included as part of the 1986 law are the National

Table 10-1 Organizations concerned with promotion of vaccine use (representative lists)

United States
    National Vaccine Program
    National Vaccine Advisory Committee
    Influenza/Pneumococcal Action Group of the American Lung Association
    American College Health Association
    National Foundation for Infectious Diseases
    Immunization Practices Advisory Committee (ACIP)
    U.S. Agency for International Development (AID)
    Academy of Pediatrics
    American Public Health Association
    American College of Physicians
Worldwide
    Expanded Program for Immunization (EPI) of the World Health Organization (1977)
    Children's Vaccine Initiative of the WHO, UNICEF, and the United Nations Development
        Program (UNDP)
    Task Force for Child Survival of the World Bank, UNDP, WHO, Rockefeller Foundation,
        UNICEF (1984)
    Pan American Health Organization
    CARE
    Project Hope

Vaccine Program and its two advisory groups, the National Vaccine Advisory Committee and the Advisory Committee on Childhood Vaccines. These groups, working closely together, are seeking to address all issues of significance in accelerating vaccine development and in expanding disease prevention by vaccine application.

It is believed by health agencies that the new vaccine initiatives to ensure procurement of supplies, to undertake public education for vaccine use, and to reduce the concerns for liability by alternatives to tort law will increase the incentive of manufacturers to re-enter the field of vaccines and to expand their research and development activities with them.

The benefits of vaccines

Much of the basis for increase in the average human lifespan from a few decades to approximately 70 years has been by control of infectious diseases. This control has been accomplished by environmental control of transmission of infectious agents, by improved nutrition, and by vaccination. Vaccines have proved to be extremely cost-effective and are obtained at a relative bargain price for the large social and economic benefits that have come from their use.

Vaccines in the United States

Case reduction Nine of the principal vaccines used in the United States include those against diphtheria, pertussis, tetanus, measles, mumps, rubella, paralytic poliomyelitis, and, recently, *Haemophilus influenzae* type B and hepatitis B. If the maximum number of cases per year prior to vaccine introduction is compared with the number of cases that occurred in 1989, the reduction in cases (the first 7 diseases) ranged from 92% for tetanus to 99.9% for diphtheria, a most remarkable achievement. It is especially worth noting that the congenital rubella syndrome, affecting as many as 20,000 newborn infants/year at its peak, was reduced to only 3 cases by 1989. And despite a resurgence of measles and rubella in 1990 and 1991 due to the failure to vaccinate children, once again they are under control as a result of interim efforts to vaccinate additional children.

No single vaccine used in the United States has been of greater benefit than that against measles. Between 1963 and 1990, the vaccine averted nearly 75 million cases of measles and prevented more than 7,000 deaths and 24,000 cases of mental retardation due to the disease.

Cost: benefit evaluations   If one calculates the total cost per year for the care and time losses from the occurrences of a disease and compares that figure with the total cost for a vaccination program, one can obtain a ratio denoting dollars saved per dollar spent.

Individually given, measles, mumps, and rubella vaccines each save, on the average, $8.77 in care and time loss for every dollar spent on their administration in the United States. With a single combined measles, mumps, and rubella dose, the savings is $14.40 per dollar spent. This amounts to nearly $1.5 billion per year.

For poliomyelitis the vaccine saves $10.30 per dollar spent; for pertussis or whooping cough, $2.10 per dollar spent. These numbers do not even take into account the suffering and death caused by the diseases.

GLOBAL USE OF VACCINES

Much progress has been made in recent years in controlling certain infectious diseases using existing vaccines. In 1974, the WHO established its Expanded Program on Immunization (EPI), which included vaccines against 6 diseases: diphtheria, pertussis, tetanus, poliomyelitis, tuberculosis, and measles. At the time the program was established, the worldwide coverage of the birth cohort with these vaccines was only 5%. By 1981, this coverage had increased to 20% worldwide; however, more than 5 million deaths occurred annually from these 6 vaccine-preventable diseases. By 1990, worldwide coverage had grown to at least 80%, with reduction of the number of vaccine-preventable deaths to 2 million, half of which were due to measles (2). This reduction was achieved as a result of an effective collaboration on the part of the WHO and related agencies, and also by the health workers who administered the vaccine programs in each country.

Global coverage for a single dose of Bacillus Calmette-Guérin (BCG) (tuberculosis vaccine) and 3 doses each of DPT and oral polio vaccine (OPV) by 1 year, one dose of measles vaccine by 2 years, and tetanus to women of the child-bearing age group have risen dramatically (2). By 1990, coverage had risen to 90% for BCG, 83% for DPT,

85% for polio, 80% for measles, and 34% for tetanus to women of child-bearing age. Although this is a remarkable accomplishment, the worldwide average figures were skewed by nearly 100% coverage in China, with its 22 million births, and by excellent coverage in Europe and the Western Hemisphere. In other parts of Asia and in Africa, rates for vaccination vary widely, ranging from 40% to 80%, depending in large part on the war status of the country in question. Despite the remarkable progress that has been made, there is much still to be accomplished.

WHO GOALS FOR IMMUNIZATION COVERAGE

In 1992, the World Health Assembly established a target for the 1990s to boost immunization coverage of the birth cohort with the 6 pediatric vaccines to 90% worldwide by the year 2000. Hepatitis B vaccine was added to the regimen for areas of moderate to high endemicity, and a goal of 90% coverage for tetanus for women of child-bearing age was established. According to the plan, measles deaths will be reduced by 95% by 1995, neonatal tetanus will be eliminated by 1995, and poliomyelitis will be eradicated globally by the year 2000 (it should be noted that the last case of poliomyelitis in the Western Hemisphere occurred in August 1991, although an outbreak of approximately 30 cases occurred in Holland in 1992 in an unvaccinated religious sect) (3).

Children's vaccine initiative

A Children's Vaccine Initiative (CVI) was created during the summer of 1990, and its aims were stated in the "Declaration of New York." This initiative was approved on September 10, 1990, at the World Summit for Children, held at the time of the General Assembly of the United Nations. The founding members of the CVI included the WHO, UNICEF, United Nations Development Program, World Bank, and The Rockefeller Foundation. The CVI was intended to address the agenda for the 1990s set forth by the World Health Assembly. Through new and improved vaccines, the CVI aims to save 2 to 3 million children from death per year—in addition to the 2 to 3 million who have already been saved by the EPI since 1980—and to save 5 to 8 million more children from disabilities.

The target for the CVI is to develop a heat-stable vaccine that can be given orally, at or near birth, on a single occasion, to confer protection against a large number of different diseases. Furthermore, it was stated that this vaccine must be affordable within the resources of the user nation. Despite its worthiness, the objective was greeted originally with great skepticism by immunologists, bacteriologists, virologists, and other scientists interested in the development of new vaccines. However, analysis shows that parts of the objective may be achievable in step-wise fashion over the next decade or two. Because each of the elements of this sweeping objective currently is not technically achievable, progress will depend to a great degree on the rate of expenditure on research and development by government agencies, universities, and pharmaceutical companies.

REFERENCES

1   **Douglas RG Jr.** The children's vaccine initiative—will it work? *J Infect Dis* 1993; 168, 269–274.

2   **World Health Organization.** *Expanded Programme on Immunization: EPI for the 1990s.* Geneva, Switzerland: WHO, 1992:1–15.

3   **Wright PF, Kim-Farley RJ, de Quadros CA, et al.** Strategies for the global eradication of poliomyelitis by the year 2000. *N Engl J Med* 1991;325:1774–1779.

Bacillary angiomatosis and *Rochalimaea* species

DAVID A. RELMAN

INTRODUCTION

Bacillary angiomatosis (BA) is an angioproliferative disease first characterized and associated with visible bacilli in 1983 (1). By the end of the 1980s, a growing number of reported cases and the consistent finding of argyrophilic bacillary structures prompted intense efforts to identify the causative agent. These efforts included more traditional culture-based methods, as well as the development of a culture-independent approach for identifying microbial pathogens directly from infected host tissues (2). The findings generated by the latter experimental approach have now been corroborated and extended by culture-based methods (3–5). Currently, the combined data implicate at least 2 organisms in the pathogenesis of BA: a novel *Rochalimaea* species (*R. henselae*) and the previously-characterized agent of trench fever (*R. quintana*), as well as the possibility of other species. The recent association of *R. henselae* with cat scratch disease (CSD) further emphasizes the clinical and biological significance of this group of rickettsia-like organisms (6,7,8,9). I review the features of BA, the basis on which these organisms have been incriminated in these diseases, and the critical features of the molecular approach by which *R. henselae*, and now other fastidious or uncultured microbial pathogens, have been identified.

CLINICAL FEATURES OF BA

In 1983, Stoler and colleagues (1) described an atypical subcutaneous infection in a 32-year-old man with the acquired immunodeficiency syndrome. The patient presented with subcutaneous nodules that were composed of proliferating endothelial cells within a framework of poorly formed capillary channels. Numerous small pleomorphic bacilli accompanied these cells within the tissue interstitium, as revealed with the Warthin-Starry silver stain and electron microscopy. This patient responded to erythromycin, despite the inability to cultivate or characterize further these organisms. In the same year, Waldo and colleagues (10) described similar tissue pathology but failed to discover bacillary structures. Reports by Cockerell and associates (11), Knobler and co-workers (12), LeBoit and colleagues (13), Koehler and associates (14), and other case studies (15,16) further characterized the proliferative cell type, expanded on the initial clinical descriptions of this syndrome, and pointed out a possible relationship between the BA organism and those seen within CSD tissues. Confusion about the etiology of this disease was reflected in its terminology— epithelioid angiomatosis (11) and disseminated CSD (14)—and in consideration of a possible neoplastic origin (11–13,15,17). Subsequent studies have led to a more complete appreciation and understanding of the clinical and histopathologic features of BA (18–22).

Epidemiology

The epidemiology of BA is still not well defined. Most data derive from retrospective analysis of selected cases. Nonetheless, more than 90% of patients with documented evidence of characteristic angioproliferative tissue pathology have been immuno-compromised individuals, and primarily those suffering from the later stages of human immunodeficiency virus (HIV) infection. Correspondingly, the majority of these patients resided in those regions of the United States and Europe where HIV infection is most prevalent. Approximately 90% of patients were men, with equal representation of Caucasians and Afro-Americans (23), and a median age of 38 years (24). As with the classic forms of CSD (25), the environmental risk factors for BA include cat bites and cat scratches (23). Insect bites, specific terrain exposure, or specific known HIV risk factors have not been significantly associated with BA.

Cutaneous manifestations

Skin and subcutaneous tissues seem to be the most common sites of BA pathology. In the majority of patients with BA, there are either cutaneous papules, plaques, or subcutaneous nodules (19,26). However, the relative ease of skin lesion detection probably introduces a bias into our perceptions of this disease distribution.

Superficial cutaneous papules are most often red, purple, or flesh-colored, and dome-shaped with a collarette of scale; however, they may be pedunculated or ulcerated and crusted. Readers are referred to numerous published color photo-graphs of these lesions (19,21,22,27). These lesions may be solitary or multiple. Lesions with similar appearance are often found on mucosal surfaces. Subcutaneous nodules may be mobile or fixed to underlying structures, including bone (14,28,29).

By gross appearance, superficial BA lesions may resemble Kaposi's sarcoma, and single lesions may resemble pyogenic granuloma or simple angioma. Cutaneous lesions of BA sometimes resolve spontaneously; however, antibiotic treatment seems to hasten this process. Evolution of these lesions often leads to persistent, hyperpigmented macules.

Visceral and systemic manifestations

Several of the first described patients with cutaneous manifestations of BA also suffered from visceral disease (11). Prior to identification of the silver-staining bacilli in these tissues, the reminiscent morphology of these organisms led investigators to diagnose these patients with disseminated CSD, even though the angioproliferative BA histology was quite distinct from the suppurative granulomatous response in classic CSD. The most frequently reported visceral sites of BA involvement are liver, spleen, lymphatic system, and bone marrow (12,30–32). Other sites of involvement that have been less frequently described include the bronchial mucosa (22,33) and the brain (34). Pleuritis, meningitis, and encephalitis have been attributed to BA based on their clear response to antibiotics initiated for documented BA elsewhere in the same patient.

Visceral BA can occur in the absence of cutaneous disease (32). The majority of patients with internal involvement manifest fever and other signs of systemic disease; however, it is often difficult to attribute these signs to BA given the frequency of other documented concurrent infections. As discussed later, the bacterial agents associated with BA can now be cultivated from blood samples. Bacteremia may be a frequent accompaniment of cutaneous and visceral disease and may occur in the absence of documented tissue pathology (3).

Histopathology

Despite similarities between this disease and other tissue lesions, the histologic features of BA are unique (19). There is a lobular proliferation of atypical plump, closely adherent (epithelioid) endothelial cells that form aggregates of capillary-like channels; an extracellular stroma that can be edematous or fibrotic; a neutrophil-predominant mixed inflammatory infiltrate scattered throughout the lesion; and variable degrees of endothelial cell necrosis with microabscess formation. Superficial BA lesions may include an epithelial collarette, enhancing their similarity to pyogenic granulomata. BA pathology is also sometimes confused with that of angiosarcoma, epithelioid hemangioma, and, most importantly, Kaposi's sarcoma; however, histologic features can be used to distinguish each of these entities and have been tabulated by various authorities (18,19).

One of the most specific diagnostic features are clumps of granular material. With hematoxylin and eosin stains, the clumps are amphophilic; with the Warthin-Starry silver stain, they are argyrophilic. These granular clumps correspond with pleomorphic bacilli measuring approximately 0.5×1.5 mm, as seen with electron microscopy (1). One cutaneous vascular lesion that can be nearly indistinguishable from BA (13) is verruga peruana, the chronic stage of human infection by the cultivatable bacterium, *Bartonella bacilliformis*, found only in South America (35). As of 1990, despite a few single isolations (36), numerous attempts to cultivate the similar-appearing bacterium in BA lesions had failed to produce consistent results (19).

In 1990, a culture-independent experimental approach for identifying microbial pathogens was developed and applied to BA tissues (2). This approach took advantage of developments in the field of molecular phylogeny, a field based on the use of genetic sequences as evolutionary clocks (37). The relevance of Bartonellosis to BA pathogenesis has been made even more apparent by elucidation of the evolutionary relationships between this organism and the causative agents of BA.

AN APPROACH TO THE IDENTIFICATION OF UNCULTURED MICROBIAL PATHOGENS

Traditional methods for identifying microbial pathogens rely on cultivation or purification of the microbial organism. For many years, the visible organisms associated with BA could not be cultivated or purified in any other manner. As a result, these organisms remained unidentified. By turning to the analysis of certain genetic sequences, molecular phylogenists have circumvented this problem. Some of their techniques can be adapted to the study of human microbial pathogens in situ.

Use of genetic sequences as evolutionary clocks: ribosomal RNA-based phylogeny

Although all genetic sequences accumulate mutations with time, some sequences accumulate these changes in a manner that renders them highly useful as evolutionary clocks (37). In the case of some of these sequences, evolutionary distance can be calculated as a function of the number of nucleotide or amino acid differences between the versions found in 2 different organisms. The most reliable and useful sequences are those that encode molecules with essential biologic function. This property ensures consistent, clock-like behavior on the sequence, regardless of the type of organism from which it is studied. The most widely used and well-tested genetic clock is the small subunit (16S in procaryotes) ribosomal RNA (rRNA) molecule (37).

On the basis of the comparison of small subunit rRNA sequences, Woese and others (37–41) have revolutionized our understanding of the evolutionary relationships among all known organisms. The universal evolutionary tree reflects these relationships and places all organisms within one of three domains: *Eucarya*, *Archaea*, and *Bacteria*. All previously characterized human bacterial pathogens belong to the last domain. By determining the 16S rRNA sequence of a previously uncharacterized bacterial pathogen, it can be placed within an evolutionary tree.

Amplification of bacterial 16S rDNA directly from diseased tissues

Enzymatic DNA amplification techniques such as the polymerase chain reaction (PCR) generate enough product to allow DNA sequence determination, beginning with as few as 1 to 10 DNA molecules (42–45). However, short DNA molecules from sequences that flank the amplification target must first be designed to serve as primers for the DNA extension step. Bacterial 16S rRNA gene (rDNA) sequences contains crucial and relevant features: interspersed highly conserved regions as well as regions of high variability (Figure 11-1). Some of the conserved sequences are common to all

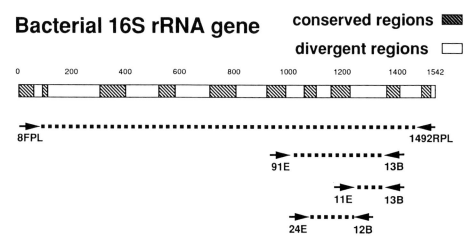

Figure 11-1   The bacterial 16S rRNA gene. During the initial PCR-based bacillary angiomatosis (BA) investigation (2), portions of the gene from uncultured BA bacilli were amplified directly from infected tissues using primer pairs, 11E + 13B and 91E + 13B. Later, a fragment corresponding to approximately 95% of the gene was amplified using primers 8FPL + 1492R (46). All these primers are homologous to conserved sequences (*hatched*) within the bacterial domain. Primers 24E and 12B were designed from variable regions of the gene and amplify fragments from members of the *Rochalimaea* genus and closely related organisms.

previously studied *Bacteria* but are not found in either of the other two domains (i.e., not found in human rRNA gene sequences) (47–50).

   With these principles in mind, an experimental approach for identifying uncultured bacterial pathogens has been developed and successfully applied to BA (2) and other diseases (51–53). Digested, frozen, or fomalin-fixed, paraffin-embedded tissue serves as substrate in PCR reactions using primers designed from known conserved regions of Bacterial 16S rDNA. These primers selectively amplify Bacterial small subunit rDNA in the presence of related human sequences. From the DNA sequence of the amplified 16S rDNA, specific PCR primers from unique regions can be designed, and the evolutionary relationships of the inferred organism can be estimated. Analysis of numerous case and control tissues is crucial to determine a specific association of the amplified sequence with the disease in question. Application of this approach to BA tissues yielded one predominant 16S rRNA sequence that corresponded to a previously uncharacterized organism.

MICROBIAL ETIOLOGY OF BA

Identification of a novel *Rochalimaea* from amplified rDNA sequences

The majority of BA tissues contain a 16S rDNA sequence that corresponds to a novel rickettsia-like organism (2). This organism is most closely-related to *Rochalimaea quin-*

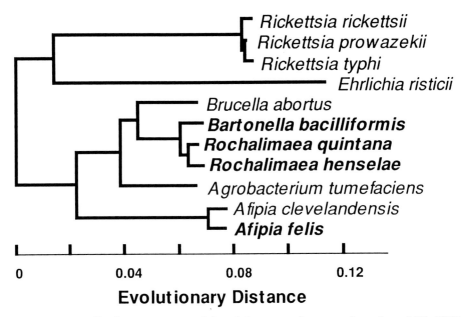

Evolutionary Distance

Figure 11-2 Evolutionary tree of the alpha-proteobacteria, based on 16S rRNA sequences. The organisms associated with bacillary angiomatosis, cat scratch disease, and *Bartonellosis* are indicated in *bold*. Evolutionary distance is proportional to the number of point mutations per sequence position. Modified from Reference (46).

tana and *Rochalimaea vinsonii* (not shown) (46) (Figure 11-2). On the basis of this analysis and the subsequent characterization of the cultivated organism (3), it has been placed within the *Rochalimaea* genus and named *Rochalimaea henselae* (4,5). An identical sequence has been detected in additional independent BA tissues (54,55). Many of the related alpha-proteobacteria are plant pathogens and intracellular symbionts, suggesting that the *Rochalimaea* may have evolved from plant-associated bacteria (56). Not surprisingly, 2 bacterial pathogens with the unusual ability to elicit an angioproliferative host tissue response, *R. henselae* and *B. bacilliformis*, are also closely related by evolutionary criteria. A recent proposal suggests the unification of the genera *Bartonella* and *Rhochlimaea*, with deletion of the latter name (57).

Sequence microheterogeneity refers to infrequent nucleotide discrepancies among different products amplified from either the same tissue digest or digests of similar tissue lesions. In the setting of PCR-based investigations of BA, 16S rDNA microheterogeneity may indicate the presence of multiple species, multiple strains, or *Taq* polymerase artifact. Although BA primers 24E and 12B (2) (see Figure 11-1) have some target specificity, they will amplify 16S rDNA templates from all of the *Rochalimaea* and perhaps from some other closely-related species; thus, PCR products should be further characterized by either Southern hybridization, restriction fragment-length polymorphisms, or DNA sequence determination. Citrate synthase gene sequences may be useful for distinguishing among cultivated rickettsia-like organisms (58); PCR-amplified fragments of this gene can be analyzed by restriction fragment-length polymorphisms.

Cultivation of *R. henselae* and its association with BA

In a serendipitous discovery, the organism now referred to as R. *henselae* was first cultivated from a number of blood samples of febrile patients (3). Isolation depended on use of the lysis-centrifugation method and prolonged incubation of blood agar plates in elevated CO_2 conditions. The 16S rRNA sequence of the isolated organism is identical to that amplified directly from BA tissues, within the range of experimental artifact (46,59). R. *henselae* has subsequently been cultivated by a number of clinical laboratories from blood and from tissue lesions of individuals with BA (29). In Oklahoma City, R. *henselae* is the third most common bacterial isolate from blood cultures that become positive after 4 days of incubation (5). However, cultivation of this organism is inconsistent from case to case and from one laboratory to another. It is also technically difficult to speciate these colonies in a definitive manner; whole-cell fatty acid analysis or citrate synthase/16S rDNA gene analysis may be required.

Other clinical syndromes ascribed to *R. henselae* (Table 11.1)

Many of the original patients from whom R. *henselae* was cultivated had no evidence of localized disease and suffered from only prolonged fever and recurrent bacteremia over a period of weeks or months (3). Relapsing or prolonged fever continues to be associated with R. *henselae* bacteremia (61). It is unclear whether the absence of apparent focal disease in this setting is more common with immunocompetent hosts, or whether the apparent absence of focal disease reflects failure to detect occult sites of tissue pathology. One such patient had lymphocytic meningitis that resolved with antibiotic treatment for the accompanying bacteremia (61). Endocarditis may accompany some cases of R. *henselae* bacteremia (62).

Peliosis is a disorder of the liver (peliosis hepatis), and occasionally of the spleen, characterized by cystic, blood-filled spaces. Historically, it has been most often associated with chronic inflammatory diseases such as tuberculosis or malignancies. In more recent years, peliosis has been diagnosed in association with visible clumps of bacilli that are indistinguishable from those seen in BA lesions (63). R. *henselae* has been cultivated from the blood of some of these patients and directly from peliosis tissue lesions (29,59,61). Bacillary peliosis probably reflects the same angioproliferative pro-

Table 11-1   Clinical
syndromes associated with
Rochalimaea henselae

Rochalimaea henselae syndrome associations
• bacillary angiomatosis
• bacillary peliosis
• bacillary splenitis
• classical cat scratch disease
• persistent or relapsing fever
• infective endocarditis
• lymphocytic meningitis (?)

cess seen in BA. In addition, *R. henselae* 16S rRNA sequence has been detected within tissue from necrotizing splenitis, in the absence of vascular proliferation (55).

OTHER CLOSELY RELATED BACTERIA AND THEIR RELATIONSHIPS TO BA

Rochalimaea quintana

R. quintana caused extensive disease during World Wars I and II, in the form of louse-borne trench fever, but had not been a known cause of disease in the United States until recently. In 1992 in the United States, *R. quintana* was isolated from BA lesions and from blood samples by cocultivation with bovine endothelial cell monolayers as well as by lysis-centrifugation techniques (29). These patients gave no history of louse exposure or rash similar to that described in patients with trench fever (64). Conversely, trench fever had not been associated with angioproliferative lesions. In retrospect, one of the BA tissues studied in the original PCR-based BA investigation had yielded a partial 16S rRNA sequence identical to that of *R. quintana*, which was ascribed to *Taq* error. The recently expanding spectrum of diseases caused by *R. quintana* now includes sustained bacteremia (5) and subacute endocarditis in HIV-seropositive individuals (65). The reservoir and vector for *R. quintana* in the United States and the relative proportion of BA cases associated with this organism remain unclear.

Bartonella bacilliformis

The similarities between the histopathology of verruga peruana and BA have been previously discussed, as well as the close evolutionary relationship between the causative organisms. *B. bacilliformis* has not been detected in association with disease acquired in the United States. Preliminary work suggests that *B. bacilliformis* may secrete an angiogenic factor (66) and induce endothelial cell proliferation (67), which raises the question as to whether the same might be true for *R. henselae*. The answer is currently unknown. Phylogenetic analysis suggests that the ability to induce angioproliferation by these 2 organisms may have been acquired from a common ancestor (46). Finally, it remains possible that this bacterium-induced angioproliferation in human tissue requires a cofactor.

Are there currently uncharacterized organisms also associated with BA?

The inconstancy of *Rochalimaea* cultivation and the recognition of 16S rDNA sequence microheterogeneity in BA tissues (2) raise the possibility that there are other species in addition to *R. henselae* and *R. quintana* that are associated with some BA cases. There are no substantial data to support this theory; however, relatively few cases of BA have been investigated using broad range (nonspecific) 16S rRNA PCR primers. Welch and colleagues (5) described the isolation of additional "*R. quintana*-like organisms" from the blood of febrile patients. It is unclear whether any of these organisms might be causal agents in BA.

RELATIONSHIPS BETWEEN *ROCHALIMAEA* SPECIES, CAT SCRATCH DISEASE, AND CATS

Cat scratch disease and *Afipia felis*

In the same year that Stoler and colleagues (1) visualized bacilli in the tissues of a patient with BA, Wear and colleagues (68) detected virtually identical organisms in a majority of classical CSD lymph nodes, using the same Warthin-Starry silver staining procedure. Five years later, English and colleagues (69) published a description of an organism that was cultivated from a similar type of CSD tissue. Despite initial indications of a similar organism in multiple CSD tissues, this bacillus could be reproducibly propagated from only one patient specimen. This organism has been characterized and named *Afipia felis* (70). Although it is an alpha-proteobacterium, it is clearly distinct from the *Rochalimaea* species (see Figure 11-2). Unpublished reports suggest that multiple CSD specimens yielded the same or a closely related group of organisms (70). Nonetheless, A. *felis* has been directly implicated in only a minority of CSD cases. A recent case report of a patient with acute meningoencephalitis and seroconversion to A. *felis* supports the concept that this organism has the potential to cause disease (71).

R. henselae and cat scratch disease

Bacterial morphology or staining properties are not usually reliable or specific features with which to identify organisms, and there are distinct phylogenetic and serologic differences between R. *henselae* and A. *felis*. Nonetheless, there may be more than a loose connection between the argyrophic bacilli seen in CSD and in BA tissues. Regnery and colleagues (6) detected a humoral response to R. *henselae* in 36 of 41 patients with "suspected CSD" and in 6 of 107 healthy control subjects. Although these results seem persuasive, there are 2 important areas of this study for which further details might be important. First, the clinical features of the patients with "suspected CSD" are crucial, especially because BA has been confused clinically with disseminated or atypical CSD for a number of years. These features remain unpublished. Second, given that cat scratches and bites are known risk factors for both CSD and BA, it is important to know whether these risks were found in comparable fractions of patients and control subjects. Healthy cat owners may be much more likely to be R. *henselae*–seropositive than non-cat owners. A second serology-based study, confirmed the findings of Regenery et al. (6), and found a significantly greater proportion of seropositive individuals among symptomatic versus asymptomatic family members. Other evidence that *Rochalimaea* species may have a role in classic CSD includes PCR analysis of cat scratch antigen preparations. All 5 skin test preparations that were analyzed in one study contained *Rochalimaea*-related 16S rDNA sequences (72). In a more recent study, PCR reactions with broad range bacterial 16S yRNA primers and 2 CSD antigen preparations only yielded sequences virtually identical to those of R. *henselae* (73). In addition, R *henselae* can be cultivated from lymph nodes with classic CSD pathology (8).

A number of questions about the pathogenesis of CSD remain unanswered. Are each of the implicated organisms sufficient alone to induce the same necrotizing granulomatous lymphadenitis? Are some cases of CSD polymicrobial infections? What

Table 11-2   Features associated with 4 related alpha-proteobacterial human pathogens

	R. henselae	*R. quintana*	*B. bacilliformis*	*A. felis*
Reservoir	Cats	?	?	Cats
Vector	?	Human louse	Sandfly	?
Syndrome associations: strong or more frequent*	BA, BP, RF, ?CSD	Trench fever	Bartonellosis	
Syndrome associations: weak or less frequent*	BS, LM,BE/CSD	BA, BE		

*Refers roughly to the relative strength or frequency of the association between the given organism and the syndrome.
BA = bacillary angiomatosis; BP = bacillary peliosis; RF = relapsing or persistent fever; CSD = cat scratch disease; BS = bacillary splenitis; LM = lymphocytic meningitis; BE = bacterial endocarditis.

role do host factors, such as the level of immune competence, have in the development of CSD? Host immune status has been postulated to have an important role in determining the development of vascular proliferation in R. *henselae* infection; yet, immunocompetent hosts can still develop this pathology (55,74). Some selected features of the organisms associated with BA, CSD, and related disorders are summarized in Table 11-2.

Cats as a reservoir for *R. henselae*

Given the epidemiologic association between cat scratches and bites and R. *henselae*–associated diseases, one would suspect that cats might be a reservoir for this organism. In support of this suspicion, R. *henselae* has been cultivated from the blood of one seropositive domestic cat on multiple occasions (7). The prevalence of bacteremia in this animal population has not yet been published; however, in one study of CSD 81% of case-associated and 38% of control cats were R. *henselae*-seropositive (19). In addition, the possibility of cat fleas serving as *Rochalimaea* vectors has not been ruled out (9).

DIAGNOSIS AND TREATMENT OF *ROCHALIMAEA*-ASSOCIATED DISEASES: CURRENT RECOMMENDATIONS

Despite the significant recent revision in our understanding of the pathogenesis of BA and CSD, relatively few practical advances have reached most clinical microbiology laboratories. The diagnosis of BA still rests heavily on microscopic tissue examination. The histopathology of this disease is sufficiently unique to allow an unequivocal tissue diagnosis in many cases (19); however, a microbiologic diagnosis will not be so easily revealed.

Culture-based methods

Attempts should be made routinely to cultivate *Rochalimaea* spp. and other potential pathogens from suspected tissue lesions (29) and from blood specimens of persistently febrile individuals (4,5,61). Specimens should be subcultured early onto appropriate eucaryotic cell monolayers (29) as well as onto appropriate solid agar plates and held for up to 3 weeks. Optimal growth occurs on brain-heart infusion agar or tryptic soy agar supplemented with 5% sheep blood or on heart infusion agar supplemented with 5% rabbit blood (4,5). Original colonies of R. *henselae* are observed after 9 to 15 days of incubation at 35°C in a 5% CO_2, humidified atmosphere. With multiple passages, the growth rate on agar increases. The organism is biochemically unreactive in commonly used assays. Colonies may exhibit 2 different morphologies, one of which includes agar invagination and twitching motility. Colony morphology may suggest *Campylobacter* or *Helicobacter* spp. Definitive speciation may require cellular fatty acid analysis or molecular genetic analysis. An immunofluorescence assay may offer an alternative approach (60). Further refinements in culture methods may be necessary before this approach becomes a practical and routine procedure in clinical laboratories.

Serologic assays

Detection of specific humoral responses to *Rochalimaea* spp. may provide helpful diagnostic information. However, there are still significant uncertainties about the specificity and interpretation of these results. Currently, there are 2 available referral sites for *Rochalimaea* spp. serologic testing. The Viral and Rickettsial Zoonoses Branch, Centers for Disease Control and Prevention, Atlanta (tel: (404) 639-1075; Fax: (404) 639-3163) offers an indirect fluorescence antibody assay for serum immunoglobulin G (IgG) directed against R. *henselae*, R. *quintana*, and *Rochalimaea elizabethae* spp. Titers of 1:64 or greater are considered evidence of infection, but data have not been provided to indicate whether the infection is ongoing. In addition, Specialty Laboratories, Inc., Santa Monica ([800] 421-7110) offers an enzyme-linked immunosorbent assay for anti-R. *henselae* IgG and IgM in serum and cerebrospinal fluid (CSF) specimens (75). The paucity of published data based on the use of these various tests in different patient populations makes it difficult to interpret these results, as well as to be able to recommend general use of these assays (particularly CSF testing). Clearly, detection of a 4-fold or greater increase or decrease in titer with paired samples would imply greater clinical significance; however, publication of additional seroprevalence studies with appropriate controls as well as species specificity data are needed.

PCR-based assays and other research techniques

For those with access to this technology, PCR-based assays offer a sensitive and specific means of identifying *Rochalimaea* and related pathogens. So far, the most specific, tested PCR primers for detecting *Rochalimaea* spp. are 24E and 12B (2). With isolated colonies, citrate synthase gene sequences can be amplified and analyzed for restriction fragment-length polymorphisms (58). Needless to say, these assays are labor-intensive and require characterization of PCR products. They are also fraught with the danger of crosscontamination. For the time being, these methods should be pursued primarily in research settings. In situ immunocytochemical techniques may become a useful option for specific identification of *Rochalimaea* spp. in tissues (76).

Treatment

Unfortunately, empiric clinical observations still form the basis of current therapeutic recommendations for BA. Most investigators favor the use of erythromycin as first-line therapy, with doxycycline as an alternative. Appropriate regimens would include erythromycin (2.0 g/day in 4 divided doses) or doxycycline (0.2 g/day in 2 divided doses). Anecdotal data suggest that there may be an increased incidence of disease relapse with the tetracyclines (4,5,59). Therapy with these agents should probably continue for at least 4 weeks; immunocompromised hosts may require substantially longer treatment courses. Parenteral administration is preferable in individuals with evidence of more serious systemic disease. These same agents are probably effective against disease caused by *R. quintana* as well. The newer macrolides, clarithromycin and azithromycin, may have activity against *R. henselae* but have not been well tested. Several reports suggest that clinical antibiotic response may not correlate with in vitro susceptibilities of *R. henselae* (8).

BA: FUTURE DIRECTIONS

Given the growing significance of *Rochalimaea* spp. and their role in disease, there are likely to be a number of areas in which important advances will be made. (a) What is the true spectrum and relative frequency of bacterial species that can be detected in BA and CSD tissues? (b) Elucidation of bacterial factors that contribute to angioproliferation in host tissues: Are cofactors required, such as herpes viruses (73,74)? (c) What are other determinants of pathogenicity in the *Rochalimaea*? (d) What is the natural ecology of the *Rochalimaea* spp. in the United States? What are the natural reservoirs? Are arthropod vectors involved? The study of BA has already led to the development of novel experimental approaches that may find multiple applications with other unrelated human diseases and syndromes.

ACKNOWLEDGMENTS

D.R. is a Lucille P. Markey Scholar, and this work was supported in part by a grant from the Lucille P. Markey Charitable Trust, and by a grant from the Director's Research Fund, Program in Molecular and Genetic Medicine, Stanford University School of Medicine.

REFERENCES

1 Stoler MH, Bonfiglio TA, Steigbigel RT, Pereira M. An atypical subcutaneous infection associated with acquired immune deficiency syndrome. *Am J Clin Pathol* 1983;80: 714–718.

2 Relman DA, Loutit JS, Schmidt TM, Falkow S, Tompkins LS. The agent of bacillary angiomatosis. An approach to the identification of uncultured pathogens (see comments). *N Engl J Med* 1990;323:1573–1580.

3   Slater LN, Welch DF, Hensel D, Coody DW. A newly recognized fastidious gram-negative pathogen as a cause of fever and bacteremia (see comments). N *Engl J Med* 1990;323: 1587–1593.

4   Regnery RL, Anderson BE, Clarridge III JE, Rodriguez-Barradas MC, Jones DC, Carr JH. Characterization of a novel *Rochalimaea* species, *R. henselae* spp. nov., isolated from blood of a febrile, human immunodeficiency virus-positive patient. *J Clin Microbiol* 1992; 30:265–274.

5   Welch DF, Pickett DA, Slater LN, Steigerwalt AG, Brenner DJ. Rochalimaea henselae spp. nov., a cause of septicemia, bacillary angiomatosis, and parenchymal bacillary peliosis. *J Clin Microbiol* 1992;30:275–280.

6   Regnery RL, Perkins BA, Olson JG, Bibb W. Serological response to "*Rochalimaea henselae*" antigen in suspected cat scratch disease. *Lancet* 1992;339:1443–1445.

7   Regnery R, Martin M, Olson J. Naturally occurring "*Rochalimaea henselae*" infection in domestic cat. *Lancet* 1992;340:557–558.

8   Dolan MJ, Wong MT, Regnery RL, et al. Syndrome of Rochalimaea henselae adenitis suggesting cat scratch disease. *Ann Intern Med* 1993;118:331–336.

9   Zangwill KM, Hamilton DH, Perkins BA, et al. Cat scratch disease in Connecticut: epidemiology, risk factors, and elevation of a new diagnostic test. *New Engl J Med* 1993; 329:8–13.

10 Waldo E, Sidhu GS, Stahl R, Zolla-Pazner S. Histiocytoid hemangioma with features of angiolymphoid hyperplasia and Kaposi's sarcoma. *Am J Dermatopathol* 1983;5:525–538.

11 Cockerell CJ, Whitlow MA, Webster GF, Friedman KA. Epithelioid angiomatosis: a distinct vascular disorder in patients with the acquired immunodeficiency syndrome or AIDS-related complex. *Lancet* 1987;2:654–656.

12 Knobler EH, Silvers DN, Fine KC, Lefkowitch JH, Grossman ME. Unique vascular skin lesions associated with human immunodeficiency virus. *J Am Med Assoc* 1988; 260:524–527.

13 LeBoit PE, Berger TG, Egbert BM, et al. Epithelioid haemangioma-like vascular proliferation in AIDS: manifestation of cat scratch disease bacillus infection? *Lancet* 1988;1:960–963.

14 Koehler JE, LeBoit PE, Egbert BM, Berger TG. Cutaneous vascular lesions and disseminated cat-scratch disease in patients with the acquired immunodeficiency syndrome (AIDS) and AIDS-related complex. *Ann Intern Med* 1988;109:449–455.

15 Angritt P, Tuur SM, Macher AM, et al. Epithelioid angiomatosis in HIV infection: neoplasm or cat-scratch disease? (letter). *Lancet* 1988;1:996.

16 Hall AV, Roberts CM, Maurice PD, McLean KA, Shousa S. Cat-scratch disease in patient with AIDS: atypical skin manifestation. *Lancet* 1988;2:453–454.

17 Brooks JJ, Fisher C. Epithelioid angiomatosis: a variant of Kaposi's sarcoma. *Lancet* 1987; 2:1214–1215.

18 LeBoit PE, Berger TG, Egbert BM, Beckstead JH, Yen TS, Stoler MH. Bacillary angiomatosis. The histopathology and differential diagnosis of a pseudoneoplastic infection in patients with human immunodeficiency virus disease. *Am J Surg Pathol* 1989;13:909–920.

19 Cockerell CJ, LeBoit PE. Bacillary angiomatosis: a newly characterized, pseudoneoplastic, infectious, cutaneous vascular disorder. *J Am Acad Dermatol* 1990;22:501–512.

20 LeBoit PE. The expanding spectrum of a new disease, bacillary angiomatosis (comment). *Arch Dermatol* 1990;126:808–811.

21 Jimenez AF, Pardo RJ, Cohen RJ, Gould EW, Penneys NS. Bacillary angiomatosis of acquired immunodeficiency syndrome: case report and literature review. *J Am Acad Dermatol* 1990;22:525–529.

22 Szaniawski WK, Don PC, Bitterman SR, Schachner JR. Epithelioid angiomatosis in patients with AIDS. *J Am Acad Dermatol* 1990;23:41–48.

23 Spach DH. Bacillary angiomatosis. *Int J Dermatol* 1992;31:19–24.

24 Tappero JW, Mohle-Boetani J, Koehler JE, et al. The epidemiology of bacillary angiomatosis and bacillary peliosis. *J Am Med Assoc* 1993;269:770–775.

25 Carithers HA. Cat-scratch disease. An overview based on a study of 1,200 patients. *Am J Dis Child* 1985;139:1124–1133.

26 Webster GF, Cockerell CJ, Friedman-Kien AE. The clinical spectrum of bacillary angiomatosis. *Br J Dermatol* 1992;126:535–541.

27 Schwartzman WA. Infections due to *Rochalimaea*: the expanding clinical spectrum. *Clin Infect Dis* 1992;15:893–902.

28 Baron AL, Steinbach LS, LeBoit PE, Mills CM, Gee JH, Berger TG. Osteolytic lesions and bacillary angiomatosis in HIV infection: radiographic differentiation from AIDS-related Kaposi sarcoma. *Radiology* 1990;177:77–81.

29 Koehler JE, Quinn FD, Berger TG, LeBoit

PE, Tappero JW. Isolation of rochalimaea species from cutaneous and osseous lesions of bacillary angiomatosis. *N Engl J Med* 1992; 327:1625–1631.

30 Schwartzman WA, Marchevsky A, Meyer RD. Epithelioid angiomatosis or cat scratch disease with splenic and hepatic abnormalities in AIDS: case report and review of the literature. *Scand J Infect Dis* 1990;22:121–133.

31 Milam MW, Balerdi MJ, Toney JF, Foulis PR, Milam CP, Behnke RH. Epithelioid angiomatosis secondary to disseminated cat scratch disease involving the bone marrow and skin in a patient with acquired immune deficiency syndrome: a case report. *Am J Med* 1990; 88:180–183.

32 Kemper CA, Lombard CM, Deresinski SC, Tompkins LS. Visceral bacillary epithelioid angiomatosis: possible manifestations of disseminated cat scratch disease in the immunocompromised host: a report of two cases. *Am J Med* 1990;89:216–222.

33 Slater LN, Min KW. Polypoid endobronchial lesions: a manifestation of bacillary angiomatosis. *Chest* 1992;102:972–973.

34 Spach DH, Panther LA, Thorning DR, Dunn JE, Plorde JJ, Miller RA. Intracerebral bacillary angiomatosis in a patient infected with human immunodeficiency virus. *Ann Intern Med* 1992;116:740–742.

35 Arias-Stella J, Lieberman PH, Erlandson RA, Arias-Stella J Jr. Histology, immunohistochemistry, and ultrastructure of the verruga in Carrion's disease. *Am J Surg Pathol* 1986; 10:595–610.

36 Schlossberg D, Morad Y, Krouse TB, Wear DJ, English CK. Culture-proved disseminated cat-scratch disease in acquired immunodeficiency syndrome. *Arch Intern Med* 1989; 149:1437–1439.

37 Woese CR. Bacterial evolution. *Microbiol Rev* 1987;51:221–271.

38 Fox GE, Stackebrandt E, Hespell RB, et al. The phylogeny of prokaryotes. *Science* 1980; 209:457–463.

39 Olsen GJ, Lane DJ, Giovannoni SJ, Pace NR, Stahl DA. Microbial ecology and evolution: a ribosomal RNA approach. *Annu Rev Microbiol* 1986;40:337–365.

40 Winker S, Woese CR. A definition of the domains *Archaea, Bacteria,* and *Eucarya* in terms of small subunit ribosomal RNA characteristics. *Syst Appl Microbiol* 1991;14:305–310.

41 Olsen GJ, Larsen N, Woese CR. The ribosomal RNA database project. *Nucl Acids Res* 1991;19(suppl):2017–2021.

42 Saiki RK, Scharf S, Faloona F, et al. Enzymatic amplification of beta-globin genomic sequences and restriction site analysis for diagnosis of sickle cell anemia. *Science* 1985; 230:1350–1354.

43 Mullis KB, Faloona FA. Specific synthesis of DNA in vitro via a polymerase-catalyzed chain reaction. *Methods Enzymol* 1987;155:335–350.

44 Saiki RK, Gelfand DH, Stoffel S, et al. Primer-directed enzymatic amplification of DNA with a thermostable DNA polymerase. *Science* 1988;239:487–491.

45 Eisenstein BI. The polymerase chain reaction. A new method of using molecular genetics for medical diagnosis. *N Engl J Med* 1990; 322:178–183.

46 Relman DA, Lepp PW, Sadler KN, Schmidt TM. Phylogenetic relationships among the agent of bacillary angiomatosis, *Bartonella bacilliformis,* and other alpha-proteobacteria. *Mol Microbiol* 1992;6:1801–1807.

47 Lane DJ, Pace B, Olsen GJ, Stahl DA, Sogin ML, Pace NR. Rapid determination of 16S ribosomal RNA sequences for phylogenetic analyses. *Proc Natl Acad Sci USA* 1985; 82:6955–6959.

48 Medlin L, Elwood HJ, Stickel S, Sogin ML. The characterization of enzymatically amplified eukaryotic 16S-like rRNA-coding regions. *Gene* 1988;71:491–499.

49 Chen K, Neimark H, Rumore P, Steinman CR. Broad range DNA probes for detecting and amplifying eubacterial nucleic acids. *FEMS Microbiol Lett* 1989;48:19–24.

50 Wilson KH, Blitchington RB, Greene RC. Amplification of bacterial 16S ribosomal DNA with polymerase chain reaction. *J Clin Microbiol* 1990;28:1942–1946.

51 Relman DA, Schmidt TM, MacDermott RP, Falkow S. Identification of the uncultured bacillus of Whipple's disease. *N Engl J Med* 1992;327:293–301.

52 Relman DA, Falkow S. Identification of uncultured microorganisms: expanding the spectrum of characterized microbial pathogens. *Infect Agents Dis* 1992;1:245–253.

53 Relman DA. The identification of uncultured microbial pathogens. *J Infect Dis* 1993 (in press).

54 Sagerman PM, Relman DA, Niroomand F, Neidt GW. Localization of Mycobacterium avium-intracellulare within a skin lesion of bacillary angiomatosis in a patient with acquired immunodeficiency syndrome. *Diagn Mol Pathol* 1992;1:212–216.

55 Tappero JW, Koehler JE, Berger TM, et al.

Bacillary angiomatosis and bacillary splenitis in immunocompetent adults. *Ann Intern Med* 1993;118:363–365.

56 Weisburg WG, Woese CR, Dobson ME, Weiss E. A common origin of rickettsiae and certain plant pathogens. *Science* 1985;230:556–558.

57 Brenner DJ, O'Connor SP, Winkler HH, Steigerwait AG. Proposals to unify the genera *Bartonella* and *Rochalima*, with descriptions of *Bartonella vinsonii* combinov., *Bartonella henslae* combinov., and *Bartonella* Elizabethae combinov., and to remove the family *Bartonellaceae* from the order *Rickettsinles*. *Int J Syst Bacteriol* 1993;43:777–786.

58 Regnery RL, Spruill CL, Plikaytis BD. Genotypic identification of rickettsiae and estimation of intraspecies sequence of divergence for portions of two rickettsial genes. *J Bacteriol* 1991;173:1576–1589.

59 Relman DA, Falkow S, LeBoit PE, et al. The organism causing bacillary angiomatosis, peliosis hepatis, and fever and bacteremia in immunocompromised patients (letter). *N Engl J Med* 1991;324:1514.

60 Slater LN, Welch DF, Min K-W. Rochalimaea henselae causes bacillary angiomatosis and peliosis hepatis. *Arch Intern Med* 1992;152: 602–606.

61 Lucey D, Dolan MJ, Moss CW, et al. Relapsing illness due to Rochalimaea henselae in immunocompetent hosts: implication for therapy and new epidemiological associations. *Clin Infect Dis* 1992;14:683–688.

62 Hadfield TL, Warren R, Kass M, Braun E, Levy C. Endocarditis caused by *Rochalimea henselae*. *Hum Pathol* 1993; 24:1140–1141.

63 Perkocha LA, Geaghan SM, Yen TS, et al. Clinical and pathological features of bacillary peliosis hepatis in association with human immunodeficiency virus infection (see comments). *N Engl J Med* 1990;323:1581–1586.

64 Vinson JW, Varela G, Molina PC. Trench fever. 3. Induction of clinical disease in volunteers inoculated with Rickettsia quintana propagated on blood agar. *Am J Trop Med Hyg* 1969;18:713–722.

65 Spach DH, Callis KP, Paauw DS, et al. Endocarditis caused by *Rochalimaea quintana* in a patient infected with human immunodeficiency virus. *J Clin Microbiol* 1993;31:692–694.

66 Garcia FU, Wojta J, Broadley KN, Davidson JM, Hoover RL. *Bartonella bacilliformis* stimulates endothelial cells *in vitro* and is angiogenic *in vivo*. *Am J Pathol* 1990;136:1125–1135.

67 Garcia FU, Wojta J, Hoover RL. Interactions between live Bartonella bacilliformis and endothelial cells. *J Infect Dis* 1992;165:1138–1141.

68 Wear DJ, Margileth AM, Hadfield TL, Fischer GW, Schlagel CJ, King FM. Cat scratch disease: a bacterial infection. *Science* 1983;221:1403–1405.

69 English CK, Wear DJ, Margileth AM, Lissner CR, Walsh GP. Cat-scratch disease. Isolation and culture of the bacterial agent. *JAMA* 1988;259:1347–1352.

70 Brenner DJ, Hollis DG, Moss CW, et al. Proposal of *Afipia* gen. nov., with *Afipia felis* spp. nov. (formerly the cat scratch disease bacillus), *Afipia clevelandensis* spp. nov. (formerly the Cleveland Clinic Foundation strain), *Afipia broomeae* spp. nov., and three unnamed genospecies. *J Clin Microbiol* 1991;29:2450–2460.

71 Drancourt M, Donnet A, Pelletier J, Raoult D. Acute meningoencephalitis associated with seroconversion to "*Afipia felis.*" *Lancet* 1992; 340:558.

72 Perkins BA, Swaminathan B, Jackson LA, et al. Case 22-1992-pathogenesis of cat scratch disease. *N Engl J Med* 1992;327:1599–1600.

73 Anderson B, Kelly C, Threlkel R, Edwards K. Detection of *Rochalimaea* henselae in cat-scratch disease skin test antigens. *J Infec Dis* 1993;168:1034–1036.

74 Cockerell CJ, Bergstresser PR, Myrie WC, Tierno PM. Bacillary epithelioid angiomatosis occurring in an immunocompetent individual. *Arch Dermatol* 1990;126:787–790.

75 Patnaik M, Schwartzman WA, Barka NE, Peter JB. Possible role of *Rochalimaea henselae* in pathogenesis of AIDS encephalopathy. *Lancet* 1992;340:971.

76 Reed JA, Brigati DJ, Flynn SD, et al. Immunocytochemical identification of *Rochalimaea henselae* in bacillary (epithelioid) angiomatosis, parenchymal bacillary peliosis, and persistent fever with bacteremia. *Am J Surg Pathol* 1992;16:650–657.

77 Guarner J, Unger ER. Association of Epstein-Barr virus in epithelioid angiomatosis of AIDS patients. *Am J Surg Pathol* 1990;14:956–960.

78 Lopez-Elzaurdia C, Fraga J, Sols M, Burgos E, Garcia MS, Garcia-Diez A. Bacillary angiomatosis associated with cytomegalovirus infection in a patient with AIDS. *Br J Dermatol* 1991;125:175–177.

Prevention of human immunodeficiency virus infection among hospital personnel

JULIE LOUISE GERBERDING

RISK ASSESSMENT FOR HEALTH CARE PERSONNEL

Risk of infection associated with a discrete exposure

The risk of acquiring human immunodeficiency virus (HIV) following a discrete occupational exposure has been the subject of more than 15 prospective studies since the acquired immunodeficiency syndrome (AIDS) epidemic was recognized (1–3). These studies evaluated personnel for the presence of HIV antibody as soon as possible after an exposure (baseline) and then for at least 6 months after the exposure (follow-up) to identify evidence of new infection temporally associated with the exposure event (seroconversion). Pooled data indicate that the current estimate of risk conferred by an HIV needlestick injury or similar percutaneous exposure is 0.2% (8 infections/3,967 exposures) (1–3). The risk associated with mucous membrane or nonintact skin contamination with infected material is too low to be quantified in these prospective studies, but it is not zero, because a small number of anecdotal reports describing infection by these routes have appeared in the literature (3). To date, no case of HIV infection has been attributed to exposure of intact skin or from exposure to blood aerosols.

Potential modifiers of exposure risk

Several factors could modify the transmission risk during individual exposure events. Most experts agree that the inoculum of virus involved in the exposure is likely to be one of the most important variables. Inoculum is dependent on both exposure volume (which usually ranges within one order of magnitude for most needlestick injuries) as well as virus titer (which varies by several logs depending on the clinical stage of illness in the source patient) (4,5). Glove materials have been shown to reduce the volume of blood transferred during simulated needlestick injuries by more than 50% and may exert a protective effect during percutaneous injuries (4). Although the effect of these variables on the magnitude of infection risk has not been quantified, it is likely that

220

superficial needle injuries caused by nonhollow suture needles contaminated from blood from asymptomatic source patients passing through gloves are less risky than those involving hollow needles from source patients with advanced AIDS. This effect may partially explain the observation that suture needle injuries have not yet been directly implicated in occupational HIV infection.

Cumulative professional risk

The number of health care providers occupationally infected with HIV in the United States is not known with certainty because reporting is apt to be incomplete. As of October 1992, the Centers for Disease Control and Prevention (CDC) had evidence of 32 documented seroconversions and 69 cases of possible occupational infection (i.e., HIV was diagnosed in health care workers with no history of other HIV risks, but a baseline negative HIV test was not available) (3). Most experts believe that the true number of infected health care providers is not likely to exceed the number known to the CDC by more than 50%. Nurses and laboratory personnel comprise the largest proportion of those with known or suspected occupational infection, but virtually all categories of health care providers appear to be at risk. The vast majority of these individuals acquired their infection during needlestick exposure to infected blood.

The cumulative risk of infection experienced by health care personnel can be estimated by the product of 3 probabilities: (a) the probability that an exposure will occur; (b) the probability that the exposure will involve HIV; and (c) the probability of infection following a discrete exposure event, as discussed. The probability of exposure varies widely among different occupational categories. In many studies, students and trainees have been shown to be at high risk for exposure (6,7). Surgical personnel, dentists, prehospital care personnel, emergency department clinicians, and labor and delivery staff are known to have a high risk of hepatitis B infection (at least prior to the availability of vaccine) and have also been shown to be at high risk for blood exposure (8–10).

The probability that the exposure will involve HIV is in large part dependent on the prevalence of HIV in the community. However, HIV prevalence can vary dramatically even in a given institution. For example, at San Francisco General Hospital, more than 25% of the adult medical patients are diagnosed with HIV, whereas the prevalence on the orthopedic surgery service is less than 6%. Hence, a medical nurse may be more likely to experience an HIV needlestick than a nurse in the surgical suite, even though the surgical nurse may sustain a greater total number of possible exposures.

EXPOSURE PREVENTION

Infection control

Awareness of HIV in the health care environment has proven to be an effective marketing strategy for implementing universal precautions. This new approach to

infection control is based on the concept that exposure to blood and other potentially infectious body fluids and tissues should be avoided, regardless of the probability that HIV or other blood-borne infection will be diagnosed in the patient
(11,12). Additional disease-specific categories of isolation (e.g., respiratory precautions, strict isolation, enteric precautions) are added when other infections are suspected or diagnosed.

Body substance precautions (BSP) is a similar system of infection control; precautions to avoid contact with blood and other body fluids and tissues are implemented for
all patients (13,14). However, in this system, additional categories of isolation are not
required. Rather, the level of protection utilized is based on the degree of contact with
potentially infectious substances anticipated during a specific procedure or patient
contact. Knowledge of specific diseases is not required to implement these precautions.
Proponents of this approach argue that BSP is easier to teach and offers a greater degree
of protection than category-specific isolation systems because appropriate precautions
can be implemented before the diagnostic evaluation is complete. This advantage is
especially relevant for prehospital care personnel and emergency clinicians. Moreover,
procedure-specific precautions can easily be developed for invasive surgical and dental
procedures.

Although the relative merits of universal precautions and BSP have been debated,
in practice, these systems of infection control afford a similar degree of protection
against HIV exposures. Both emphasize prevention of percutaneous injuries and use
of personal protective equipment (i.e., gowns, gloves, masks, eye protection) to minimize mucocutaneous exposures, and both rely heavily on motivating health care
providers to comply with the recommended behaviors. In most efficacy studies, the
frequency of blood contacts has been reduced by more than 50% when efforts to
motivate compliance with infection control standards are included in the implementation process (15–17). However, neither universal precautions nor BSP has consistently achieved a satisfactory reduction in the frequency of needlestick injury. For this
reason, prevention efforts now emphasize engineering controls to improve needle
safety for health care providers (18).

Engineering controls

Engineering controls include substituting alternative methods for performing procedures that do not require the use of needles and employing needle devices that are
designed with inherent safety features (18,19). Manufacturers have begun to appreciate
the market for these devices, and more than 300 patents have been requested in the past
5 years. Ideally, safety devices should operate passively (i.e, the safety feature should be
activated automatically when the product is used for its intended purpose). However,
most of the devices currently available do require some action on the part of the user to
engage the safety feature.

Access to a wide number of safety products has created some new issues for health
care providers. Many of these devices are currently quite expensive relative to the
traditional product, and many institutions have been reluctant to purchase them with-

out compelling evidence of efficacy in preventing injuries. Uniform evaluation standards have not been established but should include consideration of safety for health care providers as well as patients, ease of use, ease of training, and cost (20). Nevertheless, it is likely that engineered approaches to needle safety will ultimately prove to have a positive impact on the frequency of post-use needle injuries.

Percutaneous injuries sustained by health care providers while the device is being used for its intended purpose are more difficult to prevent. Dental and surgical personnel and others who perform invasive procedures are at significant risk for this type of injury. In one study of intraoperative needle injuries, palpating the suture needle tip with the index finger of the nondominant hand and using fingers to retract tissue were associated with suture needle punctures (21). Interest in developing procedure-specific interventions such as "no touch" techniques to prevent this type of accidental exposure is increasing. Use of blunt suture needles, substitution of electrocautery devices for scalpels, and redesign of tenaculums and other sharps are examples of engineered controls that may also contribute to prevention efforts.

HIV testing for infection control

The value of HIV testing as an infection control intervention remains controversial. Proponents of this approach believe that knowledge of HIV infection status will improve safety for health care personnel by allowing implementation of special infection control procedures for infected patients that are not feasible or advisable for all patients, or by motivating compliance with universal precautions. Available data do not demonstrate improved safety during surgical procedures performed on patients known to be infected, but randomized controlled trials have not been performed (8,22,23). In settings where the prevalence of HIV and other blood-borne pathogens is known to be high among surgical patients, health care personnel may be more likely to practice universal precautions and would experience little additional benefit from selectively labeling those with diagnosed infection (23). In contrast, clinicians practicing in areas where HIV is unusual may be less motivated to practice universal precautions and could selectively increase their level of protection if patients with infection were identified. Ironically, routine preprocedure testing in low prevalence locales is not likely to be cost-effective. Even at Johns Hopkins University, where HIV infection is highly prevalent among emergency patients, routine testing of elective surgical patients was abandoned because the number of undiagnosed infections detected by this program was too low to justify its continuation (24).

One major reason for not conditioning infection control on HIV test results is that many other pathogens also pose a serious risk to health care providers. Obtaining a negative HIV test result could promote a false sense of security when in fact a patient could be infectious with another blood-borne infection. This issue points out one of the most important benefits of universal infection control: protection is provided against both diagnosed and undiagnosed blood-borne infections. Adopting this generic approach is believed by most experts to provide the best margin of safety for health care providers.

POSTEXPOSURE INTERVENTIONS

An estimated 50,000 occupational exposures to HIV have occurred since the AIDS epidemic was recognized. Even with optimal infection control, it will be difficult to eliminate the opportunity for accidental exposure entirely. Postexposure interventions to reduce the risk of infection are essential, but unfortunately, there is little scientific evidence available to guide postexposure treatment decisions. The approach outlined herein is therefore based on consensus established by those experienced in the care of exposed health care personnel, but it is subject to modification if and when efficacy data become available (25).

Immediate wound care

The site of percutaneous or cutaneous exposures to blood or other potentially infected materials should be cleaned with soap and water as soon as patient safety permits. No data indicate additional benefit from application of bleach (1:100 dilution), iodophores, or other antiseptics, but their use is not contraindicated. Large wounds should be thoroughly irrigated, but incision or excision is not recommended. Contaminated mucous membranes of the mouth or nose should be flushed with clean water. Sterile saline, eye irrigants, or clean water should be used to decontaminate ocular membranes. Spontaneous bleeding is believed by many to facilitate decontamination, but no information is available to determine the value of inducing bleeding by manipulating the exposure site.

Chemoprophylaxis

Zidovudine and newer nucleoside analogues have been advocated to reduce the risk of infection after exposure (25,26). Approximately 40% of exposed health care personnel will elect this treatment when the exposure involves HIV, despite the absence of any firm data documenting efficacy (27). Zidovudine chemoprophylaxis is effective in tissue culture and in nonprimate animal models of retroviral infection (25). Experience in primate systems is limited, but no efficacy has been associated with pre-exposure or postexposure nucleoside analogue treatment of adult monkeys infected with large inocula of virus. However, preliminary studies in infant macaques infected with relatively low inocula of virus suggest that pre-exposure oral zidovudine may be efficacious (28). Postexposure experience in this model has not yet been reported.

Several anecdotes describing failure of postexposure zidovudine to prevent infection have been published. In some of these cases, drug was provided in reasonable doses in a timely manner postexposure; therefore, pharmacologic factors are not likely to explain the treatment failure (27). Resistance to zidovudine has become more widespread now that many source patients have been treated for several months. Whether acquired resistance contributes to the lack of zidovudine efficacy in prophylaxis of occupational exposures remains to be established.

Several large observational studies of zidovudine use suggest that serious objective toxicity associated with its use in healthy health care providers is rare (27,29,30). One regimen commonly used includes zidovudine (200 mg every 4 hr) for 3 days, followed by zidovudine (200 mg every 4 hr) while awake (5 times a day) for 25 more days. However, subjective intolerance with this regimen, most notably gastrointestinal complaints, headache, fatigue, and myalgia, often mandate dose reduction or treatment discontinuation.

Provision of zidovudine treatment to health care providers should not be regarded as a standard of care. Until animal or clinical data, or both, are available to determine the appropriate role for zidovudine or other antiretroviral therapies in prevention of occupational infection, treatment must be individualized and should be considered experimental (25). Those electing zidovudine should be fully informed of the uncertainties surrounding efficacy, short-term toxicity, as well as the potential for delayed toxicity. Careful hematologic and hepatic monitoring during treatment is also advised.

Immunoprophylaxis with preparations of antibody designed to provide neutralizing activity against wild-type strains of HIV is a promising approach that may be evaluated in the near future. Immune therapy is known to be effective with hepatitis B exposures and could be a sensible approach to HIV as well. However, the biology of early HIV infection is not clearly defined, and the window of opportunity wherein immunoglobulin could be efficacious is not known. Primate experiments will hopefully shed some light on this issue and provide a scientific basis for postexposure therapeutic decisions.

Follow-up care of exposed workers

HIV infection is usually diagnosed within 3 months of exposure and is associated with seroconversion illness characterized by mononucleosis-like symptoms and signs in the majority of reported cases. To date, seroconversion more than 6 months after exposure has not been documented among occupationally exposed health care providers and is likely to be extremely rare. Conventional HIV antibody testing algorithms (enzyme-linked immunosorbent assay with Western blot or indirect fluorescent antibody test confirmation) are adequate to detect most cases of infection. However, antibody titers may be below the level of detection at the onset of seroconversion illness. In this setting, performing a p24 antigen test may facilitate earlier diagnosis. If antigen testing is not available, repeating the antibody test in 2 to 4 weeks will confirm the clinical diagnosis. Gene amplification studies (polymerase chain reaction) and HIV cultures are expensive tests that have not been proved useful in the routine management of exposed health care personnel.

Compensation and insurance issues

HIV will remain an important occupational issue for at least the next decade. Employers are beginning to appreciate the need to provide adequate compensation to those who do become infected through work activities. Most employees are at least entitled to workers' compensation benefits that will help defray any medical costs associated with infection. However, these costs may not be incurred until years after infection, and policies must be established to allow coverage even if employment has been terminated. High-level professionals usually have access to supplemental disability insurance that provides income support when HIV disability occurs, but many categories of health care providers have not had access to this type of insurance or have found it to be prohibitively expensive. Students and other trainees have special needs. These individuals are not always regarded as employees and so may not be eligible for workers' compensation. Moreover, they do not have access to disability insurance. Special programs have been established at several institutions to provide HIV-related disability insurance. Ideally, coverage should continue even after students and housestaff matriculate, with a step-up in benefits commensurate with the income level achieved at the time disability actually occurs.

REFERENCES

1 Henderson DK, Fahey BJ, Willy M, et al. Risk for occupational transmission of human immunodeficiency virus type-1 (HIV-1) associated with clinical exposures. A prospective evaluation. *Ann Intern Med* 1990;113:740–746.

2 Beekmann SE, Fahey BJ, Gerberding JL, Henderson DK. Risky business: using necessarily imprecise casualty counts to estimate occupational risks for HIV infection. *Infect Control Hosp Epidemiol* 1990;11:371–379.

3 Centers for Disease Control Surveillance for occupationally acquired HIV infection—United States, 1981–1992. *MMWR* 1992;41:823–825.

4 Mast ST, Gerberding JL. Factors predicting infectivity following needlestick exposure to HIV: an in vitro model. *Clin Res* 1991; 39:381A.

5 Ho DD, Moudgil T, Alam M. Quantitation of human immunodeficiency virus type 1 in the blood of infected persons. *N Engl J Med* 1989;321:1621–1625.

6 Jones DB. Percutaneous exposures of medical students to HIV. *JAMA* 1990;264:1188–1190.

7 Mangione CM, Gerberding JL, Cummings SR. Occupational exposure to HIV: frequency and rates of underreporting of percutaneous and mucocutaneous exposures by medical housestaff. *Am J Med* 1991;90:85–90.

8 Gerberding JL, Littell C, Tarkington A, Brown A, Schecter WP. Risk of exposure of surgical personnel to patients' blood during surgery at San Francisco General Hospital. *N Engl J Med* 1990;322:1788–1793.

9 Denes AE, Smith JL, Maynard JE, Doto IL, Berquist KR, Finfel AJ. Hepatitis B infection in physicians. Results of a nationwide seroepidemiologic survey. *JAMA* 1978;239:210–212.

10 Klein RS, Phelan JA, Freeman K, Schable C, Friedland GH, Trieger N. Low occupational risk of human immunodeficiency virus infection among dental professionals. *N Engl J Med* 1988;318:86–90.

11 Centers for Disease Control Recommendations for prevention of HIV transmission in health-care settings. *MMWR* 1987;36(suppl 2S):1S–19S.

12 Centers for Disease Control Update: universal precautions for prevention of transmission of human immunodeficiency virus, hepatitis B virus, and other bloodborne pathogens in health-care settings. *MMWR* 1988;37:377–391.

13 Gerberding JL, the University of California, San Francisco Task Force on AIDS. Recommended infection-control policies for patients with human immunodeficiency virus infection: an update. *N Engl J Med* 1986;315:1562–1564.

14 Lynch P, Jackson MM, Cummings MJ, Stamm WE. Rethinking the role of isolation practices in the prevention of nosocomial infections. *Ann Intern Med* 1987;107:243–246.

15 Wong ES, Stotka JL, Chinchilli VM, Williams DS, Stuart GS, Markowitz SM. Are universal precautions effective in reducing the number of occupational exposures among health care workers? *JAMA* 1991;265:1123–1128.

16 Kelen GD, Green GB, Hexter DA, et al. Substantial improvement in compliance with universal precautions in an emergency department following institution of policy. *Arch Intern Med* 1991;151:2051–2056.

17 Fahey BJ, Koziol DE, Banks SM, Henderson DK. Frequency of nonparenteral occupational exposures to blood and body fluids before and after universal precautions training. *Am J Med* 1991;90:145–153.

18 Jagger J, Hunt EH, Bland-Elnaggar J, Pearson RD. Rates of needlestick injury caused by

various devices in a university hospital. *N Engl J Med* 1988;319:284–288.

19   **Centers for Disease Control** Occupational exposure to bloodborne pathogens; final rule. *Federal Register* 1991;56:64004–64182.

20   **Orenstein R, Reynolds L, Karabaic M, et al.** Evaluation of efficacy and cost of protective devices for the prevention of needlestick injuries among health care workers [Abstract 621]. In Program and Abstracts of the 33rd Interscience Conference on Antimicrobials and Chemotherapy. American Society of Microbiology, Washington D.C. 1993.

21   **Tokars JI, Bell DM, Culver DH, et al.** Percutaneous injuries during surgical procedures. *JAMA* 1992;267:2899–2904.

22   **Panlilio AL, Welch BA, Bell DM, et al.** Blood and amniotic fluid contact sustained by obstetric personnel during deliveries. *Am J Obstet Gynecol* 1992;167:703–708.

23   **Gerberding JL.** Does knowledge of human immunodeficiency virus infection decrease the frequency of occupational exposure to blood? *Am J Med* 1991;91:308S–311S.

24   **Charache P, Cameron JL, Maters AW, Frantz EI.** Prevalence of infection with human immunodeficiency virus in elective surgery patients. *Ann Surg* 1991;214:562–568.

25   **Gerberding JL, Henderson DK.** Management of occupational exposures to bloodborne pathogens: hepatitis B virus, hepatitis C virus, and human immunodeficiency virus. *Clin Infect Dis* 1992;14:1179–1185.

26   **Centers for Disease Control** Public health service statement on management of occupational exposure to human immunodeficiency virus including considerations regarding zidovudine post-exposure use. *MMWR* 1990;39:1–14.

27   **Takars JI, Marcus R, Culver DH, Shabel CA, McKibben PS, Bandea CI, Bell DM.** Surveillance of human immunodeficiency virus infection and zidovudine use among health care workers after occupational exposure to HIV infected blood: The CDC Cooperative Needlestick Group. *Ann Intern Med* 1993; 118:913–919.

28   **Van Rompay KKA, Marthas ML, Ramos RA, et al.** Simian immunodeficiency virus (SIV) infection of infant rhesus macaques as a model to test antiretroviral drug prophylaxis and therapy: oral 3'-azido-3'-deoxythymidine prevents SIV infection. *Antimicrob Agents Chemother* 1992;36:2381–2386.

29   **Puro V, Ippolito G, Guzzanti E, et al.** Zidovudine prophylaxis after accidental exposure to HIV: the Italian experience. The Italian Study Group on Occupational Risk of HIV Infection. *AIDS* 1992;6:963–969.

30   **Fahrner R, Beekmann S, Koziol DE, Henderson DK, Gerberding JL.** Safety of zidovudine as post-exposure chemoprophylaxis for health care workers after occupational exposure to HIV (abstract PcC 4132). Abstracts of the VIII International Conference on AIDS, Amsterdam, The Netherlands, July 1992.

Cytokine therapy of infectious diseases

MILES H. BEAMAN

INTRODUCTION

The immune system is composed of a diverse population of many different cell types (including T and B lymphocytes, natural killer [NK] cells, monocyte/macrophages, (M0) dendritic cells, Langerhans' cells, neutrophils, and mast cells) that interact with each other by the production of soluble protein mediators known as cytokines, which include interleukins [ILs], interferons [IFNs], and colony-stimulating factors (CSFs). These cytokines are produced by one type of cell and are released either locally, to positively or negatively modulate the immune functions of themselves (i.e., autocrine effects) or other cell types (i.e., paracrine effects), or into the circulation to influence the function of cells at distant sites (i.e., endocrine effects). Cytokines bind specific membrane receptors on the target cell, resulting in signal transduction and subsequent expression of cellular effects. The net effect of a particular cytokine is influenced by the amount of cytokine produced, the number of available target cells, and the density and affinity of specific cytokine receptors on their surface, as well as the presence of soluble circulating cytokine receptors (which may function as carrier molecules to assist in delivery of cytokine molecules to distant sites, or inhibitors of cytokine effects by binding free cytokine molecules and thus preventing their interaction with cell surface receptors). In addition, individual cytokines may interact with target cells to either up-regulate or down-regulate the production of other cytokines or the response of target cells to them, resulting in positive and negative feedback loops that amplify or dampen the effect of an individual cytokine. Hence, the cytokine system constitutes a complex network of individual mediators that interact with each other (1,2).

Over the last decade, great advances have been made in our understanding of the immunopathogenesis of infectious diseases, especially the role of cell-mediated responses, and it has become clear that overproduction of cytokines in response to certain infections can have deleterious effects on the host (i.e., IL-1 and tumor necrosis factor-alpha [TNF-α] in sepsis and meningitis; TNF-α in malaria), whereas in other infections, inadequate cytokine production results in impaired immune responses to certain pathogens (i.e.,

228

IFN-γ and IL-2 in lepromatous leprosy and opportunistic infections of patients with acquired immunodeficiency syndrome [AIDS]) (3–9). Many groups have initiated studies utilizing cytokines as therapeutic agents for human infections, and, although much data is preliminary and experience is currently limited, the results obtained have been very exciting and suggest great potential for these agents. I outline the breadth of experience with these therapies and identify applications with the most promise.

CYTOKINES USED IN HUMAN STUDIES

Interferon-alpha and interferon-beta

Interferons-alpha (IFN-α) and interferons-beta (IFN-β) are also known as type-1 interferons and were first recognized as inducible inhibitors of viral infection (10). It is now recognized that they represent a whole family of molecules; IFNα is produced by leukocytes (predominantly by monocytes, but also by NK cells and lymphocytes), and IFN-β is produced by fibroblasts in response to many stimuli. Both IFNs are peptides of 165–166 amino acids that share approximately 30% sequence homology and bind the same receptor (which is present on numerous different cell types) (11). Binding of a type-1 IFN to its receptor leads to signal transduction, which results in the induction of approximately 20 different proteins that have antimicrobial (including 2′,5′-oligoadenylate synthetase and indoleamine 2,3-dioxygenase), antiproliferative, and immunomodulatory properties (via enhanced expression of major histocompatibility complex [MHC] class I and II molecules) (12).

Initial clinical experience with type-1 IFNs came from studies of the treatment of malignancies, which clarified the side-effect profile of these agents. Although most experience has been with IFN-α, IFN-β appears to have similar toxicities (13). The major dose-limiting effects have been neutropenia, influenza-like symptoms (including fever, chills, myalgias, fatigue, and weakness), and elevated liver transaminase levels. Other common side effects have included anorexia, weight loss, thrombocytopenia, alopecia, and mild cognitive deficits. Most of these effects are well tolerated or are able to be controlled by nonsteroidal agents when moderate dosages of IFN (up to 18×10^6 U) are used, and they exhibit tachyphylaxis over time. Less common, but potentially serious, side effects include hypotension, cardiac dysrhythmias, and seizures; caution has been urged in the use of IFN in patients with cardiac, seizure, or psychiatric disorders (12). Another interesting observation made during studies of long-term therapy with IFN was the induction of autoantibodies that have sometimes been associated with the development (14,15) or exacerbation (16) of autoimmune disorders. Numerous reports regarding the induction of neutralizing antibodies to IFN exist, but the exact clinical significance of these observations (especially with respect to the development of resistance to therapy) is not yet fully clarified (17–21).

Interferon-gamma

Interferon-gamma (IFN-γ) is produced by the type-1 subset of CD4-positive T cells, and, to a lesser extent, NK cells and CD8-positive T cells. Biologic actions include activation of Mφ (resulting in enhanced oxidative and nonoxidative killing of intracellular pathogens), enhancement of NK-cell function as well as antibody-dependant cellular cytotoxicity and monocyte and neutrophil Fc receptor, and major histocompatibility antigen expression (22). These activities result in markedly enhanced immune responses to many infections (including toxoplasmosis, leishmaniasis, and listeriosis) *in vitro* and *in vivo* (22). This cytokine was initially evaluated as an antitumour agent in relatively high doses (>100 μg/m²/day), and toxicities were sometimes quite severe (including hypotension, heart failure, confusion, hallucinations, thromboembolism, bronchospasm, and hepatic insufficiency) (23). More recently, it has been used in lower dosages (50 μg/m², 3 times/wk SC) for the treatment of human infections with promising results, and only mild toxicities (e.g., fever, headache, chills, and localized erythema, which usually responded to acetaminophen) have been observed (23).

Interleukin-2

Interleukin-2 (IL-2) is produced by T lymphocytes and has many potent immunostimulatory effects, including activation of T cells, NK cells, and macrophages (the latter indirectly, via induction of IFN-γ and TNF-α). IL-2 was first evaluated clinically in studies of cancer patients who received high doses (up to 10^6 U/kg, administered by continuous or thrice-daily infusion), and reported toxicities have included fever and rigors, anemia, erythroderma, thrombocytopenia, weight gain, and capillary leak syndrome (24). Another toxic effect noticed in these initial trials was the high incidence of bacterial intravenous catheter–related infections (25), which appeared to be related to the use of central venous catheters (and may in some instances be prevented by the use of totally implanted catheters [26]), as well as an acquired defect of neutrophil chemotaxis induced by IL-2 (27). This neutrophil defect is probably mediated by induction of TNF-α production by IL-2 and may be prevented by concurrent administration of corticosteroids. Because the pathogens involved in these infections were usually staphylococci, prophylactic antibiotics active against gram-positive organisms were recommended during IL-2 therapy (28); recently, gram-negative infections have also been reported to occur with IL-2 therapy, and broader antibiotic cover may be warranted (29). In an attempt to minimize the toxicity of IL-2 and to enable less frequent administration, IL-2 has been covalently bound to polyethylene glycol (i.e., PEG-IL-2), resulting a much longer half-life than unconjugated IL-2 (30).

Granulocyte colony stimulating factor

Granulocyte colony stimulating factor (G-CSF) preferentially stimulates proliferation, differentiation, and activation of neutrophil precursors. Monocyte/macrophages, fibroblasts, and endothelial cells produce G-CSF in response to stimulation by endotoxin and cytokines (including TNF-α, IFN-γ, IL-1, IL-3 and GM-CSF) (31). G-CSF was first administered to patients with malignancies and chemotherapy-induced neutropenia (32) and is well tolerated with only mild toxicity (mainly bone pain, which may be successfully managed with nonsteroidal agents).

Granulocyte-macrophage colony stimulating factor

Granulocyte-macrophage colony stimulating factor (GM-CSF) is a multipotent growth factor produced by T cells, monocytes, fibroblasts, and endothelial cells after exposure to endotoxin, lectins, and cytokines (31). Its actions include induction of proliferation, differentiation, and activation of both neutrophil and monocyte precursors. As with G-CSF, GM-CSF has been used to ameliorate chemotherapy-induced neutropenia (33). Unlike G-CSF, however, GM-CSF has a broader toxicity profile (including fever, influenza-like symptoms, anorexia, elevated liver transaminase levels, localized rash, and bone pain [31]). These toxicities are rarely severe, usually respond to symptomatic treatment, and tend to decrease with continuation of therapy. Less commonly, a capillary-leak syndrome associated with thrombotic events may occur at higher dosages ($>30 \mu g/kg/day$).

Macrophage colony stimulating factor

Macrophage colony stimulating factor (M-CSF) is released from monocytes, fibroblasts, and endothelial cells in response to many different activating stimuli (31). It enhances proliferation, differentiation, and activation of monocyte/macrophages and tends to act at later developmental stages than GM-CSF. Early preparations were partially purified and induced myalgias and low-grade fevers, but more recently, pure preparations have produced minimal toxicity (34).

Interleukin-3

IL-3 is a cytokine with a very broad cell specificity and is produced by activated T cells and NK cells in response to stimulation by endotoxin, IL-1, and TNF-α (31,34). IL-3 stimulates early pluripotent marrow progenitors, resulting in increases in circulating granulocytes (which exhibit synergy with GM-CSF), monocytes, erythrocytes, basophils, and platelets (34A).

STUDIES OF CYTOKINE THERAPY OF HUMAN INFECTIONS

Viral infections

Hepatitis B virus   Hepatitis B virus (HBV) is a 42-nm enveloped DNA virus that causes acute hepatitis, which spontaneously resolves in the majority of patients. In 5% to 10% of patients infected with HBV, chronic infection ensues, which has the potential for serious sequelae, such as chronic active hepatitis, cirrhosis, and hepatocellular carcinoma (35). The pathogenesis of these sequelae involves persistent viral replication and abnormal host immune responses, although the relative contributions of each of these components are still to be established (36). It has been noted that HBV infection results in impaired IFN production by cells (37). Despite effective vaccines against this virus being available for a decade, continued transmission of this agent is occurring (especially in the third world), and there are approximately 300 million chronic carriers worldwide (35). Although therapy with IFN-α has not been shown to be effective during acute infection (38), this product has become established over the last decade as a useful agent for the treatment of chronic HBV infection.

Greenburg and colleagues (39) first described an antiviral effect (manifested by a decrease in viral DNA polymerase and e-antigen titer) induced by human leukocyte IFN-α when it was administered in relatively low doses ($6-170 \times 10^3$ U/kg/day) for a short duration (10 days to 3 months) in 4 patients with chronic HBV infection. Since then, many studies, commencing with small open-label studies (40,41) and progressing to larger controlled trials (42–44), have confirmed these findings and resulted in development of optimal regimens for treatment of this condition (35,45). IFN-α in doses of 3 to 5×10^6 U daily or three times a week for 3 to 6 months yields a response rate between 30% to 50% (usually defined as normalization of liver transaminase levels and supported in many studies by improvement in liver histology), and an initial follow-up study suggested that, in a large proportion of patients, responses are of long duration (i.e., 87% still in remission after a mean of 4.3 yr) (46). Many studies have also documented loss of e-antigen, with appearance of anti-e antibody; a quantifiable decrease in viral DNA present in serum; and an improvement in histologic scores in response to IFN-α. Successful response is often heralded by a "healing flare" with hypertransaminasemia, which is followed by loss of viral markers (45). Whether the major effect of IFN-α therapy is mediated by antiviral mechanisms or immune enhancement is still being debated (35,45), but some authors favor the latter hypothesis (47,48) in part because of the demonstration of increased numbers of infiltrating CD8+ T cells and human leukocyte antigen (HLA) class I antigen expression in hepatic lesions in response to IFN-α therapy (49). It appears that doses of IFN-α below 1×10^6 U 3 times a week (43,50,51) or treatment of less than 3 months' duration (40,51) does not reliably induce a response. Doses above 10×10^6 U 3 times a week appear to have unacceptable toxicity (40,51,52). The role of prednisone withdrawal prior to IFN-α therapy of chronic hepatitis B is not currently fully defined (43,53). Although the acute side effects of IFN-α induced by these doses are able to be tolerated by most patients, they may be more severe in patients with decompensated liver failure (45), and extreme care is advised when administering IFN-α to this subgroup of patients. As is the case in cancer patients treated with IFN, both neutralizing and non-neutralizing antibodies against IFN develop in patients infected with HBV treated with IFN, but their clinical significance is currently uncertain (54,55).

Unfortunately, response rates in Chinese patients have been relatively low (56–58), due either to the long duration of infection or the young age at which patients were infected. A preliminary report from Taiwan, however, reported response rates similar to those seen in studies using Caucasian subjects (59). Other patient subgroups shown to have suboptimal responses to IFN include children with inactive biochemistry and immunocompromized hosts (60–62). Individual responses to IFN therapy have, however, been described in members of such groups. Because studies have not been able to prospectively identify individual patients with a high likelihood of response, all patients with chronic HBV infection who have serologic and biochemical evidence of activity are currently candidates for therapy with IFN-α (63). Because of the need to treat all patients and the current cost of this product, economic considerations (rather than clinical need) are likely to dictate usage patterns. Nevertheless, a recent study from the UK concluded that the use of IFN-α for chronic hepatitis B and C was cost-effective when a hypothetical model relevant to that health system was used (64).

Small, uncontrolled studies have reported responses to IFN-β alone (65) or in combination with IFN-α (66) in chronic HBV infection; a reduction in viremia during short-course administration of combination therapy has been reported (67). Whether these regimens will be of widespread clinical use remains to be determined.

Several studies have reported an inadequate response to treatment with IFN-γ in chronic hepatitis B infection when it was used alone (68,69). Combination therapy with IFN-α and IFN-γ was inferior to IFN-α alone (70,71).

Small studies have demonstrated efficacy of IFN-α when combined with antiviral agents such as vidaribine (72), acyclovir (73), or desciclovir (73), but it is not currently clear whether these represent an improvement on the efficacy of IFN-α alone in treatment of chronic HBV infection.

Hepatitis C virus   Hepatitis C virus (HCV) was first described as part of the syndrome of non-A, non-B hepatitis and is now known to be caused by an RNA virus belonging to the flavivirus family (74). It is recognized that this virus accounts for approximately 90% of all cases of post-transfusion hepatitis (i.e., 150–300 thousand cases/yr) and 50% of sporadic hepatitis cases (i.e., 850,000–1.7 million/yr) in the United States (75,76). Approximately 50% of patients acutely infected by transfusion with hepatitis C virus will progress to chronic infection, cirrhosis will develop in 20%, and 25% of those with cirrhosis will die of hepatic failure (47,75). In addition, hepatocellular carcinoma may complicate chronic infection with hepatitis C (77).

Hoofnagle and colleagues (78) first reported a response (assessed by normalization of serum transaminase levels) of chronic non-A, non-B hepatitis to varying doses (ranging from 0.5–5 million units 3–7 times/week for 4–12 months) of IFN-α in a small open-label study. Since then, a number of randomized, controlled trials using moderate doses of recombinant or lymphoblastoid IFN-α ($2–5 \times 10^6$ U 3 times/wk for 6 months) have confirmed responses (with normalization of transaminase levels, improvement in histology, and reduction in serum viral RNA levels) in approximately 45% of patients (range, 23–70%) (47,48,75). There is evidence that the dose of IFN-α influences its therapeutic effect in HCV infection because 3×10^6 U resulted in a higher response rate than 1×10^6 U (79,80). Increasing the dose to 5 or 15×10^6 U does not, however, significantly increase response rates further. Moreover, very low dose therapy (0.25×10^6 U) is still able to induce remission in 27% of patients (81). Increasing the duration of therapy has effected a trend toward higher response rates, but this increase was not significant from standard therapy (75). Interestingly, response to IFN in chronic HCV infection (which is usually evident within 12 weeks of therapy) is manifested by rapid decrease of serum transaminase levels to normal, rather than being preceded by a "healing flare," as is observed in HBV, leading some authors to interpret that the major mechanism of IFN response in hepatitis C is an antiviral rather than an immunomodulatory effect (47,48). Also of interest was the recent observation in a small study that IFN induced a 58% response rate in human immunodeficiency virus (HIV)–infected patients who also had chronic HCV infection (82), suggesting that immunocompromised patients infected with HCV may not have impaired response to IFN.

Enthusiasm for IFN treatment of chronic HCV infection has been tempered by the observation that approximately half of patients who achieve remission will relapse (usually within 12 weeks of discontinuation of therapy), with a rebound in serum transaminase levels. Nevertheless, up to 25% of all IFN recipients will remain in remission after 6 months, and there is no current evidence that late relapses occur in this subgroup (75). If relapse occurs, patients usually respond to retreatment (75), and this response may occur with low-dose therapy (1×10^8U)(78), although there is preliminary data to suggest that second remissions are no more durable than the first (83). Therefore, retreatment of initial nonresponders may not be cost-effective. Attempts have been made to reduce the relapse rate by prolonging the duration of therapy, and there is some suggestion that this approach might be of value (84). As is the case with chronic HBV infection, there is no prospective predictor for individual response of chronic HCV infection to IFN therapy; therefore, particular patients cannot be targeted for therapy. Despite these failings, a recent cost-benefit analysis concluded in favor of IFN therapy of chronic HCV infection in the UK medical system (64).

In addition to the previously recognized acute effects of IFN-α, treatment of chronic hepatitis C may produce less common delayed effects, such as production of auto-antibodies, which may be associated with thyroiditis, hyperthyroidism (85,86), hypothyroidism (86), or type 1 diabetes mellitus (87).

Good response of chronic hepatitis C to IFN-β therapy has also been described, but no long-term studies have been reported (48).

Hepatitis D virus Hepatitis D virus (HDV) is a defective virus that requires the presence of hepatitis B surface antigen to be able to replicate; hence, hepatitis D manifests as an acute superinfection in chronic HBsAg carriers. Preliminary studies have not identified any useful activity of IFN against hepatitis D (35).

Human immunodeficiency viruses (HIV-1 and HIV-2) Infection with these retroviruses results in the development of progressive immunodeficiency characterized by a progressive reduction in circulating CD4+ T lymphocytes (88); impairment of their function (including reduced production of immunomodulatory cytokines [89,90]) and eventual development of opportunistic infections and malignancies resulted in AIDS (91). Because of the impaired production of cytokines in patients with AIDS and the reported inhibition of HIV growth in vitro induced by interferon (92), it was inevitable that cytokines would be assessed for therapeutic potential in AIDS. Enthusiasm for this approach has had to be balanced, however, by the knowledge that some cytokines (i.e., TNF-α, IL-2, IL-6, and GM-CSF) may induce enhanced HIV expression in vitro (93). All studies of cytokine therapy in AIDS reported thus far have involved HIV-1 infection; most have been small, with relatively short follow-up periods; and most have focussed on the effect of therapies on surrogate markers of disease activity (i.e., total CD4 count, viral p24 antigen, or nucleic acid quantitation by polymerase chain reaction [PCR]), which may not directly correlate with long-term outcome.

The role of IFN-α in immune responses to HIV infection is complex: Cells infected by HIV have impaired production of IFN-α (94), but HIV-infected cells induce IFN-α production in uninfected cells, although these species of IFN-α tend to have low anti-HIV activity (94). In vitro, IFN-α inhibits HIV growth predominantly at late stages in the viral life cycle (95). Somewhat paradoxically, serum IFN-α levels increase progressively with advancing HIV infection (96), but this effect probably does not result in an antiviral effect due to the down-regulation of IFN-α receptors observed in patients with AIDS (97).

The first study to suggest a role for IFN-α in HIV infection was that of Krown and associates in 1983 (98); they showed that high doses ($36-54 \times 10^6$ U/day) induced a tumor response rate of 38% in 36 patients with Kaposi's sarcoma (KS). Although subsequent studies have reported lower response rates when lower doses of IFN-α were used (99), analyses of patients with IFN-responsive KS revealed an antiviral effect, as measured by a decrease in p24 antigen level in serum (100,101), whereas nonresponders did not manifest a decrease in p24 Ag. These findings were supported by evidence of an anti-HIV effect induced by IFN-α in patients who were also infected with hepatitis B (102). In these studies, the responders tended to have earlier stages of HIV disease, with higher CD4 counts at study entry. In a study of more advanced HIV disease in patients without KS, no antiviral effect of IFN-α was found (103). Recently, the findings of a randomized placebo-controlled, double-blind study of IFN-α (35×10^6 U/d for $\geq$ 12 wk) in 34 patients with early HIV infection showed evidence of a significant antiviral effect, and follow-up revealed a reduction in opportunistic infections and mortality (104). The low response rate to IFN-α reported in patients with advanced HIV disease appears to be related to down-regulation of IFN-α receptors, and although these patients tend to have high endogenous levels of IFN-α, it tends to be of low antiviral activity. Recently, de novo HIV resistance to IFN-α has been described, which may explain why all patients do not respond to therapy with this agent (105). In addition, there is evidence from a small study that the antiviral effect of IFN-α may be of short duration (106). Low doses of IFN-α also, somewhat paradoxically, reversed HIV-related thrombocytopenia (107–109). Although uncontrolled trials have reported efficacy of low-dose oral IFN-α therapy in patients with AIDS (110–112), a recent randomized placebo-controlled, double-blind study did not confirm these findings (113).

Zidovudine (ZDV) and IFN-α exhibit synergistic activity against HIV in vitro (114). It has been demonstrated that moderate doses of IFN-α can be tolerated by HIV-infected patients if low-dose ZDV regimens are used (115–118). There is preliminary data that suggest IFN-α plus ZDV has superior efficacy to ZDV alone in asymptomatic (119) and symptomatic HIV-infected patients without KS (120,121). The addition of IFN-α to long-term ZDV monotherapy regimens appears to result in improved CD4 counts (122) and virologic stabilization in some patients (123).

Similar antiviral and antitumor responses to IFN-β ($90-180 \times 10^6$ U/day) have been observed, and the patients most likely to respond are those with early disease (124). Combination cytokine therapy with IL-2 and IFN-β has been used in HIV infection with disappointing results (125).

Even before the first isolation of HIV, IL-2 was shown to be capable of reversing some of the cellular immune defects of patients with AIDS in vitro (126). Recently, administration of IL-2 in vivo was shown to induce delayed-type hypersensitivity response in previously anergic HIV-seropositive patients (127). High-dose IL-2 monotherapy was first used in patients to treat advanced HIV disease; little or only transient responses was observed (128–131). Recently, IL-2 was administered by continuous infusion in moderate doses (up to 12×10^6 U/m^2) to patients with early-stage HIV disease receiving ZDV, and significant increases in CD4 count (132) and reduction in HIV provirus load (measured by quantitative PCR [133]) have been reported. As in studies with patients with cancer, HIV-infected patients receiving IL-2 have an increased incidence of bacterial infections (134). In an attempt to minimize toxicity from IL-2 therapy, very low subcutaneous doses of rIL-2 (180,000 U/day) and PEG-IL-2 (36,000 U/day) have been administered to a small number of patients without major toxicity and evidence of enhanced cell-mediated immunity; however, measures of viral load were not reduced (30). A recent study using higher doses of PEG-IL-2 ($1–5\ 10^6$ IU/m^2) administered to patients with early or late HIV disease showed an improvement in CD4 counts without any significant change in viral replicative markers (135).

As discussed, IFN-γ production in vitro in response to antigenic stimulation is impaired in patients with AIDS (89). IFN-γ is able to induce increased mitogenic activity in vitro in lymphocytes obtained from patients with AIDS (136). In addition, administration of IFN-γ to monocytes obtained from patients with AIDS enhances the ability of such cells to kill intracellular parasites (137). For these reasons, IFN-γ (0.3–3 mg/m^2) was administered to patients with AIDS, and early studies did not show significant responses (138). More recently, IFN-γ has been used in earlier stages of HIV infection, and, although no significant change in CD4 count was detected, HIV p24 Ag titers decreased in 6 of 9 patients, and clinical response in patients with KS was seen in 3 of 17 (139). Preliminary results from 2 other studies have shown antiviral effects of IFN-γ alone (140) or in combination with ZDV (141) in patients with AIDS. Future prospects of IFN-γ therapy may include targeted delivery of cytokine to the lung via aerosol, because systemic administration does not result in detectable cytokine levels in respiratory epithelial lining fluid (142).

Because of the myelosuppression observed in patients with AIDS, which is aggravated by therapy with ZDV, colony stimulating factors have been evaluated for efficacy in preventing neutropenia. GM-CSF (1.3×10^3 to 2×10^4 U/kg/day) was first shown to reverse AIDS-related neutropenia when administered by intravenous infusion (143), and long-term subcutaneous GM-CSF has been shown to maintain neutrophil counts for prolonged periods (144). Although GM-CSF has been shown to up-regulate HIV expression in vitro (145), this effect has not been of clinical significance in most studies. The one study that reported increased p24 antigen with GM-CSF monotherapy (146) showed that this effect was reversed by institution of ZDV therapy, suggesting that these 2 agents should probably be administered together in clinical studies. Combining ZDV with GM-CSF is also supported by in vitro evidence of synergistic antiviral activity between these 2 agents (147). A recent clinical study reported improvement in ZDV-induced neutropenia by low-dose ($10^2–10^3$ U/kg/day or 1–10 μg/kg/day SC) GM-CSF (148) in HIV-infected patients. GM-CSF (mean dose, 0.64 μg/kg/day SC) has also been used to successfully reverse neutropenia associated with concomitant ZDV and IFN-α therapy of HIV infection (149). As with studies in non-HIV–infected patients, GM-CSF produced prominent flu-like symptoms and fever, as well as local erythematous reactions.

G-CSF (3.6–7.2 μg/kg/day SC) has also been successful in ameliorating the neutropenia of ZDV and gancyclovir in HIV-infected patients, and the addition of erythropoietin improved anemia in some patients, although this regimen did not prevent the development of opportunistic infections (150). Another small uncontrolled study described useful activity of adjunctive therapy with G-CSF in patients with AIDS with neutropenia and bacterial infections (151). Toxicity due to G-CSF in these studies has been generally mild; bone pain and local discomfort are most commonly reported.

Cytomegalovirus   Cytomegalovirus (CMV) is a DNA virus that can cause potentially fatal disease in immunocompromised hosts, including neonates, transplant recipients, and patients with malignancies or AIDS (152). CMV is a recognized cause of fever and leukopenia, pneumonia, chorioretinitis, hepatitis, superinfection, and possibly graft rejection in recipients of solid-organ transplants. In 1979, Cheeseman and associates (153) reported that short-course prophylactic lymphoblastoid IFN-α (3 × 10 U twice weekly for 6 wk) delayed the onset of CMV viremia in a small study of renal transplant recipients (153). A randomized, double-blind study of renal transplant recipients receiving prolonged (14 wk) prophylaxis demonstrated a significant reduction (1/20 vs 7/22; $p = 0.03$) in clinical CMV disease in IFN-α recipients (154). Enthusiasm for treatment of CMV disease with cytokines has waned somewhat with the introduction of ganciclovir, but GM-CSF may have a useful role in ameliorating CMV and ganciclovir-induced leukopenia (155). IFN-α does not appear to be effective in treatment of established CMV pneumonia of marrow transplant recipients (156,157).

CMV retinitis is a common manifestation of AIDS that can cause blindness, and therapy with antiviral agents is often hampered by toxicity of these agents (158). For example, up to 50% of such patients cannot tolerate gancyclovir therapy due to myelosuppression (159). Recently, both GM-CSF (159,160) and G-CSF (161) have been reported to improve the myelosuppression of gancyclovir therapy in patients with AIDS with CMV infections.

Herpes zoster infections   Reactivation of latent varicella-zoster virus infection in patients with malignancies can result in disseminated disease, which may be fatal (162). High-dose IFN-α therapy in this setting has been reported to reduce the risk of dissemination (163–165), but the toxicity experienced at the highest dose (68 × 10^6 U/day) was difficult to tolerate (165). Acyclovir has since become established as the first-line agent for herpes zoster infections in immunocompromised hosts, but it is not known whether combination therapy with lower doses of IFN-α than those previously used would result in synergistic effects. Myelitis is an uncommon complication of herpes zoster infection in competent hosts; a recent case report suggested a possible role for IFN-α in management of this problem in patients unresponsive to acyclovir (166).

Herpes simplex virus   Herpes simplex virus (HSV) is a DNA virus capable of producing disseminated disease in immunocompromised hosts and neonates, as well as a devastating encephalitis in immunocompetent hosts. Less serious diseases caused by HSV (including herpes labialis, genital herpes, and keratitis) have a tendency to recurrence and result in a significant amount of morbidity worldwide. Prior to the development of effective nucleoside antiviral agents, the potential of IFN-α as an antiherpetic agent was evaluated. Topical IFN-α (1–3 × 10^7 U/mL for 7 days) was shown in a placebo-controlled study to reduce recurrences of HSV keratitis (167). Prophylactic systemic administration of IFN-α (7 × 10^4 U/kg/day for 5 days) to patients undergoing operations on the trigeminal nerve was effective in reducing viral shedding and the number of patients with herpes labialis lesions (168). IFN-α (5 × 10^5 U/kg/day for 14 days) has been shown to hasten healing of lesions and reduce viral shedding if given within 72 hours of onset of recurrence of genital herpes (169). Topical IFN-α (10^6 U/g) has been effective in reducing viral shedding and symptoms during recurrence of genital herpes (170). Topical IFN-β also appears to have efficacy in treatment of labial and genital herpes (171). Although acyclovir (ACV) has now supplanted IFN for treatment of recurrent HSV infections (172), the selection of ACV-resistant mutants during therapy has been recognized and appears to be associated with clinical failures in patients with AIDS (173). It is of interest, therefore, that a small study reported success in treatment of ACV-resistant HSV with a combination of IFN-α and trifluorothymidine applied topically (174). IFN may therefore prove a useful agent in combination regimens against ACV-resistant HSV infections.

Acyclovir has been shown to have impressive activity in HSV encephalitis (175,176). However, because encephalitis can be caused by viruses unresponsive to ACV, a definitive diagnosis of HSV encephalitis may require invasive procedures (such as brain biopsy), and because there still remains a significant mortality and sequelae rate for HSV encephalitis treated with ACV, there is some attraction for the use of combination drug therapy of viral encephalitis. A retrospective study described the combination of acyclovir and IFN-β (5 × 10^6 U/kg/day) for viral encephalitis in children and reported that a subgroup of patients (those with low-density lesions on computed tomography scan to suggest severe encephalitis) had significant reduction in mortality and sequelae over those that received monotherapy with ACV (177). This observation needs to be explored further with controlled prospective studies.

Human papilloma virus   Human papilloma virus (HPV) is one of the most prevalent sexually transmitted infections and has been associated with condylomata accuminata (genital warts), as well as the development of cervical carcinoma. IFN was first shown to enhance HPV lesions in a patient receiving systemic IFN-α for malignant disease (178). Subsequently, topical IFN was successfully used in treating condylomata accuminata (D Ikic; [179]). Since then, many studies have reported efficacy of intramuscular, intralesional, and topical IFN preparations in enhancing resolution and preventing recurrence of HPV-associated lesions (179,180,181). IFN has also been successfully employed in treatment of laryngeal HPV infections (179).

Rhinovirus infections   Although rarely the cause of serious human disease, rhinoviruses are a frequent cause of upper respiratory tract infections, which result in significant economic losses for the community. Short-course prophylaxis with intranasal IFN

$(14 \times 10^6 \text{ U})$ reduced symptoms and viral shedding during experimental rhinovirus challenge (182). Topical IFN is also effective in preventing development of clinical signs in family contacts of patients with "colds" (183, 184). Aside from the cost of this preparation, the major drawback to the use of IFN in this setting is the development of local side effects in the form of nasal stuffiness and bleeding, which limits its widespread use (185).

Bacterial infections

Prophylaxis against infections in neutropenic states   Chemotherapeutic regimens used to treat malignancies result in iatrogenic neutropenia, which can be complicated by potentially fatal bacterial or fungal infections (186). Although institution of broad-spectrum antibiotic therapy in patients with fever and neutropenia is able to improve outcome, mortality from infection remains a major cause of death in cancer patients (187). Over the last 6 years, extensive experience has been gained in the use of G-CSF and GM-CSF to reduce the duration and nadir of neutropenia, the number of febrile episodes, the incidence of mucositis, the requirement for antibiotics, the number of days hospitalized, and the incidence of confirmed infections in patients with chemotherapy-induced neutropenia (34,188–191). Less experience currently exists for the use of M-CSF, but some preliminary studies have suggested a possible role for this agent in neutropenia (31). Although G-CSF and GM-CSF appear to have similar efficacy in this setting, G-CSF has less apparent toxicity. In many of these studies, subcutaneous administration has been efficacious, with doses commencing around 5 μg/kg/day or 250 μg/m^2/day and titrated upward until target neutrophil counts were reached. In addition to reducing the morbidity of current chemotherapeutic regimens, there is hope that use of these CSFs will enable dose intensification and improve response rates to poorly responsive tumors (190). Other clinical settings where CSFs have been used to reduce the infectious morbidity of neutropenia include marrow transplantation, cyclic neutropenia, congenital neutropenia, aplastic anemia, myelokathexis, myelodysplastic/syndrome (MDS), and idiopathic neutropenia (188,189,192). Potential stimulation of malignant clones in leukemia and MDS have tempered enthusiasm for their use in these settings.

Because of the rapid onset and offset of CSF effect, cytokines with different pharmacologic kinetics have also been evaluated. IL-3 (60–500 g/m SC) has a more delayed onset on neutrophil response, but it also increases production of other cell lines (including platelets and reticulocytes) and there is in vitro evidence for synergistic activity with GM-CSF (34). IL-3 has been used as monotherapy in phase I/II studies of secondary bone-marrow failure, MDS, and aplastic anemia with encouraging multi-lineage responses (34). Sequential therapy utilizing 5 days of IL-3 followed by 10 days of GM-CSF has been used and the results obtained were similar to those with 15-day monotherapy using either agent. These observations are of interest because of the development of a fusion protein of IL-3 and GM-CSF (PIXY 321), which may reproduce the biologic activity of both cytokines (193).

Treatment of established infections in neutropenia   Because CSFs increase oxidative function of neutrophils and monocytes as well as their numbers (188), GM-CSF has recently been evaluated as an adjunct to antimicrobials in the treatment of established bacterial (194,195) and fungal infections (196); promising responses have been reported in small studies. M-CSF has also been administered (50–2,000 μg/m^2/day by infusion) to 33 bone marrow transplant recipients with invasive fungal infection (which historically has a very high mortality rate), and an impressive improvement in mortality was reported when compared with historical controls (Nemunaitis, 1991, #10851).

Chronic granulomatous disease   Chronic granulomatous disorder (CGD) is an uncommon disorder that is a heterogeneous collection of inherited diseases characterized by defective killing of ingested organisms by phagocytic cells, which results in recurrent serious bacterial and fungal infections commencing early in childhood. IFN-γ was shown to reverse some of the biochemical defects of CGD phagocytes in vitro (197). A multicenter, randomized, double-blind, placebo-controlled international study reported striking efficacy of IFN-γ (50 μg/m^2 3 times/wk) in CGD, with a significant reduction in the number of serious infections and an increase in the duration of infection-free periods in IFN-γ–treated patients (198). This regimen produced fever but little in the way of serious toxicity.

Leprosy   Leprosy is caused by *Mycobacterium leprae* and may manifest anywhere along a disease spectrum ranging from localized skin lesions with few organisms (i.e., tuberculoid leprosy) to widespread body involvement with lesions containing many millions of organisms (i.e., lepromatous leprosy). The immunopathogenesis of leprosy is complex, and in lepromatous disease there is a selective unresponsiveness to specific *M. leprae* antigens, with impairment of lymphocyte proliferation, reduced expression of HLA-DR antigens, and production of macrophage-activating cytokines (including IFN-γ and IL-2) in vitro, as well as impaired delayed-type hypersensitivity skin responses (199,200). Some of these specific immune defects were able to be reversed by administration of related mycobacterial antigens (i.e., PPD) or IL-2 (201). Because antimicrobial therapy of leprosy may involve the prolonged use of multiple drugs with recognized toxicities, researchers have sought alternative treatment strategies, including the use of cytokines.

The first cytokine evaluated in leprosy was IFN-γ; low doses (1–10 μg) were injected into lepromatous lesions, and subsequent biopsy revealed histologic conversion toward the less severe (i.e., tuberculoid) end of the disease spectrum, with a reduction in the numbers of organisms and an increase in the inflammatory exudate (202). Further studies by Cohn's group (203,204) and others (205,206) confirmed beneficial local effects of intradermal low-dose IFN-γ, as well as systemic effects attained with higher doses of intramuscular cytokine (200). In all these studies, no major toxicity was observed with such low doses of IFN-γ, but prolonged administration of 30 to 100 μg has been associated with an increased incidence of erythema nodosum leprosum, which appears to be related to increased secretion of TNF-α and may be ameliorated by thalidomide (a known inhibitor of TNF-α production in vitro) (207). In addition, some individual variability in response to IFN-γ therapy was noted. Recently, results from a small, uncontrolled study of short-course intralesional IFN-γ (10–100 μg/day for 1–3 days) did not suggest any difference after 18 months in the histologic response observed at other sites from those achieved with standard multidrug therapy, suggesting that this regimen did not offer advantages over standard therapy (208).

Cytokine therapy of infectious diseases **241**

The effect of small intralesional doses of IL-2 (1–25 μg) was studied by Kaplan and associates in 1989 (209), and it was found that a cell-mediated immune response could be induced by this agent, which was associated with a striking reduction in the bacillary index (BI) of such lesions. The effect of higher cumulative doses was evaluated in 14 Nepalese patients with lepromatous leprosy: 10 μg IL-2 administered twice daily for 8 days was able to show striking cell-mediated immune responses in lesions distant from the injection sites, as well as evidence of systemic effects reflected in enhanced lympho-cyte proliferation in response to related mycobacterial antigens (but not to M. *leprae*) (210). Also of interest was the fact that this regimen resulted in a greater reduction in BI than that seen in historical controls receiving multidrug chemotherapy alone. In these studies, local skin reactions and nontender axillary lymphadenopathy were noted with-out any major toxicity. IL-2 appears to be a somewhat more promising agent for further evaluation in leprosy than IFN-γ.

Antigen presentation appears to be impaired in lepromatous leprosy, and GM-CSF is recognized to enhance the antigen-presenting cell function of Langerhans' cells in the skin as well as to promote keratinocyte proliferation (211). For these reasons, GM-CSF (7.5–45 μg/day for 10 days) was administered to patients with intermediate-grade leprosy lesions, and, although local recruitment of Langerhans' cells and proliferation of keratinocytes was observed, no evidence of an enhanced cell-mediated immune response was noted (212).

***Mycobacterium avium-intracellulare* infections** *Mycobacterium avium-intra-cellulare* (MAI) is a major opportunistic pathogen of patients with advanced HIV disease. Such patients tend to have impaired secretion of IFN-γ in response to mycobacterial antigens in vitro (213). Recently, preliminary uncontrolled experience suggested that combined therapy with antimycobacterial agents and IFN-γ may result in enhanced reduction in bacillemia (214).

Prophylaxis against bacterial infections in severely injured patients Severely traumatized patients are at high risk of serious bacterial infections as well as abnormal immunologic function, including reduced expression of HLA-DR on monocytes and impaired production of IFN-γ (215). In vitro treatment of monocytes obtained from patients with severe injuries with IFN-γ has been shown to result in increased HLA-DR expression (216). Because of these findings, a multicenter prospective, ran-domized study was performed to evaluate the effect of IFN-γ (100 μg/day SC for 10 days) in prevention of infections in this group of patients (217). Although the rate of death or severe infections was not reduced by IFN-γ treatment, this group had a significantly higher injury severity score at study entry. This therapy warrants further evaluation to identify better dosage protocols or to identify patient subgroups with better response rates to therapy.

Protozoal infections

Leishmaniasis Leishmania is an intracellular protozoan parasite with a widespread geographic distribution that produces a spectrum of disease ranging from self-limited cutaneous lesions to disseminated visceral infection (218). This variable phenotype appears to relate to the species of infecting organisms and host factors; striking antigen-specific anergy has been described in visceral leishmaniasis. Response to standard therapy (with pentavalent antimony) may not be adequate, and significant side effects may be induced. Experimental studies have identified the critical role of IFN-γ in host defence against this parasite. IFN-γ (20–25 μg ID 3 times a week) was first evaluated in cutaneous leishmaniasis (due to *L. braziliensis guyanensis* in Brazil and *L. tropica* in Syria) by Harms and colleagues (219), who reported an improved response to this agent when compared with saline-treated control subjects. The same group subsequently compared IFN-γ (25 μg ID weekly for 5 weeks) in a controlled trial to antimonials and demonstrated a superior response to antimony (220), which suggests that higher doses of IFN-γ may be required for optimum effect.

The use of combined IFN-γ (100–400 μg/m^2/day IM for 10–40 days) and antimony for treatment of visceral leishmaniasis (VL) has been described in a study from Brazil (221). Responses in patients with VL that was previously refractory to antimony alone have been impressive (6 of 8 responded), as were the results obtained in previously untreated patients (8 of 9 responders). Combined therapy using IFN-γ (100 μg/m^2 on alternate days for 4 weeks) plus antimony had comparable cure rates when compared with therapy with antimony alone in a study of previously untreated patients with VL in Kenya, but there was a more rapid reduction in splenic parasite counts and early sterilization of splenic cultures with combination therapy (222). Further studies are currently underway to determine optimal combination regimens for therapy of VL (222).

CONCLUSIONS

The use of cytokines, alone or in combination with antimicrobial agents, represents an exciting new mode of treatment for infectious diseases and has the potential to revolutionize therapy of some difficult-to-treat infections. Although most of the studies described herein are preliminary, these agents are now established as therapy for chronic viral hepatitis and HPV infections, as well as for prophylaxis of infections in myelosuppression (and other neutropenic states) and CGD. Despite this preliminary evidence, they should ideally be used within study protocols to enable development of optimal dosage regimens and identification of patient subgroups most likely to benefit from their use. In many areas, the current costs of these agents may limit their use. They also represent very promising potential therapies for HIV infection, lepromatous leprosy, and visceral leishmaniasis, and the results of ongoing trials are eagerly awaited.

ACKNOWLEDGMENTS

Dr. Beaman is a scholar of the American Foundation for AIDS Research. The author would like to thank Dr. C. Greenfield for review of the manuscript.

REFERENCES

1 **Meager A.** *Cytokines.* Englewood Cliffs, NJ: Prentice Hall, 1991.

2 **Fernandez-Botran R.** Soluble cytokine receptors: their role in immunoregulation. *FASEB J* 1991;5:2567–2574.

3 **Kaufmann S, Flesch I.** Cell mediated immunity, immunodeficiency and microbial infections. *Curr Top Infect Dis Clin Microbiol* 1988;2:165–173.

4 **Saez-Llorens X, Ramilo O, Mustafa M, Mertsola J, McCracken G.** Molecular pathophysiology of bacterial meningitis: current concepts and therapeutic implications. *J Pediatr* 1990; 116:671–684.

5 **Scott P, Kaufmann S.** The role of T-cell subsets and cytokines in the regulation of infection. *Immunol Today* 1991;12:346–348.

6 **Grau G, Modlin R.** Immune mechanisms in bacterial and parasitic diseases: protective immunity versus pathology. *Curr Opin Immunol* 1991;3:480–485.

7 **Cohn Z, Kaplan G.** Hansen's disease, cell-mediated immunity and recombinant cytokines. *J Infect Dis* 1991;163:1195–1200.

8 **Clark I, Rockett K, Cowden W.** Proposed link between cytokines, nitric oxide and human cerebral malaria. *Parasitol Today* 1991;7:205–207.

9 **Roilides E, Pizzo P.** Modulation of host defenses by cytokines: evolving adjuncts in prevention and treatment of serious infections in immunocompromised hosts. *Clin Infect Dis* 1992;15:508–524.

10 **Isaacs A, Lindenmann J.** Virus interference. I. The interferon. *Proc R Soc Lond (Biol)* 1957;147:258–267.

11 **Borden E.** Interferons: pleiotropic cellular modulators. *Clin Immunol Immunopathol* 1992;62:S18–S24.

12 **Houglum J.** Interferon: mechanisms of action and clinical value. *Clin Pharm* 1983;2:20–28.

13 **Krown S.** Interferons and interferon inducers in cancer treatment. *Semin Oncol* 1986;13: 207–217.

14 **Ronnblom L, Alm G, Oberg K.** Autoimmunity after alpha-interferon therapy for malignant carcinoid tumors. *Ann Intern Med* 1991;115:178–183.

15 **Chazerain P, Meyer O, Kahn M.** Rheumatoid arthritis-like disease after alpha-interferon therapy. *Ann Intern Med* 1992;116:427.

16 **Conlon K, Urba W, Smith J, Steis R, Longo D, Clark J.** Exacerbation of symptoms of autoimmune disease in patients receiving alpha-interferon therapy. *Cancer* 1990;65:2237–2242.

17 **Vallbracht A, Treuner T, Flehmig B, Joester K, Niethammer D.** Interferon neutralising antibodies in a patient treated with human fibroblast interferon. *Nature* 1981;287:496–498.

18 **Jansen J, De Pauw B, Holdrinet R.** Treatment of hairy cell leukaemia with recombinant human α2-interferon. *Lancet* 1984;1:1025–1026.

19 **Von Wussow P, Freund M, Block B, Diedrich H, Poliwoda H, Deicher D.** Clinical significance of anti-IFN-α antibody titres during interferon therapy. *Lancet* 1987;2:635–636.

20 **Steiss R, Smith W, Urba W, et al.** Resistance to recombinant interferon-alpha-2a in hairy cell leukaemia associated with neutralising anti-interferon antibodies. *N Engl J Med* 1988;318:1409–1413.

21 **Figlin R, Itri L.** Anti-interferon antibodies: a perspective. *Semin Hematol* 1988;25:9–15.

22 **Murray H.** Interferon-gamma, the activated macrophage and host-defence against microbial challenge. *Ann Intern Med* 1988;108:595–608.

23 **Todd P, Goa K.** Interferon gamma-1b. A review of its pharmacology and therapeutic potential in chronic granulomatous disease. *Drugs* 1992;43:111–122.

24 **Lotze M, Matory Y, Rayner A, et al.** Clinical effects and toxicity of interleukin-2 in patients with cancer. *Cancer* 1986;58:2764–2772.

25 **Marolin K, Rayner A, Hawkins M, et al.** Interleukin-2 and lymphokine activated killer cell therapy of solid tumours: analysis of toxicity and management of guidelines. *J Clin Oncol* 1989;7:486–498.

26 **Escudier B, Lethiec J, Cosset-Delaigue M, LeClercq B, Andremont A, Nitenberg G.** Prospective trial of totally implanted catheter to prevent catheter related sepsis in patients treated with interleukin 2. Presented at the 32nd Interscience Conference on Antimicrobial Agents and Chemotherapy. Anaheim, CA, 1992.

27 **Klempner M, Noring R, Mier J, Atkins M.** An acquired chemotactic defect in neutrophils from patients receiving interleukin-2 immunotherapy. *N Engl J Med* 1990;322:959–965.

28 **Hartmann L, Urba W, Steis R, et al.** Use of prophylactic antibiotics for prevention of intravascular catheter-related infections in interleukin-2 treated patients. *J Natl Cancer Inst* 1989;81: 90–93.

29 **Hardy J, Moore J, Lorentzos A, Ellis E, Jameson B, Gore M.** Infectious complications of interleukin-2 therapy. *Cytokine* 1990;2:311.

30 **Teppler H, Kaplan G, Smith K, et al.** Efficacy of low doses of the polyethylene glycol derivative

of interleukin-2 in modulating the immune response of patients with human immunodeficiency virus type 1 infection. *J Infect Dis* 1993;167:291–298.

31 **Groopman J, Molina J-M, Scadden D.** Hematopoietic growth factors. Biology and clinical applications. *N Engl J Med* 1989;321:1449–1459.

32 **Bronchud M, Scarffe J, Thatcher N, et al.** Phase I/II study of recombinant human granulocyte colony-stimulating factor in patients receiving intensive chemotherapy for small cell lung cancer. *Br J Cancer* 1987;56:809–813.

33 **Brandt S, Peters W, Atwater S, et al.** Effect of recombinant human granulocyte-macrophage colony-stimulating factor on hematopoietic reconstitution after high-dose chemotherapy and autologous bone marrow transplantation. *N Engl J Med* 1988;318:869–876.

34 **Nemunaitis J.** Recombinant human macrophage colony stimulating factor: use for treatment of invasive fungal infections in bone barrow transplant patients In: Sonnenfeld G, Gzarniecki C, Nacy C, Byrne G, Degre M, ed. *Cytokines and resistance to non-rival pathogenic infections.* Aususta, GA: Biomedical Press, 1992:41–48.

34a **Schulz G, Krumwieh D, Oster W.** Adjuvant therapy with recombinant interleukin-3 and granulocyte-macrophage colony-stimulating factor. *Pharmacol Ther* 1991;52:85–94.

35 **Gerin J.** Treatment of viral hepatitis. *Curr Opin Infect Dis* 1992;5:806–810.

36 **Robinson W.** Hepatitis B virus and Hepatitis delta virus. In: Mandell G, Douglas R, Bennett J, ed. *Principles and Practices of Infectious Diseases.* New York: Churchill Livingstone, 1990:1204–1231.

37 **Whitten T, Quets A, Schloemer R.** Identification of the hepatitis B virus factor that inhibits expression of beta interferon gene. *J Virol* 1991;65:4699–4704.

38 **Tassopolous N, Hadziyannis S, Wright G.** A randomised-controlled trial of alpha-interferon in acute type-B hepatitis. *Hepatology* 1989; 10:576.

39 **Greenburg H, Pollard R, Lutwick L, Gregory P, Robinson W, Merigan T.** Effect of human leukocyte interferon on hepatitis B virus infection in patients with chronic active hepatitis. *N Engl J Med* 1976;295:517–522.

40 **Smith C, Weissberg J, Bernhardt L, Gregory P, Robinson W, Merigan T.** Acute Dane particle suppression with recombinant leukocyte A interferon in chronic hepatitis B virus infection. *J Infect Dis* 1983;148:907–913.

41 **Dooley J, Davis G, Peters M, Waggoner J, Goodman Z, Hoofnagle J.** Pilot study of re-

combinant human α-interferon for chronic type B hepatitis. *Gastroenterology* 1986;90: 150–157.

42 **Mazzella G, Saracco G, Rizzetto M, et al.** Human lymphoblastoid interferon for the treatment of chronic hepatitis B. *Am J Med* 1988;85(suppl 2A):141–142.

43 **Perrillo R, Schiff E, Davis G, et al.** A randomised, controlled trial of interferon alpha-2b alone and after prednisone withdrawal for the treatment of chronic hepatitis B. *N Engl J Med* 1990;323:295–301.

44 **Thomas H, Dusheiko G, Lok A, et al.** Comparative study of three doses of interferon alpha 2a in chronic active hepatitis B. In: Hollinger B, Lemon S, Margolis H, ed. *International Symposium on Viral Hepatitis and Liver Disease.* Baltimore: Williams & Wilkins, 1990: 641–642.

45 **Dusheiko G, Zuckerman A.** Therapy for hepatitis B. *Curr Opin Infect Dis* 1991;4:785–794.

46 **Korenman J, Baker B, Waggoner J, Everhart J, DiBisceglie A, Hoofnagle J.** Long-term remission of chronic hepatitis B after alpha-interferon therapy. *Ann Intern Med* 1991;114:629–634.

47 **Jacyna M.** α-interferon therapy in chronic hepatitis C infection: what have we learnt so far? *Eur J Gastroenterol Hepatol* 1992;4:703–706.

48 **Farrell G.** Treatment of chronic hepatitis C with alpha-interferon. *J Gastroenterol Hepatol* 1991;6(suppl. 1):36–40.

49 **Hayata T, Nakano Y, Yoshizawa K, Sodeyama T, Kiyosawa K.** Effects of interferon on intrahepatic human leukocyte antigens and lymphocyte subsets in patients with chronic hepatitis B and C. *Hepatology* 1991;13:1022–1028.

50 **Schalm S, Heijtink R.** Spontaneous disappearance of viral replication and liver cell inflammation in HBsAg-positive chronic active hepatitis; results of placebo vs. interferon trial. *Hepatology* 1982;2:791–794.

51 **Alexander G, Williams R.** Natural history and therapy of chronic hepatitis B virus infection. *Am J Med* 1988;85(suppl 2A):143–146.

52 **Thomas H.** Hepatitis B viral infection. *Am J Med* 1988;85(suppl 2A):135–140.

53 **Perrillo R, Regenstein F, Peters M, et al.** Prednisone withdrawal followed by recombinant interferon in the treatment of chronic type B hepatitis: a randomised controlled trial. *Ann Intern Med* 1988;109:95–100.

54 **Antonelli G, Currenti M, Turriziani O, Dianzani F.** Neutralising antibodies to interferon-alpha: relative frequency in patients treated with different interferon preparations. *J Infect Dis* 1991;163:882–885.

55 Antonelli G, Currenti M, Turriziani O, Riva E, Dianzani F. Relative frequency of non-neutralising antibodies to interferon in hepatitis patients treated with different IFN-α preparations. *J Infect Dis* 1992;165:593–594.

56 Lai C, Lok A, Lin H, Wu P, Yeoh E, Yeung C. Placebo-controlled trial of recombinant α2-interferon in chinese HBsAg-carrier children. *Lancet* 1987;2:877–880.

57 Lok A, Lai C, Wu P, Leung E. Long-term follow-up in a randomised controlled trial a recombinant α2-interferon in chinese patients with chronic hepatitis B infection. *Lancet* 1988;2:298–302.

58 Lok A, Lai C, Wu P, Lau J, Leung E, Wong L. Treatment of chronic hepatitis B with interferon: experience in Asian patients. *Semin Liver Dis* 1989;9:249–253.

59 Liaw H, Lin S, Sheen I, Chen T, Chu C. Treatment of chronic type B hepatitis in Southeast Asia. *Am J Med* 1988;85(suppl 2A):147–149.

60 McDonald J, Caruso L, Karayiannis P. Diminished responsiveness of male homosexual chronic hepatitis B virus carriers with HTLV-III antibodies to recombinant alpha-interferon. *Hepatology* 1987;7:719–723.

61 Davis G. Interferon treatment of viral hepatitis in immunocompromised patients. *Semin Liver Dis* 1989;9:267–272.

62 Brook M, McDonald J, Karayiannis P. Randomised controlled trial of interferon alfa 2a for the treatment of chronic hepatitis B virus infection: factors that influence response. *Gut* 1989;30:1116–1122.

63 Hoofnagle J. Chronic hepatitis B. *N Engl J Med* 1990;323:337–339.

64 Garcia de Ancos J, Roberts J, Dusheiko G. An economic evaluation of the costs of α-interferon treatment of chronic active hepatitis due to hepatitis B or C virus. *J Hepatol* 1990;11:S11–S18.

65 Ito S, Marutani K, Matsuo S. Changes in ultrastructure of hepatocytes and liver function test results before, during and after treatment with interferon-β in patients with HBeAg-positive chronic active hepatitis. *Dig Dis Sci* 1992;37:1260–1267.

66 Caselmann W, Eisenburg J, Hofshneider P, Rajen K. α- and β-interferon in chronic active hepatitis B. A pilot trial of short term combination therapy. *Gastroenterology* 1989; 96:449–455.

67 Caselmann W, Eisenburg J, Hofschneider P, Koshy R. Beta- and gamma-interferon in chronic active hepatitis B: a pilot trial of short-term combination therapy. *Gastroenterology* 1989;96:449–455.

68 Marcellin P, Loriot M, Boyer N, et al. Recombinant human gamma-interferon in patients with chronic-active hepatitis B: pharmacokinetics, tolerance and biological effects. *Hepatology* 1990;12:155–158.

69 Lau J, Lai C, Wu P, Chung H, Lok A, Lin H. A randomised controlled trial of recombinant interferon-gamma in chinese patients with chronic hepatitis B infection. *J Med Virol* 1991;34:184–187.

70 DiBisceglie A, Rustgi V, Kassianides C, et al. Therapy of chronic hepatitis B with recombinant human alpha and gamma interferon. *Hepatology* 1990;11:266–270.

71 Kakumu S, Ishikawa T, Mizokami M, et al. Treatment with human interferon of chronic hepatitis B. *J Med Virol* 1991;35:32–37.

72 Scullard G, Pollard R, Smith J, et al. Antiviral treatment of chronic hepatitis B virus infection. I. Changes in viral markers with interferon combined with adenine arabinoside. *J Infect Dis* 1981;143:772–783.

73 DeMan R, Schalm S, Heijtink R, et al. Long-term follow-up of antiviral combination therapy in chronic hepatitis B. *Am J Med* 1988;85(suppl 2A):150–154.

74 Choo Q, Kuo G, Weiner A, Overby L, Bradley D, Houghton M. Isolation of a cDNA clone derived from a blood-bourne non-A non-B viral hepatitis clone. *Science* 1989;244:359–362.

75 Davis G. Recombinant α-interferon treatment of non-A non-B (type C) hepatitis: review of studies and recommendations for treatment. *J Hepatol* 1990;11:S72–S77.

76 Chen Y, Bala K. Treatment of chronic hepatitis C with recombinant interferon alfa. *West J Med* 1992;156:72.

77 Villa E, Baldini G, Pasquinelli C. Risk factors for hepatocellular carcinoma in Italy: male sex, hepatitis B virus, non-A non-B infection and alcohol. *Cancer* 1988;62:611–615.

78 Hoofnagle J, Mullen K, Jones D, Rustgi V, DiBisceglie A, Peters M. Treatment of chronic non-A non-B hepatitis with recombinant human alpha-interferon: a preliminary report. *N Engl J Med* 1986;315:1575–1578.

79 Davis G, Balart L, Schiff E. Treatment of chronic hepatitis C with recombinant interferon alpha. *N Engl J Med* 1989;321:1501–1506.

80 Causse X, Godinot H, Chevalier M, Chossegros P, Zoulim F, Ouzan D. Comparison of 1 or 3 MU of interferon alfa-2b and placebo in patients with chronic non-A non-B hepatitis. *Gastroenterology* 1991;101:497–502.

81 Varagonna G, Brown D, Kibbler H, Scheuer P, Ashrefzadeh P, Sherlock S. Response,

relapse and retreatment rates and viraemia in chronic hepatitis treated with α2-b interferon. *Eur J Gastroenterol Hepatol* 1992;4:707–712.

82 Boyer N, Marcellin P, Degott C, et al. Recombinant interferon-α for chronic hepatitis C in patients positive for antibody to human immunodeficiency virus. *J Infect Dis* 1992; 165:723–726.

83 Marriott E, Quiroga J, Carreno V. Retreatment of chronic hepatitis C with interferon-α. *J Infect Dis* 1992;166:1200–1201.

84 Gomez-Rubio M, Porres J, Castillo L, Quiroga J, Moreno A, Carreno V. Prolonged treatment (18 months) of chronic hepatitis C with recombinant alfa-interferon in comparison with a control group. *J Hepatol* 1990;11:S63–S67.

85 Schultz M, Muuler R, VonZurMuhlen A, Brabant G. Induction of hyperthyroidism by interferon-α-2b. *Lancet* 1989;1:1452.

86 Berris B, Feinman S. Thyroid dysfunction and liver injury following alpha-interferon treatment of chronic viral hepatitis. *Dig Dis Sci* 1991;36:1657–1660.

87 Fabris P, Betterle C, Floreani A, et al. Development of type 1 diabetes mellitus during interferon alfa therapy for chronic HCV hepatitis. *Lancet* 1992;340:548.

88 Shearer G, Clerici M. Early T-helper defects in HIV infection. *AIDS* 1991;5:245–253.

89 Murray H, Rubin B, Masur H, Roberts R. Impaired production of lymphokines and immune (gamma) interferon in the acquired immunodeficiency syndrome. *N Engl J Med* 1984;310:883.

90 Murray H, Welte K, Jacobs J, Rubin B, Mertelamann R, Roberts R. Production of and in vitro response to interleukin-2 in the acquired immunodeficiency syndrome. *J Clin Invest* 1985;76:1959–1964.

91 Rosenburg Z, Fauci A. Immunopathogenesis of HIV infection. *FASEB J* 1991;5:2382–2390.

92 Ho D, Hartshorn K, Rota T, et al. Recombinant interferon alfa-A suppresses HTLV-III replication in vitro. *Lancet* 1985;1:602–604.

93 Poli G, Fauci A. The effect of cytokines and pharmacologic agents on chronic HIV infection. *AIDS Res Hum Retroviruses* 1992;8:191–197.

94 Francis M, Meltzer M, Gendelman H. Interferons in the persistence, pathogenesis and treatment of HIV infection. *AIDS Res Hum Retroviruses* 1992;8:199–207.

95 Gendelman H, Baca L, Turpin J, et al. Regulation of HIV replication in infected monocytes by IFN-a: mechanism for viral restriction. *J Immunol* 1990;145:2669–2676.

96 DeStefano E, Friedman R, Friedman-Kein A, et al. Acid-labile human leukocyte interferon in homosexual men with Kaposi's sarcoma and lymphadenopathy. *J Infect Dis* 1982;146:451–455.

97 Lau A, Read S, Williams B. Down-regulation of interferon α but not γ receptor expression in vivo in the acquired immunodeficiency syndrome. *J Clin Invest* 1988;82:1415–1421.

98 Krown S, Real F, Cunningham-Rundles S, et al. Preliminary observations on the effect of recombinant leukocyte A interferon in homosexual men with Kaposi's sarcoma. *N Engl J Med* 1983;308:1071–1076.

99 Mitsuyasu R. Use of recombinant interferons and hematopoietic growth factors in patients infected with human immunodeficiency virus. *Rev Infect Dis* 1991;13:979–984.

100 de Wit R, Schattenkerk J, Boucher C, Bakker P, Veenhof K, Danner S. Clinical and virologic effects of high-dose recombinant interferon-alpha in disseminated AIDS-related Kaposi's sarcoma. *Lancet* 1988;2: 1092–1093.

101 Lane H, Feinburg J, Davey V, et al. Antiretroviral effects of interferon-α in AIDS-associated Kaposi's sarcoma. *Lancet* 1988;2: 1218–1222.

102 Brook M, Gor D, Forster S, Harris W, Jeffries D, Thomas H. Suppression of HIV p24 antigen and induction of anti-p24 antibody by alpha interferon in patients with chronic hepatitis B. *AIDS* 1988;2:391–393.

103 Friedland G, Klein R, Salzman B, et al. A randomised placebo-controlled trial of recombinant human interferon-alpha 2a in patients with AIDS. *J Acquir Immune Defic Syndr* 1988;1:111–118.

104 Lane H, Davey V, Kovacs J, et al. Interferon-alpha in patients with asymptomatic human immunodeficiency virus infection. A randomised, placebo-controlled trial. *Ann Intern Med* 1990;112:5–11.

105 Edlin B, St Clair M, Pitha P, et al. In-vitro resistance to zidovudine and alpha-interferon in HIV-1 isolates from patients: correlations with treatment duration and response. *Ann Intern Med* 1992;117:457–460.

106 Edlin B, Weinstein R, Whaling S, et al. Zidovudine-interferon-α combination therapy in patients with advanced human immunodeficiency virus type-1 infection: biphasic response of p24 antigen and quantitative polymerase chain reaction. *J Infect Dis* 1992;165: 793–798.

107 Murphy K, Stein M, D'Amico R. Correction of HIV-associated thrombocytopenia

with low doses of interferon alfa. *South Med J* 1992;85:557–559.

108 Dhiver C, Poizot-Martin I, Drogoul M, Gastaut J. Long term therapy of severe HIV related thrombocytopaenia with alpha interferon. Presented at the VIII International Conference on AIDS. Amsterdam, The Netherlands, July 19–24, 1992.

109 Northfelt D, Charlebois E, Mirda M, Child C, Kaplan L, Abrams D. Continuous low-dose interferon-α therapy for HIV-related immune thrombocytopaenic purpura. Presented at the VIII International Conference on AIDS. Amsterdam, The Netherlands, July 19–24, 1992.

110 Hutchinson V, Cummins J. Low-dose oral interferon in patients with AIDS. *Lancet* 1987;2:1530–1531.

111 Koech D, Obel A. Efficacy of kemron (low dose oral natural interferon alpha) in the management of HIV-1 infection and acquired immune deficiency syndrome. *East Afr Med J* 1990;67(suppl 2):64–70.

112 Obel A, Koech D. Outcome of intervention with or without low dose oral interferon alpha in thirty-two HIV-1 serpositive patients in a referral hospital. *East Afr Med J* 1990;67(suppl 2):71–76.

113 Hulton M, Levin D, Freedman L. Randomised, placebo-controlled, double-blind study of low-dose oral interferon-α in HIV-1 antibody positive patients. *J Acquir Immune Defic Syndr* 1992;5:1084–1090.

114 Hartshorn K, Vogt M, Chou T, et al. Synergistic inhibition of human immunodeficiency virus in vitro by azidothymidine and recombinant alpha A interferon. *Antimicrob Agents Chemother* 1987;31:168–172.

115 Orholm M, Pedersen C, Mathiesen L, Dowd P, Nielsen J. Suppression of p24 antigen in sera from HIV-infected individuals with low-dose alpha-interferon and zidovudine: a pilot study. *AIDS* 1989;3:97–100.

116 Kovacs J, Deyton L, Davey R, et al. Combined zidovudine and interferon-α therapy in patients with Kaposi sarcoma and the acquired immunodeficiency syndrome. *Ann Intern Med* 1989;111:280–287.

117 Krown S, Gold J, Niedzwiecki D, et al. Interferon-α with zidovudine: safety tolerance and clinical and virologic effects in patients with Kaposi sarcoma associated with the acquired immunodeficiency syndrome. *Ann Intern Med* 1990;112:812–821.

118 Fischl M, Uttamchandani R, Resnick L, et al. A phase 1 study of recombinant human interferon-α2a or human lymphoblastoid interferon-an1 and concomitant zidovudine in patients with AIDS-related kaposi's sarcoma. *J Acquir Immune Defic Syndr* 1991;4:1–10.

119 Piazza M, Chirianni A, TullioCataldo P, et al. Combination zidovudine and interferon-α therapy in the treatment of asymptomatic HIV infection. Presented at the VIII International Conference on AIDS. Amsterdam, The Netherlands, July 19–24, 1992.

120 Frissen P, Wverling G, Centre NATE. Zidovudine and interferon-alpha versus zidovudine in symptomatic HIV-1 infection. Presented at the VIII International Conference on AIDS. Amsterdam, The Netherlands, Jyly 19–24, 1992.

121 Mildvan D, Bassiakos Y. Zidovudine and interferon-α-2a: ongoing assessment of synergy and tolerance in early ARC patients, ACTG 068. Presented at the VIII International Conference on AIDS. Amsterdam, The Netherlands, July 19–24, 1992.

122 Henrivaux P, Fairon Y, Baijot P. Addition of interferon-α-2b to previous long-term zidovudine therapy. Presented at the VIII International Conference on AIDS. Amsterdam, The Netherlands, 1992.

123 Lafeuillade A, Pelligrino P, Quillichini R. A pilot study of zidovudine and interferon-alpha for patients with biological deterioration on zidovudine monotherapy. Presented at the VIII International Conference on AIDS. Amsterdam, The Netherlands, July 19–24, 1992.

124 Miles S, Cortes HW, Carden J, Marcus S, Mitsuyasu M. Beta interferon therapy in patients with poor-prognosis Kaposi's sarcoma related to the acquired immunodeficiency syndrome. A phase II trial with preliminary evidence of antiviral activity and low incidence of opportunistic infections. *Ann Intern Med* 1990;112:582–589.

125 Krigel R, Padavic-Shaller K, Rudolph A, Poiesz P, Komis R. Exacerbation of epidemic Kaposi's sarcoma with a combination of interleukin-2 and beta-interferon: results of a phase 2 study. *J Biol Response Mod* 1989;8:359–365.

126 Rook A, Masur H, Lane H, et al. Interleukin-2 enhances the depressed natural killer and cytomegalovirus-specific cytotoxic activities of lymphocytes from patients with the acquired immune deficiency syndrome. *J Clin Invest* 1983;72:398–403.

127 McElrath M, Kaplan G, Burkhardt R, Cohn Z. Cutaneous response to recombinant interleukin-2 in human immunodeficiency virus-1 seropositive individuals. *Proc Natl Acad Sci USA* 1990;87:5783–5787.

128   Lotze M, Robb R, Sharrow S, Frana L, Rosenberg S. Systemic administration of interleukin-2 in humans. *J Biol Response Mod* 1984;3: 475–482.

129   Lane H, Siegel J, Rook A, et al. Use of interleukin-2 in patients with acquired immunodeficiency syndrome. *J Biol Response Mod* 1984;3:512–516.

130   Mann RM, Welte K, Sternberg C, et al. Treatment of immunodeficiency with interleukin-2; initial exploration. *J Biol Response Mod* 1984;4:483–490.

131   Volberding P, Moody D, Beardsley D, Bradley E, Wofsy C. Therapy of acquired immune deficiency syndrome with recombinant interleukin-2. *AIDS Res Hum Retroviruses* 1987;3:115–124.

132   Schwartz D, Skowron G, Merigan T. Safety and effect of interleukin-2 plus zidovudine in asymptomatic individuals infected with human immunodeficiency virus. *J Acquir Immune Defic Syndr* 1991;4:11–23.

133   Clark A, Holodniy M, Schwartz D, Katzenstein D, Merigan T. Decrease in HIV provirus in peripheral blood mononuclear cells during zidovudine and human rIL-2 administration. *J Acquir Immune Defic Syndr* 1992;5:52–59.

134   Murphy P, Lane H, Gallin J, Fauci A. Marked disparity in incidence of bacterial infections in patients with the acquired immunodeficiency syndrome receiving interleukin-2 or Interferon-γ. *Ann Intern Med* 1988;108:36–41.

135   Wood R, Montoya J, Kundu S, Schwartz D, Merigan T. Safety and efficacy of polyethylene glycol modified interleukin-2 and zidovudine in HIV-1 infection. A phase I/II study. *J Infect Dis* 1993:167;519–525.

136   Heagy W, Strom T, Kelly V, et al. Recombinant human gamma interferon enhances in vitro activation of lymphocytes isolated from patients with acquired immunodeficiency syndrome. *Infect Immun* 1989;57:3619.

137   Murray HW, Scavuzzo D, Jacobs JL, et al. In vitro and in vivo activation of human mononuclear phagocytes by interferon-gamma. Studies with normal and AIDS monocytes. *J Immunol* 1987;138:2457–2462.

138   Murray H. Interferon gamma therapy in AIDS for mononuclear cell activation. *Biotherapy* 1990;2:149–158.

139   Heagy W, Groopman J, Schindler J, Finberg R. Use of IFN-γ in patients with AIDS. *J Acquir Immune Defic Syndr* 1990;3:584–590.

140   Parkin J, Underhill J, Eales L, Pinching A. The use of recombinant human gamma interferon in AIDS patients: dose-related immunomodulation and prolonged survival. Presented at the VIII International Conference on AIDS. Amsterdam, The Netherlands, July 19–24, 1992.

141   Badaro R, Brites C, Moreira E, Ho J, Rocha H, Johnson W. Low dose zidovudine plus gamma-interferon in AIDS patients. Presented at the VIII International Conference on AIDS. Amsterdam, The Netherlands, July 19–24, 1992.

142   Jaffe H, Buhl R, Mastrangeli A, et al. Organ specific cytokine therapy. Local activation of mononuclear phagocytes by delivery of an aerosol of recombinant interferon-γ to the human lung. *J Clin Invest* 1991;88:297–302.

143   Groopman J, Mitsuyasu R, De Leo M, Oette D, Golde D. Effect of recombinant human granulocyte-macrophage colony-stimulating factor on myelopoiesis in the acquired immunodeficiency syndrome. *N Engl J Med* 1987;317:593–598.

144   Mitsuyasu R, Levine J, Miles S, et al. Effects of long term subcutaneous administration of recombinant granulocyte-macrophage colony stimulating factor in patients with HIV-related leukopenia. *Blood* 1988;72(suppl 1):356a.

145   Hammer S, Gillis J, Groopman J, Rose R. In vitro modification of human immunodeficiency virus infection by granulocyte-macrophage colony-stimulating factor and gamma interferon. *Proc Natl Acad Sci USA* 1986;83:8734–8738.

146   Pluda J, Yarchoan R, Smith P, et al. Subcutaneous recombinant granulocyte-macrophage colony-stimulating factor used as a single agent and in an alternating regimen with AZT in leukopenic patients with severe human immunodeficiency virus infection. *Blood* 1990;76: 463–472.

147   Hammer S, Gillis J. Synergistic activity of granulocyte-macrophage colony-stimulating factor and 3′-azido-3′-deoxythymidine against human immunodeficiency virus in vitro. *Antimicrob Agents Chemother* 1987;31:1046–1050.

148   Allan JLJ, Tessitore J, Falcone N, Galasso F, Israel R, Groopman J. Recombinant human granulocyte-macrophage colony stimulating factor amelieorates zidovudine-induced neutropenia in patients with acquired immunodeficiency syndrome/AIDS-related complex. *Blood* 1991;78:3148–3154.

149   Davey R, Davey V, Metcalf J, et al. A phase I/II trial of zidovudine, interferon-α, and granulocyte-macrophage colony-stimulating factor in the treatment of human immunodeficiency virus type-1 infection. *J Infect Dis* 1991;164:43–52.

150 Miles S, Mitsuyasu R, Moreno J, et al. Combined therapy with recombinant granulocyte colony-stimulating factor and erythropoietin decreases hematologic toxicity from zidovudine. *Blood* 1991;77:2109–2117.

151 Hegge U, Brockmeyer N, Goos M. Granulocyte colony-stimulating factor treatment in AIDS patients. *Clin Invest* 1992;70:922–926.

152 Ho M. Cytomegalovirus. In: Mandell G, Douglas R, Bennett J, eds. *Principles and Practice of Infectious Diseases*, 3rd ed. New York: Churchill Livingstone, 1990:1159–1172.

153 Cheeseman S, Rubin R, Stewart J, et al. Controlled clinical trial of prophylactic human leukocyte interferon in renal transplantation. *N Engl J Med* 1979;300:1345–1349.

154 Hirsch M, Schooley R, Cosimi A, et al. Effects of interferon-alpha on cytomegalovirus reactivation syndromes in renal-transplant recipients. *N Engl J Med* 1983;308:1489–1493.

155 Kutsogiannis D, Crowther M, Lazarovits A. Granulocyte-macrophage colony stimulating factor for the therapy of cytomegalovirus and ganciclovir-induced leukopaenia in a renal transplant recipient. *Transplantation* 1992; 53:930–932.

156 Meyers J, Day L, Lum L, Sullivan K. Recombinant leukocyte A interferon for the treatment of serious viral infections after marrow transplant: a phase I study. *J Infect Dis* 1983;148:551–556.

157 Wade J, McGuffin R, Springmeyer S, Newton B, Singer J, Meyers J. Treaatment of cytomegaloviral pneumonia with high-dose acyclovir and human leukocyte interferon. *J Infect Dis* 1983;148:557–562.

158 Jacobsen M, Mills J. Serious cytomegalovirus disease in the acquired immunodeficiency syndrome: clinical findings, diagnosis and treatment. *Ann Intern Med* 1988;108:585–594.

159 Hardy W. Combined ganciclovir and recombinant human granulocyte-macrophage colony stimulating factor in the treatment of cytomegalovirus retinitis in AIDS patients. *J Acquir Immune Defic Syndr* 1991;4(suppl 1):S22–S28.

160 Grossberg H, Bonnem E, Bulles W. GM-CSF with ganciclovir for the treatment of CMV retinitis in AIDS. *N Engl J Med* 1989;320:1560.

161 Jacobsen M, Stanley H, Heard S. Ganciclovir with recombinant metionyl human granulocyte colony-stimulating factor for treatment of cytomegalovirus disease in AIDS patients. *AIDS* 1992;6:515–517.

162 Dolin R, Reichman R, Mazur M, Whitley R. Herpes zoster-varicella infections in immunocompromised patients. *Ann Intern Med* 1978;89:375–388.

163 Merigan T, Rand K, Pollard R, Abdallah P, Jordan G, Fried R. Human leukocyte interferon for the treatment of herpes zoster in patients with cancer. *N Engl J Med* 1978; 298:981–987.

164 Merigan T, Gallagher J, Pollard R, Arvin A. Short-course human leukocyte interferon in treatment of herpes zoster in patients with cancer. *Antimicrob Agents Chemother* 1981; 19:193–195.

165 Winston D, Eron L, Ho M, et al. Recombinant interferon-alpha-2a for treatment of herpes zoster in immunocompromised patients with cancer. *Am J Med* 1988;85:147–151.

166 Nakano T, Awaki E, Araga S, Takai H, Innoue K, Takahashi K. Recurrent herpes zoster myelitis treated with human interferon alpha: a case report. *Acta Neurol Scand* 1992;85:372–375.

167 Jones B, Coster D, Falcon M, Cantell K. Topical therapy of ulcerative herpetic keratitis with human interferon. *Lancet* 1977;2:128.

168 Pazin G, Armstrong J, Lam M, Tarr G, Jannetta P, Ho M. Prevention of reactivated herpes simplex infection by human leukocyte interferon after operation on the trigeminal root. *N Engl J Med* 1979;301:225–230.

169 Pazin G, Harger J, Armstrong J, et al. Leukocyte interferon for treating first episodes of genital herpes in women. *J Infect Dis* 1987;156:891–898.

170 Friedman-Kien A, Klein R, Glaser R, Czelusniak S. Treatment of recurrent genital herpes with topical alpha interferon gel combined with nonoxynol-9. *J Am Acad Dermatol* 1986;15:989–994.

171 Glezerman G, Cohen V, Mosvshovitz M, et al. Placebo-controlled trial of topical interferon in labial and genital herpes. *Lancet* 1988;1:150–152.

172 Ho M. Interferon as an agent against herpes simplex virus. *J Invest Dermatol* 1990;95: 158S–160S.

173 Erlich K, Mills J, Chatis P, et al. Acyclovir-resistant herpes simplex virus infections in patients with the acquired immunodeficiency syndrome. *N Engl J Med* 1989;320:293–296.

174 Birch C, Tyssen D, Tachedjian G, et al. Clinical effects and in vitro studies of trifluorothymidine combined with interferon-α for treatment of drug-resistant and sensitive herpes simplex virus infections. *J Infect Dis* 1992;166:108–112.

175 Skoldenberg B, Forsgren M, Alestig K, et al. Acyclovir versus vidaribine in herpes simplex encephalitis. *Lancet* 1984;1:707–711.

176 Whitley R, Alford C, Hirsch M, et al. Vidaribine versus acyclovir therapy in herpes simplex encephalitis. *N Engl J Med* 1986; 314:144–149.

177 Wintergerst U, Behlohradsky B. Acyclovir versus acyclovir plus beta-interferon in focal viral encephalitis in children. *Infection* 1992; 20:207–212.

178 Strander H, Cantell K. Studies on antiviral and antitumour effects of human leukocyte interferon in vitro and in vivo. *In Vitro* 1974;3:49–56.

179 Trofatter KF. Interferon treatment of anogenital human papilloma virus-related diseases. *Dermatol Clin* 1991;9:343–352.

180 Weck P, Buddin D, Whisnant J. Interferons in the treatment of genital human papillomavirus infections. *Am J Med* 1988;85(suppl 2A):159–164.

181 Green I. Therapy for genital warts. In: Lupton G, Fitzpatrick J, eds. *Dermatologic Clinics, vol 10*. Philadelphia: W. B. Saunders, 1992:253–269.

182 Merigan T, Reed S, Hall T, Tyrrell D. Inhibition of respiratory virus infection by locally applied interferon. *Lancet* 1973;1:563–567.

183 Douglas R, Moore B, Miles H, et al. Prophylactic efficacy of intranasal alpha2-interferon against rhinovirus infections in the family setting. *N Engl J Med* 1986;314:65–70.

184 Hayden F, Albrecht J, Kaiser D, Gwaltney J. Prevention of natural colds by contact with intranasal alpha2-interferon. *N Engl J Med* 1986;314:71–75.

185 Douglas R. The common cold—relief at last? *N Engl J Med* 1986;314:114–115.

186 Bodey G, Buckley M, Sathe Y, Freireich E. Quantitative relationship between circulating leukocytes and infections in patients with acute leukaemia. *Ann Intern Med* 1965;64: 328–334.

187 Pizzo P, Robichaud K, Wesley R, Commers J. Fever in the pediatric and young adult patient with cancer. A prospective study of 1001 episodes. *Medicine (Baltimore)* 1982;61: 153–165.

188 Burdach S. The granulocyte/macrophage colony-stimulating factor: basic science and clinical application. *Klin Padiatr* 1991;203: 302–310.

189 Hollingshead L, Goa K. Recombinant granulocyte colony-stimulating factor. A review of its pharmacological properties and prospec-

tive role in neutropenic conditions. *Drugs* 1991;42:300–330.

190 Gabrilove J. The development of granulocyte colony-stimulating factor in its various clinical applications. *Blood* 1992;80:1382–1385.

191 Grosh W, Quesenberry P. Recombinant human hematopoietic growth factors in the treatment of cytopenias. *Clin Immunol Immunopathol* 1992;62:S25–S38.

192 Peters W. Use of cytokines during prolonged neutropenia associated with autologous bone marrow transplantation. *Rev Infect Dis* 1991; 13:993–996.

193 Williams D, Park L. Hematopoietic effects of a granulocyte-macrophage colony stimulating factor/interleukin-3 fusion protein. *Cancer* 1991;67:2705–2707.

194 Biesma B, deVries E, Willemse P, et al. Efficacy and tolerability of recombinant human granulocyte-macrophage colony-stimulating factor in patients with chemotherapy-related leukopenia and fever. *Eur J Cancer* 1990; 26:932–936.

195 Anaissie E, Legrand C, Elting L, Gutterman J, Vadhan-Raj S, Bodey G. Randomised trial of antibiotics plus granulocyte-macrophage colony-stimulating factor for febrile episodes in neutropenic cancer patients. Presented at the 30th Interscience Conference of Antimicrobial Agents and Chemotherapy. Atlanta, GA, October 21–24, 1990.

196 Anaissie E, Bodey G, Obrien S, Gutterman J, Vadhan-Raj S. Effects of granulocyte-macrophage colony-stimulating factor on myelopoiesis and disseminated mycoses in neutropenic patients with hematologic malignancies. *Blood* 1989;74(suppl 1):15a.

197 Esokowitz R, Orkin S, Newburger P. Recombinant interferon gamma augments phagocyte superoxide production and X-chronic granulomatous disease gene expression in X-linked variant chronic granulomatous disease. *J Clin Invest* 1987;80:1009–1016.

198 The International Chronic Granulomatous Disease Cooperative Study Group. A controlled trial of interferon gamma to prevent infection in chronic granulomatous disease. *N Engl J Med* 1991;324:509–516.

199 Mehra V, Modlin R. T-lymphocytes in leprosy lesions. *Curr Top Microb Immunol* 1990;155:97–109.

200 Kaplan G, Cohn Z. Leprosy and cell-mediated immunity. *Curr Opin Immunol* 1991;3:91–96.

201 Kaplan G, Sampaio E, Walsh G, et al. Influence of *Mycobacterium leprae* and its soluble products on the cutaneous responsive-

ness of leprosy patients to antigen and recombinant interleukin-2. *Proc Natl Acad Sci USA* 1989;86:6269–6273.

202 Nathan C, Kaplan G, Levis W, et al. Local and systemic effects of intradermal recombinant interferon-γ in patients with lepromatous leprosy. *N Engl J Med* 1986;315:6–15.

203 Kaplan G, Nusrat A, Sarno E, et al. Cellular responses to the intradermal injection of recombinant human γ-interferon in lepromatous leprosy patients. *Am J Pathol* 1987;128:345–353.

204 Kaplan G, Mathur N, Job C, Nath I, Cohn Z. Effect of multiple interferon-γ injections on the disposal of *Mycobacterium leprae*. *Proc Natl Acad Sci USA* 1989;86:8073–8077.

205 Samuel N, Grange J, Samuel S, et al. A study of the effects of intradermal administration of recombinant gamma interferon in lepromatous leprosy patients. *Lepr Rev* 1987;58:389–400.

206 Bottasso O, Besuschio S, Merlin V, et al. Lepromatous leprosy treated with recombinant interferon gamma: cutaneous histologic changes. *Int J Dermatol* 1992;31:813–817.

207 Sampaio E, Moreira A, Sarno E, Malta A, Kaplan G. Prolonged treatment with recombinant interferon-γ induces erythaema nodosum leprosum in lepromatous leprosy patients. *J Exp Med* 1992;175:1729–1737.

208 Mathur N, Mittal A, Mathur D, Jain S. Long-term follow-up of lepromatous leprosy patients receiving intralesional recombinant gamma-interferon. *Int J Lepr* 1992;60:98–100.

209 Kaplan G, Kiessling R, Teklemariam S, et al. The reconstitution of cell-mediated immunity in the cutaneous lesions of lepromatous leprosy by recombinant interleukin-2. *J Exp Med* 1989;169:893–907.

210 Kaplan G, Britton W, Hancock G, et al. Systemic influence of recombinant Interleukin-2 on the manifestations of lepromatous leprosy. *J Exp Med* 1991;173:993–1006.

211 Cohn Z, Kaplan G. Hansen's disease, cell-mediated immunity and recombinant cytokines. *J Infect Dis* 1991;163:1195–1200.

212 Kaplan G, Walsh G, Guido L, et al. Novel responses of human skin to intradermal recombinant granulocyte/macrophage colony-stimulating factor: Langerhans cell recruitment, keratinocyte growth and enhanced wound healing. *J Exp Med* 1992;175:1717–1728.

213 Murray H, Scavuzzo D, Chapparas T, Roberts R. T cell responses in patients with disseminated *Mycobacterium avium-intracellulare*. *Chest* 1988;93:922–926.

214 Squires K, Brown S, Armstrong D, Murphy W, Murray H. Interferon-γ treatment for *Mycobacterium avium-intracellulare* complex bacillemia in patients with AIDS. *J Infect Dis* 1992;166:686–687.

215 Livingstone D, Appel S, Wellhausen S, Sonnenfeld G, Polk H. Depressed interferon gamma production and monocyte HLA-DR expression after severe injury. *Arch Surg* 1988;123:1309–1312.

216 Hershman M, Appel S, Wellhausen S, Sonnenfeld G, Polk H. Interferon-gamma treatment increases HLA-DR expression on monocytes in severely injured patients. *Clin Exp Immunol* 1989;77:67–70.

217 Polk H, Cheedle W, Livingstone D, et al. A randomised prospective clinical trial to determine the efficacy of interferon-γ in severely injured patients. *Am J Surg* 1992;163:191–196.

218 Pearson R, de Quiroz Sousa A. Leishmania species: visceral (Kala-Azar), cutaneous and mucosal leishmaniasis. In: Mandell G, Douglas R, Bennett J, eds. *Principles and Practice of Infectious Disease*, 3rd ed. New York: Churchhill-Livingstone, 1990:2077–2085.

219 Harms G, Zwingenberger K, Chehade A, et al. Effects of intradermal gamma-interferon in cutaneous leishmaniasis. *Lancet* 1989;1:1287–1292.

220 Harms G, Chehade A, Douba M, et al. A randomised trial comparing a pentavalent antimony drug and recombinant interferon-γ in the local treatment of cutaneous leishmaniasis. *Trans R Soc Trop Med Hyg* 1991;85:214–216.

221 Badaro R, Falcoff E, Badaro F, et al. Treatment of visceral leishmaniasis with pentavalent antimony and Interferon gamma. *N Engl J Med* 1990;322:16–21.

222 Murray H, Squires K, Harms G, Rosenkaimer F. Clinical trials of interferon-γ in leishmaniasis. In: Sonnenfeld G, Czarniecki C, Nacy C, Byrne G, Degre M, eds. *Cytokines and Resistance to Non-viral Pathogenic Infections*. Augusta, GA: Biomedical Press, 1992:199–206.

Intelligent dosing of antimicrobials

CHARLES H. NIGHTINGALE
RICHARD QUINTILIANI
DAVID P. NICOLAU

INTRODUCTION

Over the last 50 years, considerable information has been obtained concerning the action of antimicrobials. This information provides a better understanding not only of how antibiotics work against micro-organisms, but also of the influence of the body on the disposition of the antibiotic and subsequently the effect of the body in modifying the drug's action against bacteria. For the major classes of antibiotics, we can correlate antibiotic efficacy with readily obtainable clinical parameters that allow us to devise appropriate dosing strategies to maximize clinical efficacy and to minimize toxicity. We review these principles and describe rational dosing regimens for antibiotics based on this information.

OVERVIEW OF THE ACTION OF ANTIMICROBIALS IN THE BIOLOGICAL SYSTEM

All antimicrobials exert their effect against bacteria via the same general mechanism (i.e., a binding to some site that is essential to the life process of the organism). In the case of beta-lactam antibiotics, this mechanism involves the penicillin-binding proteins; for quinolones, the DNA gyrase; and for macrolides and tetracyclines, the ribosomes. For this binding to occur, the drug must penetrate the cell wall, cross the cell membrane, diffuse through the periplasmic space, and find its way to its target binding site. For most antibiotics, this process involves passive diffusion; however, for some, there may also be an active transport (1–3). The transport of antibiotic from the outside of the cell to the cell's interior can thus be considered a concentration-dependent process. The effect of the human body on the disposition of the drug will therefore affect the concentration of drug that reaches the outside of the bacteria's cell wall and subsequently affect the amount of drug that reaches the site of attachment inside the bacteria. The bacteria can also affect the probability of the drug reaching its target site

252

based on the size of its water-filled channels (porins) and changes in these pores. The nature of the cell wall membrane and changes in its composition, the viscosity and composition of the periplasmic space, and the presence of beta-lactamase enzymes are additional reasons for the reduction of drug concentrations at the target site. Alterations in the nature of the binding site would also result in a reduced affinity of the antimicrobial for the target site. These are properties of the bacteria that cannot be effected by the host or by the prescribing clinician. Likewise, the inherent diffusability, the attraction to the binding site, and the strength of binding are properties of the antibiotic. Again, the prescriber cannot normally alter these properties, although the option to use a different antibiotic or variation in the dosing regimen to reduce these bacterial effects is always possible.

The ability of the drug to penetrate from the outside of the cell wall into the interior of the micro-organism and its affinity for the binding site is what we mean when we describe the "microbiologic activity" of an antibiotic against a particular pathogen. The use of the term *microbiologic activity* does not include the effect of the human body on influencing the drug's concentration at the outer bacterial wall, and, as stated, this concentration will eventually influence the amount of drug that reaches the target binding site. It follows then that defining the effectiveness of an antibiotic by its microbiologic activity only is an incomplete description of the entire process. Basing drug selection decisions on this criteria alone, as is commonly done in clinical prac-tice, can lead to incorrect conclusions and inappropriate drug choices.

For an antibiotic to effectively eradicate bacteria in the human body, it not only must bind to the appropriate site but also must occupy a sufficient number of these sites. Occupying a small number of these sites is generally not sufficient to elicit the desired antimicrobial action. Because the laws of mass action govern the number of sites occupied, the higher the drug's concentration in the micro-organism, the greater the number of sites taken over by the antibiotic. When a critical number of sites are occupied, the antibiotic will elicit its pharmacologic effect on the bacteria. Because the number of sites occupied is a function of mass action, it is related to the amount of available drug in the bacteria. For some antibiotics, attachment to the binding site is in a dynamic equilibrium (i.e., it binds and unbinds to that site very rapidly). If this is the case, the problem of having a sufficient number of sites occupied at any time is one of having sufficiently high drug concentrations. Therefore, the drug concentration in the proximity of the binding sites must exceed some value so a crucial number of sites are occupied with drug. Unfortunately, we do not know what the crucial concentration should be because we cannot easily measure this in individual bacteria. As a result, we use a surrogate marker that is believed to be proportional to this concentration (i.e., the minimum inhibitory concentration [MIC] or the minimum bactericidal concentration [MBC]). This approach provides the rationale for statements relating drug concentra-tions in the serum or tissues to the micro-organism's MIC or MBC.

An alternative possibility regarding the relationship between binding site concentra-tion in the micro-organism and serum concentrations in the body is the situation when the binding constant favors the bound state or the binding is irreversible. In such a circumstance, low concentrations of drug will in time accumulate at the binding site until the crucial number of sites are bound. If this accumulation happens quickly, then one cannot distinguish between the two mechanisms. If this accumulation happens slowly (in relationship to the dosing interval), then there will be a weak relationship between serum concentrations and the MIC or MBC and a stronger relationship to the time of antibiotic exposure.

If an antibiotic reaches its critical concentrations at the binding sites very rapidly and the binding site is critical for the survival of the micro-organism, then the micro-organism will be killed. If the necessary conditions for the death of the organism exist, the end result will be the same whether the condition came about from intravenous or oral administration of drug. The reluctance of clinicians to use oral therapy, especially in hospitalized patients, is often expressed in terms of a fear that oral therapy is less effective, but the only difference between oral and intravenous therapy is the additional step involving absorption of the drug into the body. Obviously, this absorption needs to occur rapidly and reliably if the oral dose is to produce the same effect as the intravenous dose. It follows, therefore, that for well-absorbed drugs (e.g., trimethoprim-sulfamethoxazole [TMP/SMX], metronidazole, clindamycin, cephalexin, cephradine, cefadroxil, ciprofloxacin, ofloxacin, lomefloxacin), the same eradication of bacteria in the human body can be expected in patients with normal absorptive abilities as that observed with the intravenous form of these drugs.

As described, antibiotics that rapidly bind to vital binding sites usually kill the bacteria and are termed *bacteriocidal in action*. If the binding site is not crucial for life, then the normal life cycle of the bacteria may be interrupted and the antibiotic is termed *bacteriostatic*. As a result, bacteriostatic drugs cannot kill organisms by themselves but require a second drug or the host's immune defenses to kill the organism. Inadequate concentrations of bacteriocidal drugs kill only the more sensitive portions of a population, allowing the more resistant members to survive. Most of these surviving bacteria remain in a "static" phase while the host eliminates the antibiotic, repairs damage to affected parts, or synthesizes new proteins. However, surviving bacteria can be killed by the host defense systems in this static phase or in some cases by the presence of other antibiotics. The static phase that results after exposure to bacteriostatic or bacteriocidal drugs is termed *the postantibiotic effect* (PAE) if it occurs after the drug concentrations in the body no longer exist (4,5). Some drugs elicit long PAEs against certain organisms and some elicit short or negligible PAEs. Thus, the length of the PAE is influenced by organism, choice of antimicrobial, antimicrobial concentrations, and duration of antimicrobial exposure. The presence or absence of a PAE will therefore effect the relationship between bacterial killing and pharmacokinetic parameters in the human body and will ultimately affect dosing strategies.

From this discussion, it is obvious that antimicrobial activity in the human body is related to the ability of the antimicrobial to penetrate to the appropriate binding site in the bacteria, to attach itself to that site in adequate concentrations, and to remain there for a sufficient period so that the bacteria, as it attempts to carry out its normal life functions, fails to do so. This is a description of what we define as the drug's microbiologic activity and its pharmacokinetic disposition in the body, because the body provides the concentration gradient that drives the antibiotic into the bacteria and maintains the concentration gradient over time. The two related areas of information, microbiologic activity and pharmacokinetics, define the efficacy of the antibiotic and the term describing these two areas of information together is *pharmacodynamics*

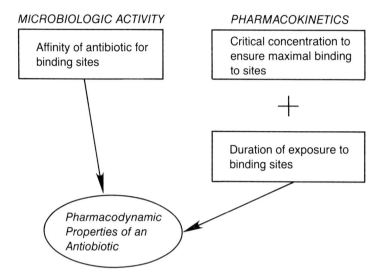

MICROBIOLOGIC ACTIVITY

PHARMACOKINETICS

Affinity of antibiotic for binding sites

Critical concentration to ensure maximal binding to sites

$+$

Duration of exposure to binding sites

Pharmacodynamic Properties of an Antiobiotic

Figure 14.1   Factors required for antibiotic action.

(Figure 14.1). As stated, it is not completely correct to choose antibiotics based solely on microbiologic properties. Likewise, it is not correct to choose antibiotics solely on their pharmacokinetic properties (e.g., long half-life). Rather, antibiotics should be evaluated based on their pharmacodynamic properties. Fortunately, there is now sufficient information to make such an analysis for the major classes of antimicrobial agents.

PHARMACODYNAMICS OF ANTIMICROBIAL AGENTS

Although antimicrobials have been available for decades, only recently has there been sufficient data to permit clinicians to select the optimal dose or dosing regimen based on the pharmacodynamic principles associated with the various antimicrobial classes. Application of these findings provides the opportunity for these agents to be utilized in a manner that promotes maximal efficacy while reducing the risk of drug-related toxicity. We discuss the pharmacodynamic principles of the major drug classes, including aminoglycosides, fluoroquinolones, beta-lactams, and glycopeptides.

Bacterial killing as a result of the exposure to a selected antimicrobial can be classified as either concentration-dependent or concentration-independent activity. Although this killing activity is a function of the chosen antimicrobial, concentration studied, and the pathogen, it is generally accepted that a given drug class will always result in the same killing profile. Although we are not yet able to measure drug concentrations directly at the site of action, we commonly use a microbiologic parameter, such as the MIC of the pathogen, as the critical value in the interpretation of these pharmacodynamic relationships.

When relating microbiologic activity and pharmacokinetics, several pharmacokinetic parameters seem to be important determinants of efficacy. The parameters of area under the serum concentration-time curve (AUC), peak serum concentration, and half-life are correlated to the MIC of the pathogen, thus producing pharmacodynamic parameters such as the AUC:MIC ratio, peak:MIC ratio, and the time the antibiotic concentration remains above the MIC (time>MIC) (Figure 14.2). Currently, it is well accepted that the time>MIC for beta-lactams and glycopeptides (e.g., vancomycin) is the predominant pharmacodynamic parameter associated with efficacy; however, for aminoglycosides and fluoroquinolones, this association has been related to the AUC, peak:MIC ratio, and the time>MIC (6–11). It is likely that all these parameters are important determinants of efficacy for the latter antimicrobials since all of these parameters are co-related. It is difficult to isolate a single pharmacodynamic relationship due to co-relation of these parameters and the impact of the study conditions on the resulting data. It is our belief, however, that the total amount of drug delivered to the micro-organism is the parameter most important in bacterial eradication.

Because the amount of drug delivered to the organism is proportional to the amount of drug delivered to the patient's body (AUC), we conclude that the AUC is the primary pharmacokinetic parameter related to efficacy. Because the AUC is a product of concentration and time, it is possible that under certain conditions the contribution of antibiotic concentration will dominate the process; under different conditions, the time above the MIC will be the major factor influencing bacterial eradication. For antibiotics that do not exhibit concentration-dependent killing and have relatively short or negligible PAEs (e.g., beta-lactam antibiotics), the time of exposure of the antibiotic contributes more to the killing process than does absolute concentration of the drug. This is not to say that concentration is not important, because the concentration in the blood drives the drug onto the micro-organism's binding sites. However, the contribution that this concentration makes to overall activity is relatively small compared with the contribution made by prolonged exposure to the drug. For this reason, we can "approximate" the relationships by saying that for beta-lactam antibiotics, the parameter that correlates with bacterial eradication is the time above the MIC. For antibiotics that exhibit dose-dependent killing, such as aminoglycosides and quinolones, and also exhibit fairly long PAEs, the contribution due to exposure time to the overall killing process is relatively small compared with the effect of concentration. We generally describe this observation using the "approximate" statement that for these drugs, peak concentration is the parameter that correlates with bacterial killing. In most clinical situations, an increase in dose also results in an increase in the AUC (e.g., an 80-mg dose of gentamicin will yield a certain AUC and serum peak level; if the dose is doubled to 160 mg, we see a doubling of the serum peak level as well as the AUC). Under these conditions, serum peak levels and AUC are co-related parameters, and either can be used to correlate with efficacy. For convenience in the clinical setting, the serum peak:MIC ratio is commonly used, as opposed to the AUC:MIC ratio. It also follows that under certain conditions, neither the peak level nor the time>MIC will predominate, and efficacy is then maximized by simultaneously increasing concentration as well as time above the MIC. In such a circumstance, only the AUC will correlate with antibiotic eradication. There are certain practical consequences to these observations and beliefs.

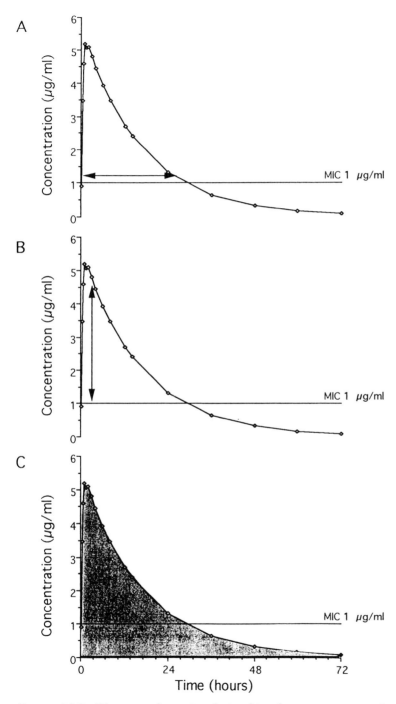

Figure 14.2 Pharmacodynamic relationship of serum concentration versus time profile to the MIC of the pathogen. (A) Time>MIC. (B) Peak:MIC ratio. (C) AUC:MIC ratio.

CONCENTRATION-DEPENDENT KILLING

The rate and extent of bactericidal activity resulting after exposure of the micro-organism to aminoglycosides or fluoroquinolones is concentration-dependent (or time-independent) (i.e., bacterial killing is dependent on the ratio [difference] between the peak drug concentration and the MIC of the pathogen) (10–13). These antibiotics tend to have relatively long PAEs, and drug activity tends to persist even after the drug is eliminated from the body. As a result, any temporal relationship between efficacy and the period that the drug concentration remains above the MIC is not observable. Stated another way, the contribution in killing of prolonged exposure of the organism to the antibiotic is relatively small compared with the contribution that high drug concentrations make to the overall killing process. Antibiotics that have concentration-dependent killing generally eradicate the organism quickly (i.e., killing is not time-dependent). These relationships were elucidated by several investigators. For example, Moore and colleagues (14,15) examined the relationship between outcome, concentration achieved in serum, and the MIC for the organism in patients treated with aminoglycosides. In these studies, a significant relationship was found between maximum concentration (C_{max}) and efficacy, and the ratio of C_{max}/MIC and efficacy. A total of 236 patients with facultative gram-negative bacterial infections were studied. The maximal peak concentration was defined as the highest level of all measured values during therapy. The mean peak level was calculated by addition of all peak levels obtained and dividing the sum by the total number of levels acquired. Of the 188 patients who had a clinical response to aminoglycoside therapy, the C_{max}/MIC average value was 8.5 ± 5.0; the 48 nonresponders had a ratio value of 5.5 ± 4.6 ($p <$ 0.00001). The group average values for the mean peak/MIC ratio were 6.6 ± 3.9 and 4.6 ± 3.6 ($p <$ 0.0001), respectively. In a study by Keating and associates (16), response rates of 57%, 67%, and 85%, respectively, were observed in neutropenic patients when the mean serum aminoglycoside concentration to MIC ratios were 1 to 4, 4 to 10, and greater than 10. These results were also similar to the finding described by Klastersky and colleagues (17). In this study of 211 cancer patients, the investigators observed that when the peak titer of bacteriostatic activity in serum was greater than 1:8, the infection was cured in more than 80% of patients.

Although not identical to the C_{max}/MIC ratio, the peak serum bacteriostatic titer is an indirect assessment of this ratio because the same parameters of maximum antibiotic concentration and organism sensitivity are required, in part, to determine the serum titer activity. These studies indicate the useful application of the peak aminoglycoside concentration to MIC ratio as a method of enhancing therapeutic outcome. By obtaining C_{max}/MIC ratios of at least 4:1 (ideally 8:1 to 12:1), clinicians can potentially augment antibacterial activity and the clinical response to therapy. In an attempt to maximize this peak:MIC ratio, the concept of once-daily aminoglycosides has evolved (18).

Currently, it appears that nephrotoxicity and ototoxicity can be reduced by employing this methodology because it results in less tissue accumulation. It should be remembered that toxicity correlates with tissue accumulation rather than with peak serum concentration. The major utility of measuring peak serum concentrations has been to determine the adequacy of dose; however, the single-daily dose should produce the desired peak:MIC ratios for susceptible pathogens. Thus, with this new method of administration, there appears little, if any, need to measure peak levels (Figure 14.3).

We have designed a once-daily aminoglycoside regimen based on the previously described pharmacodynamic principles of these agents. This method differs from that previously cited because it was developed using these principles and did not simply combine the conventional dose (mg/kg/dose) into one daily injection. Because amino-glycosides have been shown to have an optimal response rate when the peak:MIC ratio is approximately 10:1, our regimen is designed to achieve this ratio using the median MIC of the most troublesome organism (*Pseudomonas aeruginosa*; median MIC, 2μg/mL). At Hartford Hospital, we employed a 7-mg/kg dose for aminoglycosides (gentamicin, tobramycin) every 24 hours for patients with normal renal function. In patients with estimated creatinine clearances of less than 60 mL/minute, the dose is fixed at 7 mg/kg and the dosing interval is extended (19). In addition, because it is no longer necessary to obtain conventional peak and trough serum concentrations, we designed a nomogram to evaluate a single random concentration and to make subsequent dosing interval adjustments as required (Figure 14.4).

This discussion relates to the situation when the antibiotic concentration (dose) is sufficiently high enough to result in a favorable serum peak to MIC ratio. Under these conditions, peak concentration provides the greatest contribution to the killing process,

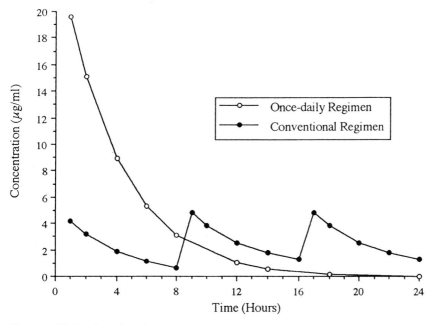

Figure 14.3 Simulated concentration versus time profile for once-daily (7 mg/kg every 24 hr) and conventional (1.5 mg/kg every 8 hr) regimens in patients with normal renal function.

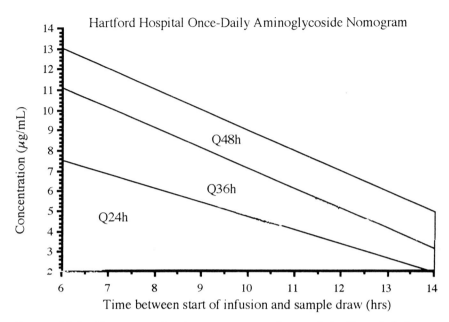

Figure 14.4 Nomogram for the accessment of once-daily (7 mg/kg) dosing.

and the statement that the important pharmacodynamic parameter to monitor is the peak:MIC ratio is essentially correct. Aminoglycosides allow dosing so that these conditions exist, which is not always the case with quinolones. When these drugs are employed in their usual clinical doses and targeted against very sensitive organisms, the peak to MIC ratio is sufficiently large so that the peak concentration is the major contributor to the killing of the organism. The time above the MIC, as in the case with aminoglycoside, is of less or negligible importance. For organisms that have higher MICs (e.g., *Pseudomonas*), the peak:MIC ratio may not be high (e.g., 2). Ideally, the dose should be increased to maximize this ratio; however, toxicity considerations prevent this increase. Under these conditions, killing will not be rapid, and the relative importance of the peak concentration to the entire process will be diminished. Likewise, slower continued killing due to lingering concentration above the MIC will become more important in organism eradication. What is described then is a situation where both peak concentration and time above the MIC are important. Integrating both these concepts is representative of the AUC because the AUC is a product of concentration and time. For this reason, it can be stated that when one cannot achieve a suitable peak:MIC ratio, then the AUC is the predominant pharmacokinetic parameter that correlates with micro-organism eradication for antibiotics with concentration-dependent killing properties.

Dosing strategies for aminoglycosides and quinolones should be to use the highest possible dose provided toxicity does not occur. This approach maximizes efficacy. In the case of quinolones when the dose cannot be increased sufficiently to yield a peak:MIC ratio of 8:1 to 10:1, then steps to increase the time above the MIC should be taken. This increase can be accomplished by using a longer half-life quinolone or by shortening the dosing interval i.e., administering an additional dose per day (1-gram every 8 hours rather than every 12 hours) whichev eventually increases the daily AUC.

One additional issue should be briefly mentioned regarding quinolones: At low concentrations, a bacteriostatic effect is observed, whereas at high concentrations, activity becomes bactericidal. Once the optimal bactericidal effect is reached, further increases in concentration result in a decrease in the bactericidal activity. This effect is believed to be due to the inhibition of RNA synthesis, which is known to preclude the bactericidal effect (20). In addition to maximizing the bactericidal activity of aminoglycosides and fluoroquinolones by optimizing the peak:MIC ratio, this resultant ratio may also prevent the emergence of resistant organisms (21).

CONCENTRATION-INDEPENDENT KILLING

Unlike aminoglycosides and fluoroquinolones, beta-lactams and vancomycin appear to have a very different bacterial killing profile. These latter agents exhibit concentration-independent (or time-dependent) killing (7,8,13,22). Apparently, once the concentration exceeds a critical value (i.e., MIC of the pathogen), killing proceeds at a zero order rate, and increasing drug concentration does not result in a proportional change in the microbial death rate. Under these conditions, a correlation between peak serum concentration is not expected. Stated another way, the contribution of the prolonged exposure to drug contributes greatly to eradication of the organism, whereas the effect of concentration is minimal. For these reasons, the predominant finding is that beta-lactam antibiotic bacterial activity in the body seems to correlate best with the time>MIC. If the dosing interval for these drugs is frequent in relationship to their half-lives, then the time>MIC will be maximized, as will bacterial eradication. As the antibiotic free period is increased, eventually a point will be reached where efficacy will begin to diminish (i.e., the dosing interval will be long relative to the time the drug concentration remains above the MIC). Unfortunately, there are little data available to clarify how long within a dosing interval the drug concentrations need to exceed the MIC of the organism. This uncertainty is probably due, in part, to the fact that traditional dosing of beta-lactam antibiotics has been in excess of what is actually required to achieve a desirable result. Schentag and colleagues (23) also found a significant relationship between the time beta-lactams remained above the MIC and the time to bacterial eradication in patients with nosocomial pneumonia.

Because beta-lactam antibiotic effectiveness is related to the time the serum concentration remains above some critical concentration, a dosing strategy for these antibiotics is to increase the serum/tissue concentrations above the MIC. Clinicians can achieve this goal by (a) using frequent dosing of the antibiotic, (b) increasing the dose of the antibiotic, (c) using an antibiotic with a long half-life, or (d) administer the antibiotic by continuous infusion. In today's economy, options a and b are generally not acceptable because they tend to unnecessarily increase the cost of therapy. In addition, increasing the dose of the beta-lactam is generally inefficient. For example, Figure 14.5 illustrates the concentration time profile for ceftazidime after a 1- or 2- gram dose.

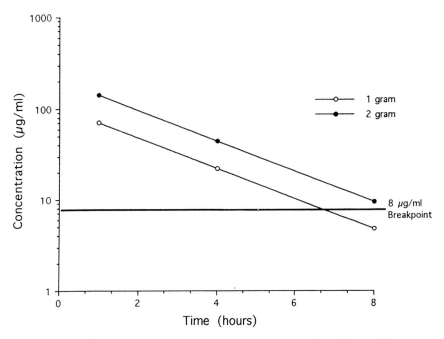

Figure 14.5 Simulated concentration versus time profile of 1 and 2 gram intravenous bolus doses of ceftazidime.

The 1-gram dose yields a time>MIC of 6.6 hours. Doubling the dose increases the time>MIC to 8.6 hours, a 30% increase. However, there is a 100% increase in the peak (not needed for efficacy), with its concurrent risk of increased side effects. There is also a 100% increase in cost. Clearly, this is not an efficient way to increase the time>MIC. Option c accomplishes the goal of maximizing the time>MIC; however, one must switch to an antibiotic with a long half-life, which may possibly result in the use of a more costly agent. Table 14.1 lists a number of formulary conversions that were successful at Hartford Hospital (i.e., resulted in the same clinical outcome using reduced dosage).

The last option (administration of the agent by continuous infusion) appears to satisfy the criteria for optimization of antibacterial activity from this class of agents because the infusion rate could be adjusted to maintain the concentration above the MIC for the entire treatment period. In addition, this mode of administration may result in a more cost-effective method of drug delivery because total daily dose (g/day), pharmacist preparation time, and nursing time would be reduced. Twenty to 40 years ago, the predominant method of dosing beta-lactam antibiotics to hospitalized patients was by constant infusion (intravenous drip).

For antibiotics with concentration-independent killing, the often-mentioned advice in package inserts that antibiotics should be given in larger and more frequent doses for infections considered to be "severe" as compared with those that are deemed "mild," makes little if any pharmacodynamic or pharmacoeconomic sense, unless the site of infection exists in a body area (e.g., cerebrospinal fluid) where the higher serum levels

Table 14.1. Formulary decisions based on the strategy of increasing the Time > MIC

Original Regimen			New Regimen		
Cephalothin,	1 gram every	4 hr	Cefazolin,	1 gram every	8 hr
Cefazolin,	1 gram every	6 hr	Cefazolin,	1 gram every	8 hr
Cefoxitin,	1–2 grams every	6 hr	Cefotetan,	1–2 grams every	12 hr
Cefamandole,	1 gram every	6 hr	Cefuroxime,	0.75 grams every	8 hr
Cefuroxime,	1.5 grams every	8 hr	Cefuroxime,	0.75 grams every	8 hr
Vancomycin,	1 gram every	6–8 hr	Vancomycin,	1 gram every	12 hr
Mezlocillin,	3 grams every	4 hr	Mezlocillin,	5 grams every	8 hr
Piperacillin,	3 grams every	4 hr	Piperacillin,	4 grams every	8 hr
Ceftazidime,	3 grams every	8 hr	Ceftazidime,	1 gram every	8 hr

may improve drug penetration. In fact, the excessively high levels should be viewed as "wasted" antibiotic, leading to unnecessary expenses through both higher acquisition costs and greater utilization of intravenous equipment and personnel, and also increasing the chances for adverse drug reactions and superinfection with multiple-antibiotic–resistant pathogens. Many of the newer expanded-spectrum beta-lactams (e.g., cefotaxime, ceftriaxone, ceftazadime) exhibit intense microbiologic activity against many gram-negative bacteria and, as a result, can often be administered in a low and infrequent dosing method. Historically, this use is even true for aqueous procaine penicillin, which in the late 1940s was given at a small 300,000 U intramuscular dose every 12 hours and still was highly efficacious in the treatment of pneumococcal pneumonia. This excellent clinical outcome was not unexpected because this dose maintains levels above its usual MIC for *S. pneumoniae* (0.02 μg/mL) for the entire dosing period. Because the time above the MIC in any dosing interval is the same whether one employs the low and infrequent dose of aqueous procaine penicillin or millions of units of penicillin given frequently and intravenously, there should be no significant differences in clinical outcome, which has been the clinical observation for decades.

It should also be remembered that the high serum levels of beta-lactam antibiotics do not drive more drug intracellularly or into "tissue," because these agents exhibit insignificant intracellular penetration. The higher serum levels merely result in similar levels in the interstitial fluid that surrounds the cells, and the same pharmacodynamic concepts that apply to serum levels also apply to the interstitial concentrations. Although there typically exists a slight lag before interstitial and serum levels attain equilibrium, there is a close parallel with beta-lactam antibiotics between drug concentration in the serum and interstitial fluid compartments. Because we are slowly coming to the realization that maximizing t > MIC is currently probably the best dosing strategy for these drugs, it is questionable whether we have made significant progress in the interim. However, considerable progress has been made with respect to the knowledge concerning pharmacodynamic interactions and their importance in dosing β-lactam since the 1940's selection. Although significant progress has been made, further research is required to characterize these pharmacodynamic interactions for a number of other important antimicrobials (i.e., clindamycin, tetracyclines, macrolides).

Despite the major constraints focused on reducing health care costs, there are many ways to reduce further cost while still providing a high standard of care for the patients. One important way is to employ scientifically sound methods of dosing antibiotics, because this type of dosing maximizes the killing of bacteria, minimizes adverse drug reactions, and accomplishes these goals with the least amount of drug and burden on expenses and ancillary services.

REFERENCES

1 **Tomasz A.** Penicillin binding protein: their role in beta lactam action and resistance. In: Root RK, Sande MA, eds. *Contemporary Issues in Infectious Diseases, New Dimensions in Antimicrobial Therapy, vol. 1.* New York: Churchill Livingstone, 1984:1–16.

2 **Bryan LE.** Mechanism of action of aminoglycoside antibiotics. In: Root RK, Sande MA, eds. *Contemporary Issues in Infectious Diseases, New Dimensions in Antimicrobial Therapy, vol. 1.* New York: Churchill Livingstone, 1984:17–36.

3 **Gibbons RJ.** Bacterial attachment to host tissues. In: Gorbach SH, Bartlett JG, Blacklow NR, eds. *Infectious Diseases.* Philadelphia: W.B. Saunders, 1992:7–17.

4 **Zhanel GG, Hoban DJ, Harding GKM.** The postantibiotic effect: a review of in-vitro and in-vivo data. *Ann Pharmacother* 1991;25:153–163.

5 **Craig WA, Gudmundsson S.** The postantibiotic effect. In: Lorian V, ed. *Antibiotics in Laboratory Medicine, ed 2.* Baltimore: Williams & Wilkins, 1986:515–536.

6 **Leggett JE, Ebert S, Fantin B, Craig WA.** Comparative dose-effect relations at several dosing interval for beta-lactam, aminoglycoside and quinolone antibiotics against gram-negative bacilli in murine thigh-infection and pneumonitis models. *Scand J Infect Dis* 1991;74:179–184.

7 **Roosendaal R, Bakker-Woudenberg IAJM, van den Berghe JC, Michel MF.** Therapeutic efficacy of continuous versus intermittent administration of ceftazidime in an experimental Klebsiella pneumoniae pneumonia in rats. *J Infect Dis* 1985;156:373–378.

8 **Ackerman BH, Vannier AM, Eudy EB.** Analysis of vancomycin time-kill studies with Staphylococci species by using a curve stripping program to describe the relationship between concentration and phamacodynamic response. *Antimicrob Agents Chemother* 1992;36:1766–1769.

9 **Dudley MN.** Pharmacodynamics and pharmacokinetics of antibiotics with special reference to the fluoroquinolones. *Am J Med* 1991;91(suppl 6A):45S–50S.

10 **Begg EJ, Peddie BA, Chambers ST, Boswell DR.** Comparison of gentamicin dosing regimens using an in-vitro model. *J Antimicrob Chemother* 1992;29:427–433.

11 **Drusano GL, Johnson DE, Rosen M, Standiford HC.** Pharmacodynamics of a fluoroquinolone antimicrobial agent in a neutropenic rat model of Pseudomonas sepsis. *Antimicrob Agents Chemother* 1993;37:483–490.

12 **Davis BD.** Mechanism of the bactericidal action of the aminoglycosides. *Microbiol Rev* 1987;51:341–350.

13 **Levison ME, Bush LM.** Pharmacodynamics of antimicrobial agents: bactericidal and postantibiotic effects. *Infect Dis Clin North Am* 1989;3:415–421.

14 **Moore RD, Smith CR, Lietman PS.** The association of aminoglycoside plasma levels with mortality in patients with gram-negative bacteremia. *J Infect Dis* 1984;149:443–448.

15 **Moore RD, Lietman PS, Smith CR.** Clinical response to aminoglycoside therapy: importance of the ratio of peak concentration to minimal inhibitory concentration. *J Infect Dis* 1987;155:93–99.

16 **Keating MF, Bodey GP, Valdivieso M, et al.** A randomized comparative trial of three aminoglycosides-comparison of continuous infusions of gentamicin, amikacin and sisomicin combined with carbenicillin in the treatment of infections in neutropenic patients with malignancies. *Medicine* 1979;58:159–170.

17 **Klastersky J, Daneau D, Swings G, Weerts D.** Antibacterial activity in serum and urine as a therapeutic guide in bacterial infections. *J Infect Dis* 1974;129:187–193.

18 **Gilbert DN.** Once-daily aminoglycoside therapy. *Antimicrob Agents Chemother* 1991;35:399–405.

19 **Nicolau DP, Quintiliani R, Nightingale CH.**

Once-daily aminoglycosides. *Conn Med* 1992; 56:561–563.

20 **Smith JT.** The mode of action of 4-quinolones and possible mechanisms of resistance. *J Antimicrob Chemother* 1986;18(suppl D):9–21.

21 **Blaser J, Stone BB, Groner MC, Zinner SH.** Comparative study with enoxacin and netilmicin in a pharmacodynamic model to determine importance of ratio of antibiotic peak concentration to MIC for bactericidal activity and the emergence of resistance. *Antimicrob Agents Chemother* 1987;31:1054–1060.

22 **Ebert SC, Craig WA.** Pharmacodynamic properties of antibiotics: application to drug monitoring and dosage regimen design. *Infect Control Hosp Epidemiol* 1990;11:319–326.

23 **Schentag JJ, Smith IL, Swanson DJ, et al.** Role for dual individualization with cefmenoxime. *Am J Med* 1984;77(suppl 6A):43–50.

Ethical issues in infectious diseases

JEROME H. KIM
DAVID T. DURACK

INTRODUCTION

The practice of medicine raises ethical issues at every turn. Thoughtful physicians recognize, debate and agonize over them. Increasing concern with medical ethics over the past 2 decades has provided opportunities for health care providers to interact with ethical consultants on the wards of major medical centers. Changes in societal views on privacy, patient autonomy, the doctor-patient relationship, and death have had extensive implications for the conduct of physicians and have made evaluation and resolution of ethical problems more difficult. The Hippocratic Oath has for centuries provided physicians with a succinct set of ethical guidelines, but the increasing complexity of medicine demands continual extension and reconsideration of the Oath, which is now only one of many bases for our personal and communal codes of ethics. This evolution of principles and practice provides the *raison d'etre* for vigorous departments of medical ethics and busy committees within hospitals, universities, and professional associations. Books, essays, and guidelines proliferate, at the risk of diluting or numbing our capacity to keep up as we should with these important issues.

Most of the major ethical issues concern medicine and society at large; they are not limited to specialties or subspecialties. Certain questions, however, are more likely to confront some physicians than others. For example, the thicket of ethical issues that has sprouted around surrogate motherhood is likely to entangle obstetricians or the infertility specialists. Infectious disease specialists are likely to encounter thorny questions involving persons carrying communicable diseases, (e.g., acquired immunodeficiency syndrome [AIDS]), conflicts of interest arising from ownership of agencies administering antimicrobials at home, or interactions with antibiotic manufacturers, including conduct of clinical trials of antimicrobial agents. Here we discuss models of physician behavior as the basis for ethical decision-making and introduce a systematic approach to identification, prioritization, and interpretation of the issues in complex ethical situations. We then discuss several cases involving problems that may arise in the clinical practice of infectious diseases.

FOUNDATIONS OF MEDICAL ETHICS

Morality is the foundation of ethical behavior. From a set of moral principles, a system of ethics can be derived. Different principles would result in different ethical models. Three prominent paradigms in medical ethics are the paternalistic model, the duty model, and the contractual model.

The paternalistic model

The first Code of Ethics (1847) of the American Medical Association (AMA) enjoined practitioners to "unite tenderness with firmness, and condescension with authority . . . to inspire the minds of their patients with gratitude, respect, and confidence." The paternalistic model places the physician in a "good parent" role, providing care, protection, counselling, and advocacy. In this model, the physician retains the decision-making authority that comes naturally to parents, whereas the patient assumes a dependent and relatively inactive role in this model.

In the United States, evolution of societal views of individual rights and superimposition of judicial constraints have made the paternalistic paradigm obsolete. It became too difficult to reconcile the father-figure role with current notions of informed consent, patient autonomy, patient activism and women's rights. The paternalistic model may survive or even thrive in societies where the physician's image remains elevated.

The duty model

Under this ethic, physicians perform services as a positive responsibility, an obligation to society, rooted in tradition and reinforced by training and education. Accomplishment of these responsibilities is a virtue. Failure to carry them out may result in loss of self-esteem, censure by the self-regulating professional society, or even legal intervention.

The duty model is attractive because it takes into account the historical and professional authority of healers in society. This is the Oslerian view of medicine as a noble profession, laden with dedication, compassion, and hard work. Physicians are by training inclined to act, and by tradition sworn to act in the best interests of the patient. The duty model is consistent with the traditional strong bonding between physician and patient. The complexity of their interactions exceeds the narrower confines of the contractual model. The duty model can be easily extended to include respect for the rights of the patient to informed consent, autonomy, and privacy.

Opposition to the duty model centers around the subservient role of the patient in what should be a balanced relationship, as well as intuitive discomfort with the somewhat elitist, militaristic, and absolutist phraseology associated with its precepts. Zuger and Miles have written: ". . . our ethical language differs enormously from past centuries . . . nor do the soldierly metaphors of the past speak clearly to our time" (1).

The contractual model

The contractual model is preferred by the legal system. An unwritten contract exists between doctor and patient, based on payment of fees in return for services. Failure to adequately provide needed services is a breach of the contract, incurring liability. In a society increasingly defined by tort law, the specific delineation of obligations and establishment of clear accountability seems easily justifiable.

Some disadvantages of the contractual system arise from its downgrading of the importance of positive human and emotional aspects of the traditional doctor-patient relationship, inability of the parties to derive generally applicable rules, and the capricious nature of our system of legal redress for medical malpractice.

No single system of medical ethics controls our decision-making behavior. Elements of all three models, and more, are combined in current practice.

APPROACH TO ETHICAL ISSUES

Approached systematically, most situations can be distilled into distinct moral issues. These issues may be in opposition. Prioritization of the issues by ethical principles, cultural norms, legal considerations, or personal attitudes permits identification of potential courses of action. It is a source of frustration for many that ethics usually cannot define which of these is the "right answer." However, we must accept that this definition is impossible because ethics do not deal in absolutes, but in ideas and relationships. Its most effective application is to define, clarify, and prioritize the issues. This approach permits consumers—physicians, patients, and their representatives—to participate in discussions of ethical issues without necessarily having any intimate knowledge of the philosophy of ethics (deontology). This approach in turn facilitates ethical decision-making in clinical practice.

There are four aspects to evaluation of an ethical dilemma: *identification, interrelation, implication, and intervention.*

Identification involves delineation of the principal issues in an ethical problem. For instance, the ethics of abortion involve the right of the fetus to life and the right of the woman to control her body and reproductive processes. This important example illustrates how the primacy of one or another moral position leads to dramatically different conclusions and actions.

Four commonly recognized ethical standards are beneficence, nonmaleficence, patient autonomy, and justice. With regard to abortion, the right of a fetus to life might be advocated on the basis of both justice and nonmaleficence.

Interrelation seeks to clarify the relationships between issues and to rank them in order of importance. Defining the relationships between conflicting or diverging issues may sometimes allow compromise along lines not apparent at first glance. For example, there is much controversy over the advisability of operative intervention in the case of lethal but surgically correctable malformations in neonates with serious chromosomal abnormalities. The issues here are: the right of the infant to life (justice); the right of the infant to life of reasonable quality (beneficence); the right of the infant to appropriate medical care (nonmaleficence); the rights of parents to make decisions in the best interest of their children (autonomy); and the interest of the state in protecting the lives of all its citizens (justice). Although resolution of these complex problems could be abdicated to the judicial system, recent emphasis on quality of life and the central responsibility that parents bear as a result of any decision favor a determination by the parents. They could make the decision after counselling by physicians, clergy, and social workers, allowing a reasonable compromise between the rights of an afflicted newborn and the interests of society.

Implication is an assessment of the consequences of actions based on ethical precepts. For example, concern over conflict of interest might lead to a ban on sponsorship of lecturers by pharmaceutical companies. The implication of this moral decision could be the loss of dissemination of useful medical information to health care providers, possibly to the disadvantage of patients. The Federal ban on the receipt of honoraria by employees of the government, also intended to avoid conflict of interest, has negative implications for recruitment and retention of scientists and physicians. Clearly, understanding the implications of an ethical decision requires some prior knowledge of the courses of action that might result.

Intervention involves application of the ethical analysis to the situation in question, which could take the form of action or inaction. Examples of interventions are taking a decision to transplant a liver into a patient with alcoholic cirrhosis, replacing a heart valve in an intravenous drug addict, switching off ventilatory support, or acceding to a request that no extraordinary means be used to sustain life.

It may be helpful to go through the exercise of applying these "four Is" to the analysis of several cases that might arise in the practice of infectious disease.

Case reports

Case 1 A 46-year-old homeless man lives an active and independent life on the streets of New York City. One night in a shelter for the homeless, he coughs up some blood. The next morning he is sent to an Emergency Room where a chest radiograph shows upper lobe cavities. Sputum smears are heavily positive for acid-fast bacteria. He is referred to a public Infectious Diseases Clinic, where he is found to be human immunodeficiency virus (HIV)–negative and is started on supervised treatment. One month later, despite being compliant with treatment, he has a persistent, productive cough with smear-positive sputum. The organism is now known to be a multidrug-resistant strain of *Mycobacterium tuberculosis* (MDRTB). He could infect many others. He says that he is willing to continue treatment but adamantly refuses hospitalization, saying that if any attempt is made to commit him he will disappear and not return for further treatment. He seems to be sane and competent.

The situation is difficult. Ethical, legal, and practical aspects all must be weighed. The ethical conflict centers on whose rights come first—the patient's or society's? The legal question is, *can* he be committed to inpatient care? If so, the practical question is, how can we compel him to enter the hospital and stay there.

Patients' rights are fundamental to codes of medical ethics. Confidentiality, privacy, freedom of choice between alternative treatments, informed consent, and redress for harm due to negligence are rights that are transgressed easily and often. Such rights must be scrupulously protected, even at the cost of allowing patients to make decisions that seem unwise or even self-injurious. Yet, there are limits. Most societies have "set their canon 'gainst self-slaughter," indicating that the patient's right to act self-destructively is not absolute. Nevertheless, an individual may refuse treatment under most circumstances. Two possible exceptions exist: when the patient is mentally ill or incompetent, and when there is danger to others. For this patient with MDRTB, does the clear and present danger to society outweigh the patient's rights and freedoms?

Another legal issue is whether his endangerment of others, if he refuses isolation, constitutes a crime. The answers may vary from state to state, according to local laws. In New York, where this patient lives, commitment for tuberculosis is sanctioned. To achieve this commitment, documentation is required, after which a police officer can arrest a resisting patient and take him or her to a hospital. The question of criminality is more murky. In at least two recent cases, an HIV-positive person was convicted of attempted murder or manslaughter for actively exposing others to HIV infection. Our MDRTB patient, who probably represents a greater danger to others than these rare psychopaths, is not willfully trying to infect others. He is not yet a criminal, but could become one if he resists a legitimate commitment order.

In the past, fear of contagion has often led to ostracism, exclusion from social contact, or worse. Leper colonies, pest houses, quarantine stations, and tuberculosis sanatoria come to mind. Some of these infection control measures were logical or effective; many were not. In any case, it seems to be established that society may in its own interest violate the wishes of individuals, presumably based on the principle of the greatest good for the greatest number. Patients may harm themselves, up to a point, but may be coerced to prevent them harming others. The obvious problem is, where do we draw the line between advising and arresting the patient? We do not incarcerate patients with influenza, even though the infection is highly communicable and kills far more people in the United States in an average year than tuberculosis. Application of society's right to protect itself from infectious diseases, we must concede, often has been arbitrary and inconsistent. Nevertheless, because this patient's MDRTB could infect and kill unwitting passers-by, we conclude that from an ethical point of view, he may be committed. From a public health point of view, he should be committed.

Case 2 A 35-year-old woman who has used illicit injected drugs for many years has had three episodes of infective endocarditis and has undergone valve replacement. She now has a paravalvular leak suspected to be associated with an intracardiac abscess, and heart failure has developed. Valve replacement surgery is clearly indicated. The patient now requests surgery, saying that she will stop using illicit drugs. Should this patient be offered valve replacement?

The indication for surgical intervention is clear. Under normal circumstances, surgery would be offered. She has no relative contraindications, such as HIV infection. The patient has a right to appropriate, efficacious medical care, and the physician has an obligation under the duty model to provide it if possible.

There is, however, overwhelming evidence that her pattern of antisocial, self-destructive behavior will continue. She is a proven liar who has shown no evidence of trying to stop injected drug use in the past. She has proven on many occasions to be unreliable, manipulative, deceptive, and noncompliant with medical advice and treatment. For example, during the last episode of endocarditis, she used illicit drugs while in the hospital and signed out against medical advice after only 8 days of treatment. She has repeatedly refused to enter, or dropped out of, drug rehabilitation programs. She is a prostitute who is frequently in trouble with the law and has visited emergency rooms many times for overdoses and other drug-related problems. She has no remaining peripheral veins for antibiotic treatment, and for at least 4 weeks after surgery will require a central venous access line that she likely will use for injection of illicit drugs. The surgery will be very expensive and probably futile because she will infect her new prosthetic valve within a short time.

The consumption of health care resources for little long-term benefit seems neither right nor practical. Her choice to continue the abuse of injectible drugs is an extreme manifestation of her right to autonomy and self-determination, even if this includes self-destructive behavior. The interests of society, in this case to limit costs and to control criminal behavior, can be opposed to her rights of autonomy and appropriate care. The ethics of the Hippocratic era, when many fewer effective treatments were available, would have permitted inactivity in hopeless cases when good judgment determined that further treatment would be ineffective.

A study of the implications of each right is instructive. If surgery is not performed, her condition will worsen and she will die. If surgery is performed, she will most likely be cured but will likely return with a new episode of prosthetic valve endocarditis later. If the usual criteria for valve replacement were followed, she could, in the course of her lifetime, receive multiple prosthetic valves. Society has, however, stated its clear opposition to her behavior and its aversion to her continued abuse of its medical beneficence. The final implication of her right to autonomy is the assumption of personal responsibility. Within the mandates of society, she may be held accountable for her choice.

The implications of her right to choose hold her answerable for the consequences. Society, represented by the physicians managing her case, must decide at what level accountability should be required. Many physicians would not offer this patient valve replacement, citing futility or conservation of costly resources for "more deserving" patients. Others would replace her valve, pointing out that our medical system frequently lavishes expensive and often futile treatment on patients with other terminal or self-induced diseases. Intervention in this case is likely to be limited to conservative treatment. Her infection and heart failure can be treated medically, even though her prognosis is poor and early death is likely.

Case 3   A 55-year-old man who contracted HIV infection 8 years ago as a result of blood transfusions during a previous admission for trauma presents with severe angina. He continues to have angina despite treatment, and coronary arteriograms reveal total occlusion of the left main coronary artery with minimal backfill. Coronary bypass surgery is indicated, but the attending cardiothoracic surgeon declines to operate, citing the patient's HIV status.

On the side of the patient the issues involved include: the right to freedom from discrimination (justice); the right to accessible, effective care (nonmaleficence); and the right to choose a doctor (autonomy). The surgeon can claim, conversely, that they should be able to operate without undue risk to self, the right to refuse to enter any therapeutic relationship, and the right to refer patients to other physicians for personal or unstated reasons. Within the contractual model of behavior this decision is acceptable, so long as the patient's condition is not an emergency and would not be materially worsened by delay. Contracts imply mutual consent, and refusal to enter the contract obviates any claim by the other party. Within the duty model, these issues are clearly defined. The obligation to any infected patient would be assumed despite any potential personal hazard. The current AMA Code of Ethics prohibits rejection of patients on the grounds of personal risk to the care provider, which is consistent with the original (1847) AMA Code of Ethics. Historically, many physicians deserted their patients during times of pestilence. In contrast, Athenian physicians died while caring for plague victims in 430 BC, as did Ricketts and Prowazeki while studying typhus in the early 20th century. Willingness to care for patients in the face of personal risk has been characteristic of the profession in Europe and America since the mid-nineteenth century. Today, this ethic may be endangered. The open rejection described and the results of confidential polls both indicate that currently there may be significant barriers to performance of surgery on HIV-infected patients.

We discuss the implications of this problem from the position taken by the duty model because the contractual model permits the refusal to initiate a contract. The aggregate implication of the patient's rights would require physicians to care for infected patients. There is a finite risk of infection from exposure to the blood of HIV-infected individuals. The average surgeon is highly exposed to blood and body fluids, and certain subspecialists are likely to suffer needlesticks. The finding that prior knowledge of HIV status does not necessarily decrease percutaneous exposure to blood increases the reluctance of some surgeons to operate on HIV-positive patients regardless of the disclosure of serologic status. The economic impact of HIV on an infected surgeon can be substantial; the refusal of several hospitals to allow HIV-infected surgeons to operate further complicates the situation.

In application, the rigid demands of the duty model are mitigated by several circumstances. First, the ethical standards are voluntary, and moral authority is seldom exercised. Second, despite the rule that patients must not be deserted, substitution of another health care provider is acceptable in nonemergency cases. Third, the growing popularity of the contractual model—with its prerequisite, mutual consent—provides a ready mechanism for an unwilling physician to avoid what some would define as a duty. Under the contractual model, if a substitute surgeon who is willing to operate can be identified, the ethical dilemma could be circumvented.

Case 4   A 24-year-old, HIV-infected, asymptomatic man, with a CD4 count of 550, is participating in a single-product trial of a new, non-nucleoside reverse transcriptase inhibitor. An increase in his mean corpuscular volume to 105 fL triggers a screening test for zidovudine, which is positive. The patient is confronted. He admits to the use of zidovudine, D4T, and a host of other nontraditional medications that he obtains from a buyers' club. He is told that, in accordance with protocol guidelines, he will be discontinued from the study. He demands to be kept in the trial, saying that he knows that others in the trial are similarly violating the protocol. He notes that several friends have refused to enter trials of new drugs because of constraints imposed by research objectives, the inconvenience of clinic visits, and the feeling that the collection of information has priority over the prolongation of life.

The conduct of basic and clinical research in HIV has been dramatically affected by public advocacy and patient activism. The traditional model of scientific-clinical investigation has been accelerated. FDA approval of drugs has become more rapid; a parallel track that affords infected patients unprecedented access to investigational drugs has been created. Patient activism has led to the creation of buyers clubs that function in an unregulated fashion, providing investigational drugs and nonallopathic medications, from traditional oriental remedies to new age nostrums. Activists have chided the biomedical community for slow progress in developing effective treatments for HIV infection, criticizing the emphasis on basic science at the expense of clinical therapeutics. Under signs such as "Silence = Death," activist presence at AIDS conferences has become formidable.

From the patient's perspective, the right to autonomy guarantees free choice between medical therapies, whereas the right to life includes the right to obtain and use investigational drugs prior to release. By extension, the "slow" pace of medical research permits the aggressive, extramedical pursuit of novel therapies. The perceived ambivalence of the government and basic scientists to the plight of HIV-infected patients justifies AIDS activism. From the investigator's point of view, protocol violations that eliminate the patient from the study invalidates important data. High drop-out rates might prevent establishment of significant differences. In a more general sense, surreptitious use of other reverse transcriptase inhibitors devastates the validity of the collected scientific information—from CD4 counts, p24 antigen levels, and onset of AIDS, to molecular analyses of reverse transcriptase resistance. It interferes with the ethical principle of beneficence; no good can come out of a study that has been invalidated by protocol violations. To a lesser extent, the nonmaleficence principle is also violated. The investigator cannot anticipate the effect of interactions with other antiretroviral drugs; a negative impact on survival might be masked by improvement induced by surreptitious agents. Pooling of investigational drugs among participants in randomized studies, availability of investigational drugs from underground sources, and abandonment of randomization diminish the ability of medical research to answer the critical questions of HIV infection and pathogenesis. Without knowledge of the effects, beneficial and untoward, of new pharmaceuticals, prescribing physicians are violating two fundamental Hippocratic ethics: ". . . to help, or at least, to do no harm." Ethicists have debated the relative importance of beneficence (doing good) versus avoiding maleficence (*primum non nocere*), but neither may be accomplished if the scientific method is compromised by intimidation.

The implications of patient activism are manifest in the proliferation of buyers' clubs and the availability of many unconventional treatments. Such therapies from rectal ozone to intravenous infusion of nonsterile crude vegetable decoctions, have sometimes been cruel, expensive, and unscrupulous deceptions. While recognizing that the right to individual autonomy does allow self-destructive behavior, the medical community has a duty to protect unsuspecting patients, whenever possible, from dangerous and ineffective medications. The failure of clinical trials because of inability to recruit an adequate number of patients or excessive patient drop-out benefits neither the understanding of HIV nor HIV-infected patients.

Within the context of current law, the sale of unlicensed medications in the United

States is illegal. Physicians have a responsibility to discourage the use of ineffective or dangerous therapies by their patients. Clinical trials should answer the critical questions of HIV therapy definitively, expeditiously, and compassionately. In common with patients and investigators, society at large also has a vital interest in the successful conduct of such studies. Patients should recognize that progress in medical research never seems rapid enough for the afflicted, but that progress can only really be made with a thorough understanding of the disease and useful demonstrations of therapeutic efficacy. This patient should be dropped from the trial, in favor of others who are willing to adhere to the agreed-upon protocol.

SUMMARY

Ethical behavior is an essential component of professional life. Developments in medical science continually test society's concepts of right and wrong, of virtue and morality. Ethical conflicts will be played out in public with greater frequency and intensity. Physicians will be challenged to maintain high standards of ethical conduct despite the pressures that personal preference, society, and government may exert. We do not present neat solutions to ethical conflicts, but we describe a framework for understanding models of physician behavior and outline an approach to the analysis of problems.

ACKNOWLEDGMENT

The opinions expressed herein are those of the authors and should not be construed to reflect the views of the Department of Defense, Department of the Air Force, Department of the Army, or the United States Government.

REFERENCE

1   **Zuger A, Miles SH.** Physicians, AIDS, and occupational risk: historic traditions and ethical obligations. *JAMA* 1987;258:1924–1928.

SUGGESTED READINGS

Ad Hoc Committee on Medical Ethics, American College of Physicians. American College of Physicians Ethics Manual. Part I: history of medical ethics, the physician and the patient, the physician's relationship to other physicians, the physician and society. *Ann Intern Med* 1984;101:129–137.

Ad Hoc Committee on Medical Ethics, American College of Physicians. American College of Physicians Ethics Manual. Part II: research, other ethical issues, recommended reading. *Ann Intern Med* 1984;101:263–274.

Callahan D. Special article. Shattuck Lecture—contemporary biomedical ethics. *N Engl J Med* 1980;302:1229–1233.

Chapman CB. The definition and teaching of the medical ethic. *N Engl J Med* 1979; 301:630–634.

Clouser KD. What is medical ethics? *Ann Intern Med* 1974;80:657–660.

Clouser KD. Medical ethics: some uses, abuses, and limitations. *N Engl J Med* 1975; 293:384–387.

Durack DT, Andriole VT, Hornick RB, Karchmer AW, Marier RL, Quie PG (IDSA Ethics Committee). Infectious Diseases Society of America guidelines for ethical conduct by members and fellows. *J Infect Dis* 1993; 167:S1–S2.

Edelstein L. In: Temkin O, Temkin CL, eds. *Ancient Medicine.* Baltimore: The Johns Hopkins University Press, 1967.

Fischl MA, Olson RM, Follansbee SE, et al. Zalcitabine compared with zidovudine in patients with advanced HIV-1 infection who received previous zidovudine therapy. *Ann Intern Med* 1993;118:762–769.

Gillon R. Medical oaths, declarations, codes. *Br Med J* 1985;290:1194–1195.

Haynes BF. Scientific and social issues of human immunodeficiency virus vaccine development. *Science* 1993;260:1279–1286.

Seedhouse D, Lovett L. *Practical Medical Ethics.* New York: John Wiley & Sons, 1992.

Stolley PD. The hazards of misguided compassion. *Ann Intern Med* 1993;118:822–823.

Index

If the letter "**t**" appears at the end of the page number, it refers to a **table**. If the letter "**f**" appears at the end of the page number, it refers to **a figure or illustration.**

A

Abbott Laboratories Diagnostic Division, 105
Abscesses
  and clarithromycin, 69
  and diabetic foot infection, 5
Access to medical care, 270–273
Acinetobacter species, 5
Acquired immunodeficiency syndrome (AIDS). *See*
  AIDS
Actinomyces, 151
Active transport, 252
Activism, patient, 267, 272–274
Acute-Kare, 174
Acyclovir
  for herpes simplex virus infections, 238
  and human herpesvirus 6 (HHV-6), 164
  with IFN-α, 233
  for varicella-zoster infections, 237
Adenosine triphosphate (ATP), 483
  dependence, 85
Advantage Microbiology Center, 105
Advisory Committee for Immunization Practices
  (of CDC)–, 197
Advisory Committee on Childhood Vaccines,
  201
Aerosols
  blood, 220
  for cytokine delivery, 236
Afipia species, 210, 213, 214
Agar
  Blood, 211, 214, 215

brain-heart infusion, 214
glucose-cysteine blood, 152
heart infusion, 214
tryptic soy, 214
Agar dilution method, 103, 104, 105t
Agrobacterium tumefaciens, 210f
AIDS (acquired immunodeficiency syndrome)
  with bacillary angiomatosis, 205
  and cytokines, 229
  and cytomegalovirus infection, 237
  epidemic, 220, 224
  and human herpesvirus 6 (HHV-6), 159
  medical ethics of, 266
  and Mycobacteriam avium complex, 56, 71–72,
  76
Airborne transmission of pathogens, 170
Alanine aminotransferase, serum (ALT), 123, 124,
  125, 126, 131, 133, 134, 135, 136
Albumin, 60, 136
Alcohol abuse
  and hepatitis C virus infection, 126, 127, 129
  and splenic abscess, 25
  and sporotrichosis, 145
Alpha-proteobacteria, 210, 210f, 214t
ALT. *See* Alanine aminotransferase, serum (ALT)
American Academy of Pediatrics (AAP), 197, 199
American College of Physicians, 197
American Medical Association (AMA), 267
American Type Culture Collection (ATCC), 104,
  114
Amidomethylcoumarin, 111

Amikacin, 150
Amino acids, 229
Aminoglycosides
  for diabetic foot infections, 7, 8
  dosing of, 260, 260f, 261
  for MRSA, 180, 182, 183
  regimen, 259
  resistance to, 116–117
Aminotransferase, serum alanine (ALT), 123, 124,
    125, 126, 131, 133, 134, 135, 136
Ammonium compounds, quarternary, 178
Amodiaquine, 96
Amoxicillin and macrolides, 64, 65, 65t, 74, 75
Amoxicillin-clavulanic acid treatment, 73, 74
Amphotericin B
  for hepatosplenic candidiasis, 43
  for nodular lymphangitis, 146, 148
Ampicillin
  and macrolides, 55, 62, 65, 66, 66t, 74, 75
  resistance, 115
Ampicillin-clindamycin treatment, 10
Ampicillin-sulbactam treatment, 8–9, 10
Amputation
  in diabetic foot infections, 12, 14f, 15, 18, 19
  of lower extremity, 1
Amputation, guillotine, 1, 12, 19
Anaerobic bacteria
  in foot infections, 3, 5, 7
  and macrolides, 64
  and splenic abscess, 28
Anergy, antigen specific, 242
Aneurysm, mycotic, 31
Angiomatosis, bacillary
  agent of, 43
  clinical features, 205–208
  histopathology, 207–208
  and Rochalimaea species, 205–219
Angiomatosis, epithelioid, 206
Angiosarcoma, 207
Anhydroerythromycin, 52
Anopheles, 81, 82f, 83, 83f, 97
  gene alteration, 100
  reduction of vector capacity, 100
  transfection of eggs, 100
Anopheles arabiensis, 89
Anopheles dirus, 92
Anopheles funestus, 89
Anopheles gambiae, 89, 92, 93
Anopheles nili, 92
Anti-e, 232
Antibiograms, 110
Antibiotics
  broad-spectrum non-nephrotoxic

  for foot infections, 7, 8
  delivery of to infected tissues, 2
  duration of treatment
    in foot infections, 10
    in splenic abscess, 42
  empirical therapies for foot infection, 8
  exposure time, 254
  MLS, 184
  for splenic abscess, 40–41
Antibodies
  against CSP, 84
  against hepatitis C virus, 125, 126, 129–130,
    132, 134
  against Staphylococci, 151
Antibodies, maternal
  to human herpesvirus 6 (HHV-6), 161
Anticoagulants, oral, 63
Antigen fluorescence studies, 68
Antigens, fungal, 146
Antihistamines, 181
Antimicrobial activity, factors, 254–255, 255t
Antimicrobial susceptibility testing, 103–119
Antimicrobial susceptibility testing systems, rapid
  automated, 103–112
  incidence of, 104–105, 105t
  potential advantages, 112–113
  potential disadvantages, 113–114
  potential problems in the detection of resistance,
    114–117
Antimicrobials
  action of, 252–255
  administration at home, 266
  clinical trials of, 266, 272–274
  concentrations at target site, 253
  concentration-dependent killing, 258–261, 259f
  dosing of, 252–265
  effects of concentration, 255
  pharmacodynamics of, 255f, 255–257t
  toxicity, 258
Antimonials, pentavalent, 148–149, 242
Antisepsis against MRSA, 174–175
Antivirals, new, 137
Anuric patients, 181
Aralen (Chloroquine), 95t
Archaea, 208
Argyrophylic bacillary structures, 205, 207
Armed Forces Epidemiological Board, 197
Arterial occlusive disease, 15
Arterial reconstruction, 19, 20
Arteriography
  in management of foot ischemia, 15
  and splenic abscess, 31
Arteriosclerosis and medical ethics, 271–272

Arthritis, 145
Artificial intelligence, 113
Aspartate aminotransferase (AST), 125
Aspergillus species
    and hepatosplenic candidiasis, 43
    and splenic abscess, 27
Asteroid inclusion bodies, 145–146
ATB-plus System, 105, 106t
ATCC, 104, 114
Atovaquone, 99
AuC, 256, 257f, 260
AuC:MIC ratio, 256
Aureobassidium pullulans
    and splenic abscess, 27
Autoantibodies, 229
Autobac System, 105
Autoimmune disorders, 229
Automicrobic System (AMS), 105
Autonomic neuropathy, 2
Autonomy of patient, 266, 267, 268, 270, 271,
    273
autoSCAN-W/A, 105
Azalides, 53. *See also* Macrolides
Azithromycin. *See also* Macrolides
    for Rochalimaea henselae infections, 216
    for nodular lymphangitis, 148, 150
Aztreonam, 10, 116

B

B-cells, 160, 161, 228
Bacillary angiomatosis
    epidemiology, 206
    identification of pathogens, 208–211
    research areas proposed, 216
Bacillary angiomatosis, agent of, 43
Bacillary index, 241
Bacillus Calmette-Guérin (BCG) vaccine,
    202
Bacitracin, 176, 178
Bacteremia
    and bacillary angiomatosis, 207, 211, 212
    in foot infections, 10
    and macrolides, 74
    and MRSA, 183
    and splenic abscess, 25, 28, 40
    therapy changes due to sensitivity studies, 112
Bacteria (domain), 208, 209
Bacterial infections, cytokine therapy for, 239–242
Bactericidal action, 254, 261
Bactericidal activity, 2
Bacteriophage types, 179
Bacteriostatic action, 254, 261

Bacteroides fragilis
    and diabetic foot infections, 5, 8, 9
    and macrolides, 54, 54t
Bacteroides species
    and diabetic foot infections, 5, 7, 8, 9, 10
    and resistance to macrolides, 57
Bar coding, 110
Barium sulfate contrast studies, 31
Bartonella bacilliformis, 207, 210, 212, 214t
Bartonellosis, 208
BASF Wyandotte, 111
Baxter Diagnostics, Inc., 105
BCG vaccine, 202
Beneficence principle, 268
Beta-blockers, 96
Beta-lactam-allergic patients, 72, 74
Beta lactam antibiotics
    detection of, 115–116
Beta-lactam antibiotics
    for community-acquired pneumonia, 75
    dosing strategy, 261–263
    expanded-spectrum, 263
    extended spectrum (ESBL), 116
    for foot infections, 8
    mechanism of action, 252
    for MRSA, 181
    for nodular lymphangitis, 149
    pharmacokinetics, 256
    for streptococcal pharyngitis, 74
Beta-lactamase-producing isolates, 65
Beta-lactamase production, 55
Beta-lactamase resistance detection, 115
Beta-lactamase-stable drugs, 74
Betadine, 174
Biaxin. *See* Clarithromycin
Bilirubin, serum, 124, 136
Biochemical test cards, 106
Biologics, defined, 193
bioMerieux, France, 105
bioMerieux Vitek, 105
Biopsy
    in diabetic foot infections, 5, 16, 17
    liver, 126, 130–131
    in nodular lymphangitis, 145, 147, 148, 156
Black fungi (dematiaceous), 142, 151
Blastomyces dermatiditis
    and splenic abscess, 27
Blastomyces dermatidis
    and nodular lymphangitis, 142, 150, 152
Bleach, 224
Blood
    exposure to, 123
    processing for RNA studies, 132

Blood culture
  and splenic abscess, 36–37
Blood cultures
  in foot infections, 7
Body substance precautions (BSP), 222
Bone infection, 3
Bone involvement
  in nodular lymphangitis, 156
Bone scans, triple-phase, 16, 18
Bone specimen culturing, 17
Bordetella pertussis and macrolides, 54, 55t, 73t
Borrelia burgdorferi
  and macrolides, 55
  and splenic abscess, 27
Botanical materials, handling of
  and atypical mycobacterial infections, 152
  and Nocardia infection, 149, 152
  and sporotrichosis, 143, 152
Botryomycosis, 151
Breast feeding, 162
Bronchitis and macrolides, 65–67, 66t, 73t, 74–75
Brown-Hopps stain, 151
Brucella abortus, 210f
Brucella species, 27
Burkitts lymphoma, 163
Burn units, hospital, 170, 172, 178
Buyers clubs, drug, 272–274

C

Campylobacter diarrhea, 52, 75
Campylobacter jejuni, 55, 56t
Campylobacter species, 215
Candida albicans, 43
Candida species, 27, 43
Candidate experimental vaccine, 194
Candidiasis, 43
Carbamazepine, 63
Carbohydrate metabolism, control of, 11
Carcinoma
  cervical, 238
  hepatocellular
    and chronic HCV infection, 128–129
    and hepatitis B virus, 231
    and hepatitis C virus, 120, 126, 233
Carriage of MRSA, elimination of, 176–179
Case studies, 268–274
Cat scratch disease (CSD)
  agent of, and splenic abscess, 27
  disseminated, 206
  and nodular lymphangitis, 142, 152
  and Rochalimaea species, 205, 206, 211t, 213–214

Catheter infections, IV, 230
Cats
  and Rochalimaea henselae, 213–214
  and sporotrichosis, 143–144
  and tularemia, 152
CBER. See Center for Biologics Evaluation and Research (CBER)
CD4− cells, 164
CD4+ cells, 234
CD8+ cells, 164, 232
CD4 count, 164, 235, 236, 272, 273
CD4++ (helper) T cells, 87, 161
Cefaclor, 62, 66, 66t, 67, 67t, 69, 73, 74
Cefadroxil, 62, 69, 254
Cefamandole, 263t
Cefazolin, 8, 263t
Cefotaxime, 116, 263
Cefotetan, 263t
Cefoxitin, 8, 263t
  for nodular lymphangitis, 150
Cefpirome, 181
Ceftazidime, 116
  dosing of, 261, 262f, 263, 263t
Ceftriaxone, 263
Cefuroxime, 263t
Cell wall membrane of bacteria, 253
Cellulitis, 69, 75
  of foot, 3, 8, 11
Center for Biologics Evaluation and Research (CBER), 195, 196, 197, 198
Centers for Disease Control and Prevention (CDC), 104, 120, 123, 127, 197, 215, 221
Cephalexin, 8, 69, 73, 74, 75, 254
Cephalosporin/beta lactamase inhibitors, 116
Cephalosporin-clindamycin treatment, 9
Cephalosporins, 74, 104, 115, 116
  for MRSA, 181
  for nodular lymphangitis, 149
Cephalothin, 263t
Cephradine, 254
Cerebrospinal fluid testing, 215
Chancriform lesions, 150
Charcot's changes, 15–19
Chemoprophylaxis
  of HIV virus infection, 224–225
  of malaria, 81, 84, 94, 95t, 95–97
  in neutropenia, 239
Chemotaxis, 2
Chemotherapy, 23, 26, 45
Children's Vaccine Initiative (CVI), 203
Chimpanzee research, 120, 122, 123, 125, 130, 131, 160

Chimpanzees, 161
Chiron Corporation, 120
Chlamydia pneumoniae, 54, 55t, 65
Chlamydia species, 68
Chlamydia trachomatis, 55, 56t, 70, 73t
Chlamydial infections, genital, 70, 72, 75, 76
Chloramphenicol, 152
Chlorhexidine, 174, 178
Chlorhexidine-gluconate-alcohol (Hibiclens), 174
Chloroquine
    resistance to, 84, 85, 93, 94, 95–97
    side effects, 96
Chloroquine (Aralen), 95t, 97, 98, 98t
Chloroquine efflux, 85, 86
Chromomycoses (chromoblastomycoses), 142, 151
Chronic fatigue syndrome, 163
Cincinnati, University of, Hospital, 180
Ciprofloxacin, 8, 18, 73, 254
    for MRSA, 178, 182
    for nodular lymphangitis, 148
Circulation to foot, 15
Circumsporozoite protein (CSP), 83, 87
Cirrhosis
    and hepatitis B virus, 231
    and hepatitis C virus, 126, 129, 130, 135, 233
    and splenic abscess, 25
Citrate synthesis gene sequences, 210, 211, 215
Citrobacter freundii, 104
Citrobacter species, 115
Clarithromycin. *See also* Macrolides
    for nodular lymphangitis, 148, 150
    for Rochalimaea henselae infections, 216
Clavulanate, 116
Clindamycin, 8, 254, 263
    for MRSA, 182
Clinical testing and trials of vaccines, 194–196
Clinical trials
    of antimicrobials, 266
    failure of, 272–274
    of macrolides, 63–72
    "ramdomization" scheme, 66
Clofazimine, 56, 71
Clostridium difficile, 27
Clostridium perfringens, 54, 54t
Clostridium species, 1, 5
    and splenic abscess, 27
Cloxacillin, 8
$C_{1/max}$/MIC, 258
Cobas Bact System, 105, 106t
Coccidioides immitis, 142, 150, 156
Code of Ethics (AMA), 267, 272
Colitis, pseudomembranous, 62

Collagen vascular disorders, 25
Colonization by MRSA, 171
Committee on Infectious Diseases (of American Academy of Pediatrics), 197
Compensation of infected workers, 225–226
Computerized tomography (CT)
    and diabetic foot osteomyelitis, 16
    and splenic abscess, 23, 26, 30, 32–35, 34f, 36f, 38, 41, 42, 43, 44f, 44–45
Concentration-dependent killing of microbes, 258–261, 259f
Concentration-independent killing of microbes, 261–264
Condoms, 136
Condylomata acuminata, 238
Confidentiality, 269
Congestive heart failure, 12
Conjunctivitis, 181
Contaminated surfaces, 172
Coronary artery disease, 20
Corticosteroids, systemic, 25
Corynebacterium diphtheriae, 27
Corynebacterium species, 6, 9
Cotrimoxazole, 147, 149
Coumermycin, 183
Cowpox virus, 142, 152
Coxiella burnetii, 68
Crepitus, 3
Cryoglobulinemia, essential, type II or III, 126
Cryotherapy, 148
Cryptococcus neoformans, 142, 150
CT. *See* Computerized tomography (CT)
Curettage, 5
Cyclosporine, 63
Cysticercosis, 143
Cytoadherence, 87
Cytochrome P450 microsomal enzyme system, 59, 63
Cytokine therapy, 228–251
    of bacterial infections, 239–242
    of protozoal infections, 241–242
    recommendations for use, 242
    of viral infections, 231–239
Cytokines. *See also* IL, IFN, TNF, G-CSF, GM-CSF, M-CSF
    and hepatocarcinogenesis, 129
    inadequate production of, 228–229
    mechanism of action, 228
    overproduction of, 228
    and pathogenesis of malaria, 84, 87, 100
    use in human studies, 229–231
Cytomegalovirus, human (CMU)
    cytokine therapy for, 237

Cytomegalovirus, human (CMV)
  and human herpesvirus 6, 159, 162, 163, 164
  vaccine, 192
Cytotoxic (CD8+) T cells, 87, 130

D

Daptomycin (LY 146032), 181
Debridement, 11, 12, 14f, 15, 18, 19
Declaration of New York, 203
DEET, 97
Dengue vaccine, 192
Densitometer, 107
Dermatitis, chronic, 171
Desciclovir, 233
Diabetes mellitus, 25
Diabetic osteopathy, 15–19
Dicloxacillin, 8, 73, 75
Digoxin, 63
Dihydrofolate reductase (DHFR), 85
Diphtheria
  and macrolides, 72
  vaccine, 199, 201
Disk diffusion tests for antimicrobial susceptibility,
    103, 104, 105t
DNA
  of human herpesvirus 6, 160
  of Marick's disease virus, 160
  plasmid or chromosomal, 179
  recombinant complementary (cDNA), 125, 129
  ribosomal, 208, 209, 210, 212, 213
  viral, 232
DNA gyrase, 183, 252
DNA probes, 118, 179
Doctor-patient relationship, 266
Domains of organisms, 208
Dosing of antimicrobials, 177, 252–265
Doxycycline
  for bacillary angiomatosis, 216
  for genital chlamydial infections, 70
  for nodular lymphangitis, 150
Doxycycline (Vibramycin)
  for malaria, 95t, 96
Drainage
  percutaneous, of splenic abscess, 23, 38–40, 39t,
    41, 45
Drug buyers clubs, 272–274
Drug infusion, 99
Drug resistance
  genetic locus, 85
  in malaria, 84–86, 86t, 93–95
Drug users, intravenous
  and hepatitis C virus, 123

  medical ethics and, 269, 270–271
  and MRSA, 180, 182
  and splenic abscess, 25, 26, 28
D4T, 272
DTP vaccine, 199, 202

E

Edema, 12
Education and feedback (staff), 178
Efflux pump, 57
Eikenella corrodens, 27
ELA, 197
Electrophoresis, 179
ELISA assays, 121, 125, 128, 129, 131, 132,
    134
Embolization, therapeutic, 25
Empyema, 30, 40
Encephalitis, 207, 238
Endocarditis
  in diabetics, 10
  and medical ethics, 270–271
  and MRSA, 181, 182, 183
  and Rochalimaea species, 212
  and splenic abscess, 26, 30, 31, 34, 42
Endonucleases, 179
Endothelial cell monolayers, bovine, 212, 214
Endotoxin, 231
Enoxacin, 182
Entameba histolytica
  and macrolides, 73t
  and splenic abscess, 27
Enteric pathogens, 55, 56t
Enterobacter species, 115
Enterobacteriaceae, 8–9, 104, 116
Enterococci
  and diabetic foot infections, 6, 9
  and macrolides, 53, 58
  and resistance to macrolides, 57
Enterococcus species, 117
Enzyme-linked immunosorbent assay (ELISA as-
    says), 121, 125, 128, 129, 131, 132, 134
Enzymes
  plasmid-mediated, 116
Epidemiological reports, 110
Epstein-Barr virus (EBV), 159, 160, 161, 162, 163
  vaccine, 192
Ergotamine, 63
Erythema nodosum leprosum, 240
Erythrocyte cycle, asexual
  of Plasmodium, 84
Erythromycin. *See also* Macrolides
  for diabetic foot infections, 8

Erythromycin
 for bacillary angiomatosis, 205, 215
ESBL, 116
Escherichia coli
 and diabetic foot infection, 8
 and macrolides, 55, 56t
 and splenic abscess, 26
Escherichia faecalis, 54t
Escherichia faecium, 54t
Establishment License Application (ELA),
 197
Ethambutal
 and macrolides, 71
 for nodular lymphangitis, 150
Ethical issues, 266–275
 case studies, 268–274
 evaluation, 268–269
 prioritization, 268
Ethical standards, 268
Ethics, Code of (AMA), 267, 272
Ethics, medical
 approach to, 268–274
 models, 267–268, 272
Eucaria, 208
Evolutionary tree of alpha-proteobacteria, 210,
 210f
Exanthem subitum, 159, 162–163
Expanded Program on Immunization (EPI) of
 WHO, 202
Extramedullary hematopoeisis, 43
Eye infection, 145

F

Facultative gram-negative bacilli, 3, 5
False resistance, 114–117
False susceptibility, 114–117
Fansidar. *See* Sulfadoxine/pyrimethadine (Fansidar)
Fatty acid analysis, whole-cell, 211, 215
FDA. *See* Food and Drug Administration (FDA)
Federal Vaccine Injury Compensation Program,
 199
Felty's syndrome, 25
Fetid smell, 3, 7
Fever
 in diabetic foot infection, 3, 7
 and Rochalimaea species, 211t
Fibroblast cell line, human diploid lung MRC5,
 160
Fibroblasts, 60
Fish-handler's disease, 147
Five-fluoro-orotic acid dehydrogenase, 99

Flaviviruses, 121, 233
Fleroxacin, 182
Fluconazole, 43
Fluctuant collections, 7
Fluorogenic compounds for microbial growth detec-
 tion, 104, 111
Fluorogenic reader, 109
Fluorogenic-substrate hydrolysis, 109
Fluorometric reader, 110, 111–112
Fluoroquinolone-clindamycin treatment, 9
Fluoroquinolones
 for bacterial simusitis, 74, 75
 dosing of, 258–261
 for MRSA, 182
 for nodular lymphangitis, 148, 150
 pharmacokinetics, 256
 for tuberculosis, 55
Folliculitis, 69
Food and Drug Administration (FDA), 1, 104,
 105, 106, 115, 134, 195, 196, 197
Foot
 bony prominences, 2
 circulation to, 15
 ischemia of, 3
Foot care, unskilled, 2
Foot infections
 classification, 3
 diabetic
  antimicrobial treatment, 7–10, 18
  clinical presentations, 2–4
   factors, 2–3
  entry for infection, 5
  microbiology, 5–7, 6t
   practical approach, 7
  osteomyelitis in, 15–19
  pathogenesis, 2
  surgical management, 10–15
  team approach, 19–20
 nosocomial, 5
Foot ulcers, 1, 3, 5
 classification and treatment, 11, 11t, 12t
 healing, 8
 neuropathic. *See* Mal perforans
 probing, 18
Fosfomycin, 183
Francisella tularensis, 142, 151–152
Free-tissue transfers, 12
Freedom of choice of treatments, 269
Fungal splenic abscesses, 27–28
Fungi
 dematiaceous (black), 142, 151
 and nodular lymphangitis, 150
Fusidic acid, 178, 180, 182, 183

G

G-CSF. *See* Granulocyte colony stimulating factor
(G-CSF)
Gallium scan
and diabetic foot osteomyelitis, 16
and splenic abscess, 31–32, 34
Ganciclovir
for HIV virus infection, 237
for human herpesvirus 6 (HHV-6), 164–165
Gangrene, 1, 3
Gas formation in infections, 3, 7, 10
Gastrointestinal infections, 70
Genetic clocks, 208
Gneetic locus of drug resistance, 85
Genital chlamydial infections, 70, 72, 75, 76
Genital warts, 238
Genome
of CMV, 160
of hepatitis C virus, 121–122, 122f, 133
of human herpesvirus 6 (HHV-6), 160
Gentamicin
for diabetic foot infections, 10
for MRSA, 176, 183
for nodular lymphangitis, 152
regimen, 259
resistance to, 117, 174
Giemsa stain, 148
Glioblastoma cells, 160
Globulin, immune, 129, 136
Glomerulonephritis, membranoproliferative,
126
Gloves, 175
Glucantime, 149
Glucose 6-phosphate dehydrogenase (G6PD) defi-
ciency, 97
Glycopeptides, 180–181, 256
Glycoproteins, alpha 1-, 60
GM-CSF. *See* Granulocyte-macrophage colony
stimulating factor (GM-CSF)
Gonococcus, 192
Gowns, 175
G6PD deficiency, 92
Gram-negative aerobes, 26, 41
Gram-negative bacilli
in diabetic foot infections, 7
facultative, 3, 5
and macrolides, 53, 64
and mupirocin, 177
and rapid susceptibility testing, 106, 109
Gram-negative bacteria, 263
facultative, 258
Gram-positive bacilli, 106
Gram-positive bacteria, 106, 109

Gram-positive cocci
and diabetic foot infections, 5, 8, 9
and macrolides, 53
and splenic abscess, 40
Gram stains, 151
Granulocyte colony stimulating factor (G-CSF).
See also Cytokines and Cytokine therapy
for cytomegalovirus, 237
for HIV, 236
in human studies, 230
for neutropenia, 239
Granulocyte-macrophage colony stimulating factor
for neutropenia, 239
Granulocyte-macrophage colony stimulating factor
(GM-CSF). *See also* Cytokines and Cytokine
therapy
for cytomegalovirus, 237
for HIV, 234, 236
in human studies, 231
for leprosy, 240
Granuloma
fish-tank, 147
pyogenic, 206, 207
Granuloma formation, 143, 147, 149, 150
Granulomatous disorder, chronic (CGD), 240
Growth curve, microbial, 109
Growth factors, tissue, 11
Growth rate comparisons, 104
Guillotine amputation, 1, 12, 19

H

H$_2$-blockers, 70
Haemophilus ducreyi, 55, 56t
Haemophilus influenzae
and macrolides, 53–54, 54t, 58, 64, 65, 66, 67,
68, 73t, 75
and splenic abscess, 27
vaccine, 192, 199, 202
Haemophilus parainfluenzae, 67
Halofantrine, 86
Hammer toe deformity, 1
Hands, transmission via, 170
Hartford Hospital, 259, 260f, 262
HBsAg. *See* Hepatitis B surface antigen (HBsAg)
Healthcare workers
as MRSA reservoir, 171
risk of HIV infection, 221, 272
Heart failure, congestive, 12
HeLa cells, 161
Helicobacter pylori
and macrolides, 55, 56t, 70, 75
vaccine, 192

Helicobacter species, 215
Helper (CD4++) T cells, 87, 161
Hemangioma, epithelioid, 207
Hematologic malignancies, 23, 26
Hematopoeisis, extramedullary, 43
Hematoxylin and eosin stain, 151, 207
Hemodialysis, 25
Hemodialysis patients, 180
Hemoglobinopathy, 25, 26
Hemolysis
    and malaria, 99, 99t
    and primaquine, 97
Hemophiliac patients, 123
Hepatitis
    and human herpesvirus 6 (HHV-6), 163
    non-A, non-B, 120, 122, 123, 125, 129, 132,
        233
    non-a, non-B
        post-transfusion, 120, 121, 122, 126, 127, 128
    post-transfusion, 122, 233
Hepatitis A and B infections, 120, 129
Hepatitis A virus, 121
Hepatitis B surface antigen (HBsAg), 122, 128,
        130, 234
Hepatitis B virus, 121, 127, 130, 162
    cytokine therapy for, 231–233, 235
    infection risk, 221
    vaccine, 199, 202, 203
Hepatitis C virus
    antibodies against, 125, 126, 129–130, 132, 134
    antigens, 125, 128, 129, 131
    and chronic liver disease, 120–141
        counseling and follow-up of patients, 135–136
        diagnostic methods, 131–134
        pathology, 130–131
        treatment, 134–135
    cytokine therapy for, 233–234
    epidemiology, 122–124
    genome structure and organization, 121–122,
        122f, 133
    immune response to, 129–130
    perinatal transmission of, 124
    post-transfusion infection with, 123
    proteins, 131
    sexual transmission of, 123–124, 136
    transmission of, 122–124
    vaccine, 192
    virology, 120–122
Hepatitis C virus infection
    clinical manifestations, 124–129
    community-acquired, 123–124, 136
    death rate, 127, 128
    pathology, 130–131

potential infectiousness of patients, 136
and primary hepatocellular carcinoma, 128
progression to chronic lever disease, 131
severity in Japan, 126
Hepatitis D virus
    cytokine therapy for, 234
Hepatitis delta virus, 130
Hepatitis E virus (HEV), 121
    vaccine, 192
Herpes simplex virus, 159
    cytokine therapy for, 237–238
    vaccine, 192
Herpes viruses
    and bacillary angiomatosis, 216
Herpesvirus, human, 6 (HHV-6), 159–169
Hexachlorophene (Phisohex), 174, 178
Hexobarbital, 63
Hibiclens, 174
Hippocratic Oath, 266
Histocompatability molecules, major (MHC), 229
Histoplasma capsulatum, 142, 150
HIV-associated syndromes, 43–45
HIV infection
    antibody testing algorithms, 225
    chemoprophylaxis of, 224–225
    cytokine therapy for, 234–237
    exposure prevention, 221–223
    and hepatitis C, 233
    medical ethics and, 269–270
    postexposure intervention, 224–226
    prevention of, 220–227
    risk assessment, 220–221
    seroconversion illness, 225
    and splenic abscess, 23, 26, 43–45
    an sporotrichosis, 145
HIV virus, 162, 163
    and bacillary angiomatosis, 206
    and subacute endocarditis, 212
    testing for, 223
    transcription and gene expression
        and human herpesvirus 6 (HHV-6), 164
    vaccine, 192
Holoendemic malaria, 80
Honoraria, 269
Horses, 151
Hospital personnel, 220–227
Hospital rooms, 175–176
Human B-lymphotropic virus (HBLV), 159
Human herpesvirus 6 (HHV-6), 159–169
    antigenic variation, 165
    antiviral theraphy, 164–165
    coinfection with, 164
    epidemiology, 161–162

Human herpes virus 6 (*cont.*)
　host range, 161
　immunity to, 165
　infection and disease, 162–164
　infection of cells, 160–161
　rersearch areas, 165
　structure, 160
　vaccine, potential, 165
Human immunodeficiency virus. *See* HIV
Human leukocyte antigen (HLA), 232, 240, 241
Humidifier, ultrasonic, 110
Hydroxychloroquine, 96
Hydroxyl radicals, 129
Hydroxyzine, 181
Hyperendemic malaria, 80
Hyperglycemia, 2, 3
Hyperparasitemia in malaria, 99, 99t
Hypoendemic malaria, 80
Hypogammmaglobulinemia, 25
Hypotension, 181

I

IFN-α. *See* Interferon α
IFN-β. *See* Inteferon β
IFN-γ. *See* Interferon γ
IL-1. *See* Interleukin 1
IL-2. *See* Interleukin 2
IL-3. *See* Interleukin 3
IL-6. *See* Interleukin 6
Imipenem
　false resistance to, 116
　for nodular lymphangitits, 149
Imipenem-cilastin treatment, 8–9, 10
Immune globulin, 129, 136
Immune system, 228
Immunity to human herpesvirus 6 (HHV-6), 165
Immunization
　to HIV virus (projected), 225
　to malaria, 100
　WHO goals, 203
Immunocompromised individuals
　and atypical mycobacteria, 150
　and bacillary angiomatosis, 206, 216
　and cytomegalovirus infection, 237
　and herpes simplex virus infection, 237
　and IFN therapy, 232
　and M. marinum infection, 147
　and nodular lymphangitis, 156
　and sporotrichosis, 145
　and varicella-zoster infections, 237
Immunofluorescent assay, 159, 215
Immunoglobulin G (IgG), 163, 215

Immunoglobulin M (IgM), 125, 163
Immunosuppressed individuals
　and human herpesvirus 6, 163, 165
　and splenic abscess, 23, 26, 27, 30, 31, 45
Impetigo, 69
in vitro testing of vaccines, 194
in vivo testing of vaccines, 194
IND application, 195, 196
Indium-111-labeled leukocyte imaging
　and diabetic foot osteomyelitis, 16, 18
　and splenic abscess, 31–32, 34
Infarction, splenic, 24, 25, 26
Infection, pedal, 1
Infection control, 221–223
Infectious Diseases Society of America,
　197
Infectious mononucleosis, 25
Influenza virus vaccine, 199
Informed consent, 267
Infusion reactions, 180–181
Injured patients, 241
Injuries, percutaneous, 220, 222, 223
Inoculum preparation, 107, 111
Insulin, 2, 11
Insurance of workers at risk, 225–226
Interfacility transfer of pathogens, 179–180
Interferon α
　for cytomegalovirus, 237
　for hepatitis B, 232
　for hepatitis C, 134–136, 233–234
　for herpes simplex infections, 238
　for HIV, 235, 237
　in human studies, 229
　for leishmaniasis, 242
　for Mycobacterium avium-intercellulare infec-
　　tions, 241
　for severely injured patients, 241
　for varicella-zoster infections, 237
Interferon β
　for hepatitis B, 234
　for herpes simplex virus infections, 238
　for HIV, 235
　in human studies, 229
Interferon γ, 230
　in AIDS, 229
　for chronic granulomatous disorder, 240
　in hepatitis C, 129
　for HIV, 236
　in human studies, 229–230
　in lepromatous leprosy, 229, 240–241
　for leprosy, 240
　in malaria, 87
　toxicities, 230

Interferon α, β, and γ. *See also* Cytokines and
  Cytokine therapy
Interferons
  for human papilloma virus infection, 238
  for rhinovirus infections, 238–239
Interferons, type 1, 229
Interleukin-1
  in meningitis, 228
  in sepsis, 228
Interleukin-2
  in AIDS, 229
  for HIV, 234, 236
  and human herpesvirus 6, 159, 161
  in human studies, 230
  for lepromatous leprosy, 229, 240–241
  for leprosy, 240–241
  toxicities, 230
Interleukin-3
  in human studies, 231
Interleukin-6
  for HIV, 234
  in malaria, 87
Interleukin-1, -2, -3, and -6. *See also* Cytokines
  and Cytokine therapy
Intestinal obstruction, 30
Investigative New Drug (IND) application, 195, 196
Iodophores, 224
Iowa City Veterans Administration Medical Center,
  179
Ischemia
  of foot, 3
  management of, 15
Isolation of patients, 175–176, 176f
Isoniazid
  for MAC infection, 71
  for nodular lymphangitis, 150
Itraconazole, 146

J
Johns Hopkins University, 223
Joints, infection of, 3
Justice and medical ethics, 271

K
Kala azar, 148
Kaposi's sarcoma
  and bacillary angiomatosis, 206, 207
  and HIV infection, 235
Ketoacidosis, 10
Ketoconazole, 146, 149
Kinyoun stain, 146, 150

Klebsiella pneumoniae, 27
Klebsiella species, 8, 116

L
Labeling of vaccines, 197
Lactobacillus species, 27
Lariam (Mefloquine), 95t
Lectins, 231
Legionella pneumophila, 54, 55t, 65, 68, 73t, 75
Legionnaire's disease, 68, 72, 75
Leishmania brasiliensis, 148, 242
Leishmania mexicana, 148
Leishmania species, 142, 148–149, 152
Leishmania tropica, 148, 242
Leishmaniasis
  cytokine therapy for, 230, 241–242
  and nodular lymphangitis, 148–149
Leprosy, 229
  IL-2 therapy for, 240–241
Leukemia
  and CSF's, 239
  and hepatosplenic candidiasis, 43
  and human herpesvirus 6 (HHV-6), 163
Liability, 268
  product, 198–199
Life support and medical ethics, 269
Limb salvage, 15
Lincosamides
  mechanism of action, 183–184
  and resistance to macrolides, 57
Linear regression, 109
Lipopeptides, 181
Lipoteichoic acid, 181
Listeria monocytogenes, 54, 54t, 73t
Listeriosis, 230
Liver disease, chronic, and hepatitis C virus, 120–
  141
  counseling and follow-up of patients, 135–136
  diagnostic methods, 131–134
  pathology, 130–131
  treatment, 134–135
  virology, 120–122
Liver fibrosis, 134
Liver inflammation, 128–129
Liver-spleen scans, ^{99m}Tc, 31–32, 34
Lomefloxacin, 254
Long-term care facilities, 179–180
Lowenstein-Jensen culture media, 146
Lupus erythematosus, systemic, 163
Lyme disease vaccine, 192
Lymphangitis, nodular, 142–158, 144f–145f,
  153t–155t

Lymphangitis, nodular (*cont.*)
  common pathogens, 143
  common sites of infection, 142
  differential diagnosis, 143
Lymphangitis in foot infections, 11
Lymphocytes, peripheral blood (PBL), 162
  phytohemoagglutinin (PHA)-stimulated, 159
Lymphomas
and human herpesvirus 6 (HHV-6), 163
  and splenic abscess, 31, 33
Lymphproliferative disorders, 159, 163
Lysis-centrifugation method, 211, 212
Lysosomes, 60

M

M-CSF. *See* Macrophage colony stimulating factor
Macrobroth dilution method, 103
Macrolides. *See also* Azithromycin,
  Clarithromycin, and Erythromycin
  activity against bacterial pathogens, chlamydiae,
    and mycoplasma, 53–55, 54t, 55t, 148, 150
  activity against pathogens of sexually transmitted
    disease, 56t
  activity against respiratory pathogens, 55t
  activity against spirochetes, mycobacteria, and
    toxoplasma, 55–57
  adverse reactions, 62, 72
  bactericidal effects, 58
  chemistry, 52–53
  clinical uses, 63–72
  and community-acquired pneumonia, 67t, 67–
    69, 75, 76
  cost, 72–74, 74t, 76
  distribution in tissues and extravascular fluids,
    60t, 60–61
  drug interactions, 63
  effect of inoculum size, 58
  effect of pH, 58
  effect of serum, 57
  indications and usual dosage, 72, 73t, 76
  mechanism of action, 183, 252
  metabolism and elimination, 59–60
  new, advantages over erythromycin, 72, 73t
  oral availability, 58–59
  pharmacodynamic interactions, 263
  pharmacokinetic properties, 58–62, 59t, 74
  pharmacokinetics in pediatric patients, 62
  potential role, 74
  resistance mechanisms, 57
  for Rochalimaea henselae infections, 216
  transfer to fetus and into milk, 61
  use in clinical practice, 72–76

  use in pregnancy, 63
  in vitro activity, 53–58
Macrophage colony stimulating factor (M-CSF).
    See also Cytokines and Cytokine therapy
  in human studies, 231
  for neutropenia, 239
Macrophages
  macrolide toxicity to, 57
  and resistance to malaria, 87
Magnetic resonance imaging
  in diabetic foot osteomyelitis, 17, 18
  and splenic abscess, 30
Mal perforans, 3, 4f, 10, 11
Malaria
  biologic factors, 81–87
  cerebral, 84, 99, 99t
  chemoprophylaxis, 81, 84, 94, 95t, 95–97
  counseling for travelers, 95
  drug resistance, 84–86, 86t
    distribution, 93–95
    genetic locus, 85
  and expatriate travelers, 81
  future strategies, 99–100
  geographic factors, 87–92, 88t
  holoendemic, 80
  host factors, 86–87
  hyperendemic, 80
  hypoendemic, 80
  immune responses, 86–87
  incidence, 80
  inoculation rate, 92
  intensity of transmission, 92–93
  life cycle, 81–84, 82f–83f
  limniting vector-human contact, 97
  mesoendemic, 80
  mortality, 81
  non-immune hosts, 83
  parasite determinants of the outcome of infec-
    tion, 84–86
  prevention, 81, 95–97
  prevention of relapse, chemoprophylaxis for, 97
  and renal failure, 84
  semi-immune persons, 81, 83, 84
  and splenic abscess, 23, 25
  treatment, 97–99, 98t
  vaccine, 192
Manufacturing of vaccines, 194, 196
Marek's disease virus, 160
Marrow tranplantation
  chemoprophylaxis in, 239
  and cytomegalovirus pneumonia, 237
Mass action, laws of, 253
Maximum concentration/MIC ratio (C_{max}/MIC),
  258

MBC. *See* Minimum bacterial concentration
McDonnell-Douglas Corp., 106
McFarland barium sulfate turbidity standard, 107,
    111
Mdr-like genes in Plasmodium falciparum, 85
Measles vaccine, 199, 201, 202, 203
Medications, nonallopathic, 271–274
Medications, nontraditional, 271–274
Medications, unlicensed, 274
Mediterranean populations, 97
Mefloquine, 85, 96, 98t
    resistance to, 86, 94
Mefloquine (Lariam), 95t
Megakaryocytes, 160
Meglumine antimoniate (Glucantime), 149
Meiosis, 83
Melioidosis, 27
Meningitis
    and bacillary angiomatosis, 207, 211t
    due to MRSA, 181
    meningococcal, vaccine, 199
    in sporotrichosis, 145
Meningococcus B, 192
Meningoencephalitis, 213
Merozoite surface protein-1 (MSP-1), 87
Mesoendemic malaria, 80
Metastatic infections, 2
    in diabetics, 2, 10
Methicillin, 53
Methicillin resistance, 117
Methicillin resistance
    in Staphylococcus aureus, 170–191
Methylumbelliferyl, 111
Metronidazole, 10, 254
Mezlocillin, 263t
MIC. *See* Minimum inhibitory concentration
    (MIC)
Microbiologic activity, 253–255, 255f
Microbiology
    of diabetic foot infections, 5–7, 6t
    of splenic abscess, 26–28, 27t
Microcuvettes. *See* Reagent cards
Microdilution tests, broth, for antimicrobial suscep-
    tibility, 103, 104, 105t
Microdilution trays, 109
Middlebrook culture media, 146
Minimal-dose regimens, 177
Minimum bactericidal concentrations (MBC),
    174–175, 253, 254
Minimum inhibitory concentration (MIC), 104,
    107, 111, 114, 117, 174, 178, 181, 253, 254,
    258, 260, 261, 263
Minocycline
    for MRSA, 182, 183

for nodular lymphangitis, 147, 149
    for toxoplasmosis, 57
MLS antibiotics, 184
MLS resistance, 57
Monkeys, 161, 224
Monobactams, 116
Mononucleosis, infectious, 163
Montenegro leishmanin skin test, 148
Moraxella catarrhalis, 54, 54t, 58, 64, 65, 67
Morganella morganii, 27
Morganella species, 115, 116
Mosquito coils, 97
Motilin receptor, putative, 62
Motor neuropathy in foot, 2
MRSA. *See* Staphylococcus aureus, methicillin-
    resistant (MRSA), nosocomial
Mueller-Hinton media, 111, 117
Mumps vaccine, 199, 201, 202
Mupirocin, 177
Muscle flaps, 12
Mutants, stably derepressed, 115
Mycetoma, 151
Mycobacteria
    and macrolides, 55
    and splenic abscess, 27
Mycobacteria, atypical
    in nodular lymphangitis, 150, 152, 156
Mycobacterium avium complex (MAC), 56, 71–
    72, 76
Mycobacterium avium-intracellulare
    cytokine therapy of, 241
    and nodular lymphangitis, 142, 150
Mycobacterium-avium intracellulare
    and splenic abscess, 27, 43–45
Mycobacterium chelonae
    and macrolides, 56, 76
    and nodular lymphangitis, 142, 150
Mycobacterium fortuitum
    and macrolides, 56, 76
Mycobacterium kansasii, 142, 150
Mycobacterium leprae
    cytokine treatment for, 240
    and macrolides, 76
Mycobacterium marinum
    and nodular lymphangitis, 142, 146–148, 152,
    156
    skin testing for, 147
Mycobacterium tuberculosis
    and macrolides, 55, 56
    and medical ethics, 269–270
    and nodular lymphangitis, 142
    and splenic abscess, 27, 43–44
Mycoplasma pneumoniae, 54, 55, 65, 68, 68t, 73t
Myelodysplasia, 239

Myelokathexis, 239
Myeloproliferative disorders, 25

N

NANB hepatitis. *See* Hepatitis, non-A, non-B
National Aeronautics and Space Administration
  (NASA), 106
National Center for Health Statistics, 127
National Childhood Vaccine Injury ACT of 1986
  (NCVIA), 199
National Committee for Clinical Laboratory Stan-
  dards (NCCLS), 103, 104, 114, 117
National Institutes of Health (NIH), 120
National Vaccine Advisory Committee, 201
National Vaccine Program, 200–201
Natural killer (NK) cells, 228, 229, 230
NCCLS, 103, 104, 114, 117
NCVIA, 199
Necrosis
  in foot infections, 1, 11
  liver, 131
Necrotizing infection, 10
Needle aspiration of infected tissue, 5, 36
Needle injuries, 221, 222, 223
Needles and needle devices, 222–223
Negligence, 269
Neisseria gonorrheae, 55, 56t, 70, 73t
Neoplastic lesions, metastatic nodular, 143
Nephelometer, 115
Neuro-osteoarthropathy, 15–19
Neuroblastoma cells, 160
Neuropathy, 2, 10, 15
Neutropenia, chemotherapy-induced, 230, 239–
  240
Neutrophilic reaction, 143, 149
N,N-diethylmetatoluamide (DEET), 97
Nocardia asteroides, 149
Nocardia brasiliensis, 149
Nocardia species
  and nodular lymphangitis, 142, 149, 156
  and splenic abscess, 27
Non-A, Non-B hepatitis (NANB). *See also* Hepati-
  tis C virus
Non-A, non-B hepatitis (NANB). *See* Hepatitis,
  non-A, non-B
Nonallopathic medication, 271–274
Nonmaleficence principle, 268, 271, 273
Nontraditional medications, 271–274
Nose in transmission of pathogens, 170
Nosocomial infections
  of foot, 5
  Staphylococcus aureus, methicillin-resistant
    (MRSA), 170–191

Novobiocin, 178, 182, 183
Nucleocapsids, 160

O

Ofloxacin, 73, 254
  for MRSA, 182
Oligonucleotide primer, 132–133
Ommaya reservoir infections, 181
Organ transplantation
  and human herpesvirus 6 (HHV-6), 163–164
  and splenic abscess, 23, 25, 26, 45
Organisms, domains of, 208
Organon-Teknika, 105
Osteomyelitis
  definition, 18–19
  in diabetic foot infections, 7, 14f, 15–19
Osteopathy, diabetic, 15–19
Oxacillin, 117
Oxygen tension, transcutaneous
  in management of foot ischemia, 15
  reduced, 1
Ozone, rectal, 273

P

p-chloro-m-xylenol (Acute-Kare), 174
Papilloma virus, human
  cytokine therapy for, 238
  vaccine, 192
Parasitemias, symptomatic asexual in malaria, 84
Patents for vaccine, 199
Patient activism, 267, 272–274
Patient rights, 268–273
PCR. *See* Polymerase chain reaction (PCR) assays
Peak:MIC ratio, 256, 257f, 258, 259, 260, 261
Pefloxacin, 182
Peliosis, bacillary, 211, 211t
Penicillin
  aqueous procaine, 263
  benzathine B, 55
  oral semi-synthetic penicillinase-resistant, 8
  resistance to, 104
  for streptococcal pharyngitis, 74
Penicillin-allergic patients, 72
Penicillin-binding proteins, 252
Penicillin V, 62, 63, 65, 75
Penicillin VK, 64t
Pentamidine, aerosolized, 44
Pentamidine isethionate, 149
Pentostam, 148
Percutaneous injuries, 220, 222, 223
Periostitis, 19

Peripheral vascular disease
  in diabetics, 1, 2
Periplasmic space, 253
Peritonitis, 30
Permethrin, 97
Pertussis
  and macrolides, 72
  vaccine, 192, 199, 201, 202
Pfizer Diagnostics, 105
PFs25 antigen, 87
Phagocytes, 60, 61
Phagocytosis, 2
Pharmaceutical companies, 269
Pharmacodynamics of antimicrobials, 255f, 255–257, 257f
Pharmacokinetics of antimicrobials, 254–255, 255f, 256
Pharmacy-link program, 110
Pharyngitis, streptococcal, 63–64, 64t, 65, 73t, 74
Phase control testing of vaccines, 195–196
Phenolics, 178
Phenytoin, 63
Phisohex, 174
Phosphonoacetic acid, 164
Phosphonoformic acid, 164
Phylogenetic analysis, 210, 210f, 212
Phytohemagglutinin (PHA), 161
Picornaviruses, 121
Piperacillin, 263t
PIXY 321 (protein), 239
PLA, 195, 197
Plant-associated bacteria, 210
Plantar ulcers, 3
Plasmid GNAB, 174
Plasmids, 57
Plasmodium
  distribution, 88t
  life cycle, 81–84
Plasmodium falciparum, 81, 83, 84, 85, 86, 87, 88, 88t, 89, 90, 91, 92, 95, 96, 97, 98, 99
  chloroquine-resistant (CQ^r)
    distribution, 93, 94, 95–97
    treatment, 98
  Fansidar-resistant, 94
  quinine-resistant (Qn^r) and quinidine-resistant (Qd^r), 94
Plasmodium malariae, 84, 87, 88, 88t, 89, 90, 91, 92, 95, 98
Plasmodium ovale, 82f, 84, 87, 88, 88t, 89, 90, 95, 97, 98
Plasmodium vivax, 82f, 84, 85, 87, 88, 88t, 89, 90, 91, 92, 95, 97, 98
Pleural effusion, 40
Pleuritis, 207

Pluronic, 111
Pneumococcus vaccine, 192, 199
Pneumocystis carinii
  and macrolides, 76
  in splenic abscess, 43–44, 44f
Pneumocystosis, disseminated, 44
  Pneumonia
  atypical, 68, 68t, 75
  community-acquired
    and macrolides, 67t, 67–69, 75, 76
  cytomegalovirus, 237
  and macrolides, 73t
  nosocomial, 261
Point prevalence survey, 173
Poliomyelitis vaccine, 199, 202, 203
Polyamine pathway, 99
Polyethylene glycol, 230
Polymerase chain reaction (PCR) assays, 85, 123, 125, 126, 133, 135, 136, 208, 209, 209f, 210, 212, 213, 215, 225, 234
Polymicrobial infection, 5, 8
Porins, 253
Porphyria cutanea tarda, 126
Postantibiotic effect (PAE), 254, 256, 258
Postexposure interventions, 224–226
Postsplenectomy sepsis syndrome, 38
Potassium iodide, saturated solution (SSKI), 146
Povidone-iodone (Betadine), 174, 178
Prednisone, 232
Premarket approval (PMA) from FDA, 104, 105, 106
Pressure sensation, cutaneous, 1
Primaquine, 97
Privacy of patient, 266, 267
Product License Application (PLA), 195, 197
Prognosis, poor, and medical ethics, 270–271
Proguanil (Paludrine), 95t, 96–97
Protein binding, serum, 60
Proteins
  of hepatitis C virus, 131–132
  penicillin-binding, 252
Proteus mirabilis
  and diabetic foot infection, 8
  and splenic abscess, 27
Proteus species, 116
  indole-positive, 115
Proteus vulgaris, 27
Prothrombin time, 125, 136
Protozoal infections, therapy, 241–242
Providentia species, 115
Pseudoallescheria boydii, 151
Pseudomonas aeruginosa
  and aminoglycoside regimen, 259

Pseudomonas aeruginosa (*cont.*)
  and antimicrobial sensitivity testing, 104, 114, 116
  and diabetic foot infections, 5
  and macrolides, 54, 54t
  and splenic abscess, 26
Pseudomonas fluorescens, 177
Pseudomonas pseudomallei, 27
Pseudomonas species
  and aminoglycoside dosing, 260
  and antimicrobial susceptibility testing, 115
  and splenic abscess, 27
Pseudomycosis, bacterial, 151
Pulmonary edema, 99, 99t
Purine salvage pathway, 99
Pyrethroid-based insect sprays, 97
Pyrimethamine
  resistance to, 84, 85
  for toxoplasmosis, 57

Q

Qinghaosu, 99
Quality of life, 268
Quinidine, 98, 98t
  resistance to, 85
Quinidine efflux, 85
Quinine, 98, 98t
  resistance to, 84, 85
Quinine efflux, 85, 86t
Quinine resistance and quinidine resistance distribution, 94
Quinolones
  dosing of, 260–261
  mechanism of action, 252
  for MRSA, 182, 183

R

Radiography
  in osteomyelitis of foot, 15–16, 18
  and splenic abscess, 24, 30–31
Radiometer America, Inc., 105
"Randomization" scheme in clinical trial, 66
Reagent cards, 106, 107t, 108f
Recombinant immunoblot assay (RIBA), 132, 133, 134, 135, 136
Red man's syndrome, 181
Refusal of treatment, 270
Rehydrator/inoculator, RENOK, 111
Renal disease, underlying, in diabetics, 7
Renal failure in malaria, 84, 99
Renal impairment, 60

Renal insufficiency, 181
RENOK rehydrator/inoculator, 111
"Reservoir" effect, 61
Residual bacteria, 9
Resistance, false, 114–117
Respiratory synctial virus (RSV) vaccine, 192
Respiratory tract infections, 72, 75
Restriction enzymes, 179
Retinitis, cytomegalovirus, 237
Reverse transcriptase (RT), 132–133, 272, 273
Rhinovirus infections, 238–239
RIBA, 132, 133, 134, 135, 136
Ribavirin, 135
Ribosomes
  and action of antibacterials, 252
  and resistance to macrolides, 57
  and streptogramins, 183
Rickettsia-like organisms, 205, 209, 210, 210f
Rickettsia species, 210f
Rifabutin, 56
Rifampin
  for MAC infections, 71
  for MRSA, 177, 178, 180, 182, 183
  for nodular lymphangitis, 147, 150
Rights of patient, 268–273
Risk assessment for HIV infection, 220–221
Risk factors for acquisition of MRSA infection, 173t
Risk of infection, 221
  ethics of, 272
RNA
  of hepatitis C virus, 121, 123, 125, 126, 128, 131, 132, 135
  studies
    processing blood for, 132
  synthesis, 261
RNA, ribosomal, 179, 208, 212
RNA probes, 179
RNA synthetase, 177
Robotic mechanism, 110
Rochalimaea henselae, 205, 209–212, 210f, 212, 213–214, 214t, 215, 216
Rochalimaea quintana, 209, 210, 210f, 212, 214t, 215, 216
Rochalimaea species
  and bacillary angiomatosis, 205–219
    diagnosis and treatment, 214–216
    clinical syndromes, associated, 211t, 211–212
    evolutionary tree, 210, 210f
Rochalimaea vinsonii, 210
Roche Diagnostics, 105
Rockefeller Foundation, 203
Rodents, 148

Rooms, hospital, 175
Roseola infantum, 162–163
Rotavirus vaccine, 192
RS232 interface, 107
Rubella syndrome, congenital, 202
Rubella vaccine, 199, 201, 202

S

Salivary glands, 162
Salmonella species
    and macrolides, 55
    and splenic abscess, 28
Salmonella typhi, 56t
    and splenic abscess, 28
San Francisco General Hospital, 221
Sandflies, 148
Sarcoidosis, 163
Scandinavia, 152
Schistosomiasis vaccine, 192
Sensititre Fluorogenic System, 105, 106t
Serratia marcescens
    and anitmicrobial sensitivity testing, 104
    and splenic abscess, 27
Serratia species
    and antimicrobial sensitivity testing, 115
Serum concentration-time curve. *See* AuC
Sexually-transmitted diseases
    hepatitis C, 136
    and macrolides, 72, 73t
Shigella flexneri
    and macrolides, 56t
    and splenic abscess, 27
Shigellae, 55
Sickle-cell disease, 80
Sinusitis, bacterial, 64–65 65t, 73t, 74, 75
Sixth disease, 162–163
Sjögren's syndrome, 163
Skin and soft-tissue infections, 69t, 69–70, 72, 73t,
    75
Skin fissuring, 2
Skin grafts, 12
Skin hydration, abnormal, 2
Skin testing
    for Leishmania, 148
    for Mycobacterium marinum, 147
Smell, fetid, 3, 7
Soaps, antiseptic, 174
Sodium chloride content in growth media, 116–
    117
Sodium fusidate, 178
Specialty Laboratories, Inc., 215
Spectrophotometer, 110

Spleen and resistance to malaria, 87
Splendore-Hoeppli reaction, 146
Splenectomy
    and splenic abscess, 38, 39, 42, 43
Splenectomy
    and resistance to malaria, 87
Splenic abscess
    clinical manifestations, 28–30, 29t
    complications, 30
    definitions, 23–24
    diagnosis, 30–37
    diagnostic microbiology, 36–37
    emerging syndromes, 43–45
    incidence, 24
    microbiology, 26–28, 27t
    pathogenesis, 24–26
    predisposing conditions, 25t, 25–26
    prognosis factors, 42–43
    treatment, 37–42
Splenic cultures, 242
Splenic cysts, pre-existing, 25
Splenic infarction, 42
Splenitis, bacillary, 211t, 212
Splenocutaneous fistula, 30, 40
Sporothrix schenckii, 142, 143–148, 156
Sporotrichoid lymphangitis
    defined, 142
    typical presentation, 142
Sporotrichosis
    geographic distribution, 144
    and nodular lymphangitis, 142, 143–148
Sporozoite rate, 92, 93
Staphylococci
    coagulase negative
        and microbial sensitivity testing, 114, 117
    coagulase-negative
        and diabetic foot infections, 9
        and hepatosplenic candidiasis, 43
        and macrolides, 53, 54t, 65
    coagulase-positive, 65
    and diabetic foot infections, 8
    and IV catheter infections, 230
    and macrolides, 57, 58, 72
    oxacillin-resistant, 116, 117
    and splenic abscess, 26
    vaccine, 192
Staphylococcus aureus
    and antimicrobial susceptibility testing,
        117
    in foot infections, 5, 6, 8, 9, 10
    hematogenously seeded, 10
    and macrolides, 53, 54t, 58, 64, 67, 68, 69, 73t,
        75

Staphylococcus aureus (*cont.*)
  methicillin-resistant (MRSA)
    community-acquired, 180
  methicillin-resistant (MRSA), nosocomial, 170–191
    antibiotic theapy, 180–184
    control measures, 174–179
    epidemiology, 170–172
    reservoirs, 172
    resistance to chlorhexidine, 174
    risk factors for acquisition, 173t
    in special setting, 179–180
    surveillance of, 172–174
    virulence, 172
  and nodular lymphangitis, 142, 151
  and splenic abscess, 26, 28, 40
Staphylococcus epidermidis, 6
Staphylococcus haemolyticus, 180
Steroids, 99
Stevens-Johnson syndrome, 96
Stibogluconate sodium (Pentostam), 148
Streptococci
  aerobic, 5, 7, 9
  anaerobic, 54, 54t
  and diabetic foot infections, 5, 7, 8, 9
  group B
    and diabetic foot infections, 5, 8
    vaccine, 192
  and macrolides, 53, 72
  and mupirocin, 177
  and nodular lymphangitis, 142
  and resistance to macrolides, 57
  and splenic abscess, 26
  viridans
    in diabetic foot infections, 6, 9
    and macrolides, 65
Streptococcus agalactiae, 53, 54t, 69
Streptococcus pneumoniae, 263
  and macrolides, 53, 54t, 58, 64, 65, 67, 68, 73t, 75
  and resistance to macrolides, 57
Streptococcus pyogenes, 53, 54t, 58, 63, 64, 69, 73t, 75
Streptogramin B, 57
Streptogramins, 183
Streptomycin, 152
Streptomycin resistance, 117
Subcommittee on Anitmicrobial Susceptibility Testing, 103
Sulfadiazine
  for nodular lymphangitis, 149
  for toxoplasmosis, 57
Sulfadoxine/pyrimethamine (Fansidar), 96, 98t
  resistance to, 84, 94

Sulfamethoxazole, 147, 149
Sulfonamide, 73t
Sulfur granules, pathognomonic, 149
Superinfection, 263
Surfaces, contaminated, 172
Surgical management of foot infection, 10–15
Surveillance for pathogens, 170, 172–174
Susceptibility, false, 114–117
Susceptibility test cards, 106, 107f, 108f
Susceptibility testing, antimicrobial, 103–119
Susceptibility testing systems, antimicrobial, rapid automated, 103–112
  incidence of, 104–105, 105t
  potential advantages, 112–113
  potential disadvantages, 113–114
  potential problems in the detection of resistance, 114–117
Susceptibility tests, antimicrobial
  broth microdilution, 103
  disk diffusion, 103, 104
Synergimycins (streptogramins). *See* Streptogramins
Synergistic effect (between bacteria), 9
Synovial involvement, 148, 156

T

T-cell tropic viruses, 159
T cells, 87, 122, 129, 130, 159, 160, 161
  and cytokines, 229, 230, 231, 232, 234
  and IFN-γ, 229
TAAS system, 105
Tachyzoites, 57
Taq polymerase artifact, 210, 212
Task Force on Adult Immunization (of American College of Physicians), 197
Technicon Instruments Corp., 105
Teichoplanin, 181, 182
Tenaculums, 223
Tenosynovitis
  in M. marinum infection, 147
  in sporotrichosis, 145
Tenosynovitis, mycobacterial, 143
Tetanus vaccine, 199, 201, 202, 203
Tetracycline
  for malaria, 98t
  for nodular lymphangitis, 152
Tetracyclines, 55, 73t, 75, 263
  and antibacterial activity, 252
  for bacillary angiomatosis, 216
Thalidomide, 240
Theophylline, 63, 74
Ticarcillin-clavulanate treatment, 9
Time>MIC values, 256, 257f, 261, 262, 263
Tinea pedis, 2

Tissue culture, 7
Tissue growth factors, 11
Tissue necrosis, 1
Tissue necrosis factor-α (TNF-α), 230. *See also*
    Cytokines and Cytokine therapy
    for HIV, 234
    im malaria, 228
    for leprosy, 240
    for malaria, 87
    in meningitis, 228
    in sepsis, 228
TMP/SMX. *See* Trimethoprim-sulfamethoxazole
    treatment (TMP/SMX)
TNF-α. *See* Tissue necrosis factor-α (TNF-α)
Tobramycin, 259
Tolerability profile of vaccines, 196
Tort law, 268
Toxicity, system, 1
Toxoplasma gondii, 55, 57
Toxoplasmosis, 76, 229
Toxoplasmosis, cerebral, 61
Transaminase, liver, 229, 232, 233
Transcutaneous oxygen tension, 1, 15
Transfer of pathogens, interfacility, 179–180
Transfusion, exchange, 99
Transmission
    of MRSA, 170–172
    of virus, 122–124
Transplantation and medical ethics, 269
Trauma
    and botryomycosis, 151
    to foot in diabetics, 15
    and splenic abscess, 24, 25, 26
Trench fever, 212
Treponema pallidum
    and macrolides, 55, 73t
    and nodular lymphangitis, 142
Triazolam, 63
Triclosan, 178
Trifluorothymidine, 238
Trimethoprim, 147, 149
Trimethoprim-sulfamethoxazole treatment (TMP/
    SMX), 73, 74–75
    action of, 254
    for MRSA, 178, 182
Tuberculosis
    and medical ethics, 269
    and peliosis, 211
    vaccine for, 192, 202
Tularemia, 151–152
Tumor necrosis factor α (INF-α), 84
Turbidity standard, McFarland barium sulfate, 107,
    111
Typhoid, 23, 25

U

Ulceration, foot, 1
Ulcers, foot, 1, 3, 5
    classification and treatment, 11, 11t, 12t
    healing, 8
    neuropathic. *See* Mal perforans
    probing, 18
Ultrasonography, 26, 32, 33f, 35f, 41, 42, 43, 44,
    45
UNICEF, 203
United Nations, 203
United Nations Development Program, 203
United States Department of Health and Human
    Services, 19
Unlicensed medications, 273–274
Ureaplasma urealyticum, 55, 56t, 70
Urinary tract infections
    and macrolides, 75
    polyvalent, vaccine for, 192

V

Vaccine, candidate experimental, 194
Vaccine initiatives, U.S.A., 200
Vaccines
    defined, 193
    development of, 192–204
        advances affecting 192
        as a business venture, 198
        incentives to, 200
        patents, 199
        phase control testing, 195–196
        process research and development, 196–197
        regulatory control of, 195
        research leading to, 193–195
    heat-stable, 203
    live-virus, 194
    mandated and nonmandated, 199
    now in research or development, 192–193
    product licensure and postlicensure, 197–198
    promotion of, 200–201, 201t
    T-cell for HCV, potential for, 130, 136
    testing of, 194–195
    use of, global, 202–203
Vancomycin, 256
    for diabetic foot infection, 10
    dosing of, 263t
    dosing strategy, 261
    for MRSA, 172, 176, 180–181, 182, 183
    tolerance to, 180
Vancomycin resistance, 117, 172
Varicella-Zoster virus, 159
    cytokine therapy for, 237
    vaccine, 192

Vascular disease, peripheral, 1
Vascular insufficiency, 1, 2
Vascular reconstructive surgery, 15
Vegetable decoctions, infusion, 273
Vein bypass grafting, autogenous, 15
Verruga peruana, 207, 212
Veterans Administration (VA) Hospitals, 171, 179
Vibramycin (Doxycycline), 95t
Vibratory sensation, absence of, 1
Vidaribine, 233
Viral infections
 cytokine therapy for, 231–239
 of tissue culture cells, 164
Viremia, 123, 126, 130, 133, 134
Virginiamycin M and S, 183
Virulence of MRSA, 172
Vitek System, 105, 106t, 106–109, 107f, 108, 111

W

WalkAway System, 105, 106t, 109–112, 110f, 111f
Warthin-Starry silver strain, 205, 207, 213
Warts, genital, 238
Web space
 infection in, 3
 skin fissuring in, 2

Western blot test, 225
Whooping cough. *See* Pertussis
World Bank, 203
World Health Assembly, 203
World Health Organization (WHO), 198, 202, 203
World Summit for Children, 203
Wound care, 224
Wound infection, 69

X

Xanthomonas maltophila, 114

Y

Yeasts, 106
Yersenia enterocolitica, 27

Z

Zidovudine
 for HIV virus infection, 235, 236, 237, 272
 for prophylaxis of HIV virus, 224
Ziehl-Neelsen stain, 146, 149, 150
Zithromax. *See* Azithromycin